Cambridge Studies in Cognitive and Perceptual Development

Series Editors
GIYOO HATANO[†]
University of the Air, Chiba, Japan

KURT W. FISCHER
Harvard University, Cambridge, Massachusetts

Advisory Board
Gavin Bremner, *Lancaster University, United Kingdom*
Patricia M. Greenfield, *University of California, Los Angeles*
Paul Harris, *Harvard University, Cambridge, Massachusetts*
Daniel Stern,[†] *University of Geneva, Switzerland*

The aim of this series is to provide a scholarly forum for current theoretical and empirical issues in cognitive and perceptual development. As the twenty-first century begins, the field is no longer dominated by monolithic theories. Contemporary explanations build on the combined influences of biological, cultural, contextual, and ecological factors in well-defined research domains. In the field of cognitive development, cultural and situational factors are widely recognized as influencing the emergence and forms of reasoning in children. In perceptual development, the field has moved beyond the opposition of "innate" and "acquired" to suggest a continuous role for perception in the acquisition of knowledge. These approaches and issues are all reflected in the series, which also addresses such important research themes as the indissociable link between perception and action in the developing motor system, the relationship between perceptual and cognitive development and modern ideas on the development of the brain, the significance of developmental processes themselves, dynamic systems theory, and contemporary work in the psychodynamic tradition, especially as it relates to the foundations of self-knowledge.

Titles in the Series

continued after the index

The Dyslexia Debate

Julian G. Elliott
Durham University

Elena L. Grigorenko
Yale University

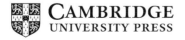
CAMBRIDGE
UNIVERSITY PRESS

CAMBRIDGE
UNIVERSITY PRESS

32 Avenue of the Americas, New York, NY 10013-2473, USA

Cambridge University Press is part of the University of Cambridge.

It furthers the University's mission by disseminating knowledge in the pursuit of education, learning, and research at the highest international levels of excellence.

www.cambridge.org
Information on this title: www.cambridge.org/9780521135870

First published 2014

Printed in the United States of America

A catalog record for this publication is available from the British Library.

Library of Congress Cataloging in Publication Data
Elliott, Julian, 1955– author.
The dyslexia debate / Julian G. Elliott, Elena L. Grigorenko.
   p. ; cm. – (Cambridge studies in cognitive and perceptual development ; 14)
Includes bibliographical references and index.
ISBN 978-0-521-11986-3 (hardback : alk. paper) – ISBN 978-0-521-13587-0 (paperback : alk. paper)
I. Grigorenko, Elena L., author.   II. Title.   III. Series: Cambridge studies in cognitive perceptual development ; 14.
[DNLM: 1. Dyslexia – diagnosis.   2. Child Development.   3. Child Psychology. WL 340.6]
RJ496.A5
618.92'8553–dc23   2013036080

ISBN 978-0-521-11986-3 Hardback
ISBN 978-0-521-13587-0 Paperback

Contents

Preface

In every country and in every language, a significant proportion of children struggle to master the skill of reading. Whereas many children gradually overcome their initial difficulty and acquire functional literacy, there is a significant proportion of children who continue to encounter decoding difficulties throughout their childhood and whose problems, although not necessarily with decoding per se, persist into adulthood. As these individuals struggle to cope with the changing demands of school and wider life, the hardship and difficulties that typically result are often incapacitating, undermining, and distressing. Given such a scenario, it is understandable that there is often a strong desire on the part of these individuals, their families, and their teachers for some form of clinical diagnosis that can help explain the reasons underpinning these problems and that can indicate, and secure, effective forms of intervention.

It is hardly surprising, therefore, that the term most frequently used to describe this phenomenon – referred to here as developmental dyslexia – has such a strong resonance. For many, the term describes a biologically based condition that, importantly, can serve to remove any impression others may have that reading problems are a consequence of low intelligence or an impoverished environment. It is widely believed that once developmental dyslexia (hereafter, dyslexia) is diagnosed, appropriate specialized interventions can be set in place that have proven success in addressing this condition. Concomitantly, it is feared that a failure to diagnose this condition will result in erroneous understandings of the underlying problem and the continued operation of an inappropriate educational diet. The natural desire for such a label can also be heightened by the (often very true) belief that gaining this may be a necessary means to acquire additional resources of one kind or another.

For several decades, however, others have sought to challenge the scientific rigor and educational utility of this construct. Criticisms have focused on the misleading, yet widespread, belief that there is consensual understanding on the part of researchers and clinicians as to the nature and features of dyslexia, that the condition differs from other forms of reading disability, and that it is possible to describe its biological and cognitive origins in ways that can guide powerful educational and clinical practices. Such critics complain that, too often, valuable resources are consumed by expensive and time-consuming diagnostic procedures when these are better utilized for providing early intervention to all children who struggle to learn to read.

In voicing such concerns, critics have sought recognition of the need for a more sophisticated analysis of the relevance and utility of the dyslexia construct itself. Somewhat paradoxically, however, the questions that have been posed as a result have often been oversimplified and fail to represent the principal concern. Thus, the key question – Is dyslexia a scientifically rigorous construct that has meaningful value for research and educational/clinical practice? – has too often been transmogrified into the unhelpful and misleading "Does dyslexia exist?" This gross misrepresentation of the core issue has often resulted in significant media interest and widely reported commentaries from public figures who, on one hand, have been dismissive of the needs of those who speak of the problems resulting from their dyslexia or, on the other hand, have proven eager to offer their personal biography to testify to the existence of the dyslexic condition. In the case of research scientists (psychologists, neuroscientists, geneticists) who work in highly specialized areas that examine the acquisition of typical and atypical reading skills, such debate has sometimes been perceived as introducing nonessential complexity that serves as an unwelcome distraction from detailed and sustained pursuit of particular scientific inquiries. However, failing to acknowledge the conceptual and definitional complexity of the core construct runs the risk of each discipline producing highly esoteric and recondite knowledge that operates primarily within a narrow disciplinary silo and whose practical applications are unclear.

This book represents a response to growing recognition that the key issues behind the debate about the construct of dyslexia (hereafter, the dyslexia debate) need to be highlighted and considered in detail. To achieve this, it takes each of the core disciplines in turn and considers what they tell us about the nature and underpinnings of typical and atypical reading. In so doing, they shed light on the question as to whether dyslexia should be conceived as a condition that is synonymous to, or different from, reading disability. In the light of this, the book then examines issues relating to assessment of and intervention for difficulties with the acquisition of reading skills. A key issue for intervention concerns whether there is value in examining underlying cognitive processes that are widely considered to be markers of dyslexia or, alternatively, whether it is preferable to focus primarily on core academic skills. Finally, in light of our examination of all of these issues, we reflect on the value of the dyslexia construct and recommend a way forward that is designed to reduce unnecessary complexity, ensure commonality of understanding, and concentrate resources on the provision of timely and appropriate intervention for all who struggle to learn to read.

Many of the specific disciplinary issues discussed in this book are complex and draw on rather specialized language and technical terminology. For this reason most readers will encounter work in one or more disciplines that, initially at least, is likely to prove challenging. This may be exacerbated, or perhaps aided, by our very deliberate decision to offer a comprehensive set of references that provides an encyclopedic overview of the available literature. However, while gaining a full and detailed grasp of all the issues is likely to require further independent reading, it is hoped that the contents of this book will enable the reader to grasp key issues in the dyslexia debate. Relevance and implications of the work across these disciplines for resolving the dyslexia debate will become clear to the reader.

In preparing this book, we have sought advice from very many scholars. We wish to thank all of them for their help and guidance. In so doing, we would like to express our particular gratitude to Dorothy Bishop, Jack Fletcher, Robert Fulbright, Fumiko Hoeft, Brahm Norwich, Keith Stanovich, Lee Swanson, Mei Tan, and Frank Vellutino. We also thank Magge Gagliardi for her assistance with the illustrations and colleagues at Cambridge University Press for their support, faith, and patience. Of course, all errors and misunderstanding are our own.

Foreword

by Frank Vellutino, University at Albany, New York

In any area of scientific inquiry, a comprehensive text discussing recent advances in both theory and research is always a welcome addition to the existing literature. Of course, such a text must also provide historical perspective in order for the reader to fully appreciate the importance and relative impacts of new findings in the field, in terms of whether or not such findings provide support for the theories that generated them and whether or not they can or have been replicated. Finally, such a text must provide a critical and relatively unbiased analysis of the theories discussed in the text and research findings related to those theories. Elliott and Grigorenko's book, *The Dyslexia Debate*, in my opinion, satisfies all three criteria. It is the latest in a series of texts focusing on issues surrounding the origin of difficulties in acquiring early literacy skills that were published during the 19th, 20th, and 21st centuries.

Chapter 1 of the book focuses on the multitude of definitions and descriptions of dyslexia as a term used in reference to developmental reading difficulties. The reader who is unfamiliar with the relevant literature will be immediately struck by the utter lack of consensus regarding whether dyslexia is little more than a descriptive and somewhat misleading label for early reading difficulties or a neuropsychological construct with well-established construct validity. After providing a brief account of early work done in the study of developmental reading difficulties, the chapter focuses on current definitional issues and thoroughly discusses the controversy surrounding a number of definitions of dyslexia, including (1) discrepancy-based definitions such as the traditional IQ-achievement discrepancy and the discrepancy between reading and listening comprehension; (2) definitions based on response to intervention; and (3) definitions based on causal explanations such as visual deficits and language-based deficits. It becomes painfully clear by the end of Chapter 1 that questions and issues associated with the definition of dyslexia and synonymous terms such as reading disability and specific reading disability will be with us for some time.

Chapter 2 discusses hypothesized explanations of early reading difficulties, implicating cognitive deficits as causes of such difficulties: phonological deficits, visual and auditory deficits, rapid naming deficits, working memory deficits, and a variety of others that have been proposed over the years. After reviewing the vast literature concerned with the cognitive deficits discussed in this chapter, it is concluded that no single causal hypothesis can explain early and protracted reading difficulties and that the origin of such difficulties must surely be multifaceted, although it is acknowledged that the largest amount of variance on measures of reading ability can be explained either by phonological deficits alone or by phonological deficits combined with other deficits.

Chapter 3 contains two broad sections. The first provides detailed descriptions of the structural and functional aspects of the brain in relation to normal and abnormal reading ability and discusses results from studies using post mortem, neuroimaging, and other functional procedures to illustrate brain-reading relationships that have been documented. The discussion is divided into four different categories: (1) studies of brain activation patterns in typical adult readers; (2) studies of brain activation patterns in typically developing pre-readers; (3) studies of brain activation patterns in atypical as compared with typical readers; and (4) studies of brain activation patterns in atypical readers before and after remedial intervention. Results provide reasonably strong support for reliable brain-reading relationships in the populations evaluated. However, the authors correctly point out that the theoretical significance and practical implications of such findings are unclear and are likely to remain so for some time to come, given that research in this area of inquiry is in its infancy.

The second section of the chapter provides a historic tracing of work done addressing the question of whether "reading disability" has a genetic basis. It is asserted, at the outset, that despite initial challenges to the view that reading disability "is a condition whose pathogenesis involves hereditary factors," there is increasing evidence that "the malfunctioning of the brain system that supports reading may be caused by multiple deficiencies in corresponding genetic machinery." The discussion distinguishes between two types of studies assessing genetic links to reading and reading disability: heritability and relative risk studies where siblings and other family members are evaluated for susceptibility to reading disability using performance measures such as reading and reading-related tasks (e.g., phonological tasks); and "molecular studies" where genetic material (DNA) is obtained in addition to such performance measures. The discussion makes it clear that although considerable progress has been made establishing a genetic link to individual differences in reading ability, this work is yet in the initial stages of validation, and the facts, as we know them, do not yet have meaningful practical application.

Chapter 4 focuses on issues surrounding assessment of the causes of early reading difficulties as well as on instructional approaches to preventing and remediating such difficulties. The chapter is organized around four related questions: (1) What is the most effective (i.e., evidence-based) means of teaching reading from an early age? (2) How can we best identify young children at risk of word-reading difficulties and use this information to prevent later problems? (3) What can be done to help those who are resistant to initial intervention? (4) Is there anything special about specialist dyslexia teaching that is particularly effective for a subgroup of poor readers? These questions are thoroughly addressed, and it is generally concluded that structured, comprehensive, and individualized reading instruction is the only defensible approach to correcting early and protracted reading difficulties as compared with alternative approaches that have questionable validity and no empirical support (e.g., visual and auditory training activities, visual-motor activities, tinted lenses, etc.), in addition to reading intervention. Special emphasis is made on the importance of adopting a preventive approach to early reading difficulties that seeks to identify children at risk of reading difficulties as early as possible, in order to provide them with the intervention necessary to remove impediments to reading skills acquisition.

Chapter 5 is the concluding one, and after summarizing issues and problems associated with the lack of consensus regarding the definition, cause(s), and remediation of dyslexia and following the discussion of the tension between the "science and politics" of dyslexia as a neuropsychological construct, the authors assert that the term has engendered unnecessary confusion in the field and has long since passed its usefulness for scientific and practical purposes. As a consequence, they strongly recommend that "dyslexia" be discarded as a term used to refer to early and long-term reading difficulties and that the term "reading disability" be used in reference to such difficulties in its stead.

In my opinion, this is an excellent text that should be read by researchers and practitioners on both sides of the dyslexia debate. The topics are important and will no doubt be of interest to both sets of professionals. They are discussed thoughtfully and even-handedly and with an appropriate amount of detail. Moreover, the text is clearly written, although a few sections in the neurobiological and genetics chapter will present many readers with some degree of challenge, especially those who are not familiar with the technology and procedures used by researchers in these two areas of inquiry. Yet, scholars on each side of the dyslexia debate are likely to have disparate views regarding the central question addressed in this text, which, of course, is the construct validity of dyslexia as a term used to refer to developmental reading difficulties. Those who question the construct validity of dyslexia will find much to like in this text and are likely to applaud the authors' suggestion that the term be discarded as a label for reading difficulties having a biological and genetic origin. Those who do not question the construct validity of dyslexia will find much to quarrel with in this text and will no doubt eschew the authors' suggestion that it be discarded as a label for developmental reading difficulties. My own biases are aligned with those of the authors. I have long argued that the term should be abandoned in scientific and practical applications because I have found that in scientific applications, the number of definitions of dyslexia can be roughly equated with the number of theories of dyslexia and in practical applications the number of definitions of dyslexia can be roughly equated with the number of commercially available interventions designed to remediate reading difficulties said to be caused by dyslexia.

For example, multisensory-type reading interventions, as initially designed by Samuel Orton and Anna Gillingham, were said to circumvent and compensate for optical reversibility ("seeing letters backwards") and other visual perceptual problems that were hypothesized by Orton (1937) to be caused by a developmental lag in hemispheric dominance. When it became clear from research evaluating Orton's theory that optical reversibility was not a psychologically real phenomenon, and when evidence began to accumulate suggesting that most reading difficulties are likely caused by language-based deficits (e.g., phonological deficits) rather than visual perceptual deficits, the raison d'être for Orton-Gillingham-type multisensory interventions eventually became the need to circumvent and compensate for language-based deficits that were said to cause early reading difficulties rather than optical reversibility and other visual perceptual deficits. Similarly, a study conducted by Tallal (1980) produced results suggesting that developmental reading difficulties are caused by a disorder in auditory temporal order perception that impairs speech perception, thereby defining dyslexia as a nonverbal auditory processing disorder rather than a visual or language-based disorder. These findings were never replicated. Yet, despite the paucity of support for Tallal's theory, a computer software program (Fast ForWord) was subsequently developed and promoted as an intervention that remediates temporal order perception deficits as the root cause of difficulties in acquiring literacy skills. At present, however, there is little more than testimonial support for the efficacy of this program in remediating early literacy difficulties.

The literature is replete with similar instances wherein the definition of dyslexia changes in accordance with different practical and/or scientific biases. Therefore, I strongly support the authors' suggestion that the term be discarded in both the scientific and practitioner communities. However, I am not sure their suggestion that the term "reading disability" be substituted for "dyslexia" will eliminate the type of confusion caused by the latter term. After all, "reading disability" and related terms such as "specific reading disability," "disabled readers," "reading disorder," "learning disability," and "specific learning disability," have all been closely associated with the term "dyslexia" and are probably loaded with as much excess meaning as dyslexia. Therefore, I would like to see all such terms jettisoned from the relevant literature as well as from the lexicons of researchers and practitioners and more neutral terms such as "reading difficulties," "learning difficulties," "atypical reader(s)," and "struggling readers" used instead. But, as opined by the authors, I rather doubt that this will happen anytime soon, given the entrenched nature of the more traditional terms.

In sum, Elliott and Grigorenko's text makes an important contribution to the literature concerned with the acquisition of skill in reading and impediments to the acquisition of skill in reading. The questions it addresses and the issues it discusses are clearly and incisively articulated, and the review of work done in the field is comprehensive and informative. It should be read by all those interested in the causes and correlates of early reading difficulties, especially scholars conducting research in this area of inquiry and practitioners working with struggling readers.

1   What is dyslexia?

Introduction

In January 2009, a British Member of Parliament, Graham Stringer, caused something of an international storm by questioning the validity of the concept of dyslexia. Unlike the majority of critiques that have questioned the conceptual and diagnostic utility of this construct (e.g., Elliott & Gibbs, 2008; Stanovich, 1994), his criticisms, written on his website (http://www .manchesterconfidential.co.uk/News/Dyslexia-is-a-myth [retrieved October 5, 2013]), were far more direct and accusatory. Describing dyslexia as "a cruel fiction . . . no more real than the 19th century scientific construction of 'the æther' to explain how light travels through a vacuum," he argued that the reason why so many children struggled with literacy was because they had been failed by the education "establishment." Rather than admitting that poor instruction was at fault, he argued, a brain disorder called dyslexia had been invented. For Stringer, "to label children as dyslexic because they're confused by poor teaching methods is wicked. . . . The sooner it is consigned to the same dustbin of history, the better" (ibid.). In response, the Chief Executive of the British Dyslexia Association stated on the association's website: "Once again dyslexia seems to be making the headlines for all the wrong reasons. It is frustrating that the focus should be on whether dyslexia exists or not, when there is so much evidence to support that it does" (http://dyslexiaaction.org.uk/ news/mp%E2%80%99s-claims-dyslexia-cruel-fiction [retrieved October 5, 2013]).

As this response acknowledges, questions about the existence or otherwise of dyslexia have raged periodically for many years. At first glance, this seems rather puzzling, as fascination with unexpected reading difficulties in individuals with high levels of intelligence and sound eyesight has been expressed for centuries (Shaywitz, 2005), and the topic has been extensively researched across a variety of disciplines.

Although the first account of "word-blindness" was produced in 1676 by the physician John Schmidt, much of the early published work appeared in the latter part of the nineteenth century, a time when an inability to learn to read first became a medical concern (Campbell, 2011). Early investigations were largely concerned with examining difficulties that had been acquired as a result of some form of brain trauma. In 1872, Sir William Broadbent reported the case of a man who, following a head injury, lost the capacity to read, despite being able to write with little difficulty. Although he had good conversational skills and extensive vocabulary, he struggled to name objects presented to him. Broadbent asserted that the reading failure was a result of this more general difficulty in naming objects. Five years later, Kussmaul (1877) reported on the case of an adult patient with no apparent disabilities other than severe reading difficulties. Kussmaul coined the term "word-blindness" to describe the inability to read text despite sound eyesight, intelligence, and speech.

The term "dyslexia" was first used in 1887 by Rudolf Berlin, a German ophthalmologist, to describe a particular form of word-blindness found in adults, which, he argued, was caused by brain lesions. Berlin contended that severe damage would result in alexia, a total inability to read, whereas partial damage would most likely result in dyslexia, a significant difficulty in decoding written symbols. Here, the focus was on the effect of a physical trauma of some kind, "acquired dyslexia," rather than that which develops naturally from a young age, "developmental dyslexia," the focus of almost all of the dyslexia literature.

The idea that "word-blindness" could be a developmental as well as an acquired condition came somewhat later. As Shaywitz (2005) notes, this is unsurprising as the suddenness of an acquired loss is considerably more salient than the more subtle picture of unfolding developmental difficulties. In 1896, a paper on "congenital word-blindness" by a British physician, W. Pringle Morgan (1896), described a child of fourteen years of age who had failed to learn to read despite normal intelligence and good eyesight. Noting the boy's other abilities, he observed: "The schoolmaster who has taught him for some years says that he would be the smartest lad in the school life if the instruction were entirely oral" (p. 1378). Morgan described two generations of one family with six cases that had strikingly similar symptoms and opined that the problem was congenital, involving a defective ability to store visual impressions of words.

Morgan's paper acted as a stimulus for a flurry of case studies, most notably by a Scottish ophthalmologist, James Hinshelwood, who gathered data on several cases involving both acquired and congenital word-blindness. The children he reported on in a classic text, *Congenital Word-Blindness* (Hinshelwood, 1917), were typically male (as were the majority of similar cases of this period [Stephenson, 1904]), intelligent, had sound eyesight, and performed well on oral tasks.

Following an autopsy on a patient whose progress he had monitored for several years, Hinshelwood (1902) located the cause of reading disability in the angular gyrus. He suggested that the primary disability was visual memory for words and letters and advocated one-to-one training designed to increase visual memory as the preferred form of intervention. Noting the embarrassment and ridicule often experienced by poor readers in the classroom, he commented:

It is a matter of the highest importance to recognise as early as possible the true nature of this defect, when it is met with in a child. It may prevent much waste of valuable time and may save the child from suffering and cruel treatment. When a child manifests great difficulty in learning to read and is unable to keep up in progress with its fellows, the cause is generally assigned to stupidity or laziness, and no systematised method is directed to the training of such a child. A little knowledge and careful analysis of the child's case would soon make it clear that the difficulty experienced was due to a defect in the visual memory of words and letters; the child would then be regarded in the proper light as one with a congenital defect in a particular area of the brain, a defect which, however, can often be remedied by persevering and persistent training. The sooner the true nature of the defect is realised, the better are the chances of the child's improvement. (Hinshelwood, 1902, cited in Shaywitz, 2005, pp. 21–22).

In their historical account of learning disabilities – a term that includes a number of specific areas of problematic functioning, including reading disability – Hallahan and Mercer (2001) observed that groundbreaking work largely shifted from Europe to the United States during the 1920s. With the increasing trend toward mass education and the issues that resulted in conjunction with the dissemination of the idea of universal literacy (Grigorenko, 2011), many researchers found themselves with the responsibility not only of understanding and explaining children's academic and behavioral difficulties but also of taking a lead in assessment and remediation techniques, particularly in relation to reading disabilities (Hallahan & Mock, 2003).

Leading clinical researchers at this time were Samuel Orton and Grace Fernald. Fernald was a clinician who employed a multisensory approach for those with reading difficulties and sought to evaluate the success or otherwise of her techniques by maintaining detailed case records of her clients' progress. Despite the rather anecdotal mode of evaluation, still largely the case for multisensory approaches today, such techniques have an intuitive appeal and continue to be popular among specialist dyslexia teachers (see Chapter 4). Orton, Fernald's contemporary, was a neurologist who became best known for his work on educational intervention, in particular multisensory approaches and an emphasis on phonics. Orton attempted to understand the origins of reading difficulties, introducing a number of ideas that added to contemporary understandings. Like his intellectual predecessor, Hinshelwood, he was interested in areas of the brain that might be influential but believed those other than the angular gyrus were involved. He suggested that reading difficulties were primarily the result of poor cerebral dominance in which the nondominant hemisphere stored a different representation to that of the dominant one. This explained the common tendency for cases to exhibit letter and word reversals, and the use of mirror reading and writing. To reflect a shift from an emphasis on purely visual deficits, Orton recommended that the term "word-blindness" should be replaced by "strephosymbolia," which in Greek means "twisted." His work proved highly influential and promoted much theorizing on various visual mechanisms held to be responsible for reading difficulties.

Early research pioneers sought to understand a condition that continues to pose significant problems for many individuals and challenges to those who seek to help them. Their puzzlement over the particular problems encountered by a small number of children would appear sufficient to refute any suggestion that dyslexia/reading disability is merely the consequence of poor teaching. Since then, more than a century of research activity has provided incontrovertible evidence that some children experience particular difficulties that render the reading process highly problematic. The original belief of these early clinicians that the difficulty was caused by a visual pathology has now been largely rejected in favor of language-based origins (see Chirkina & Grigorenko, in press, for details of similar conclusions that were arrived at rather earlier in the Soviet Union), although, interestingly, the conception of dyslexia as essentially a visual problem is still widely held by the general public (Christo, Davis, & Brock, 2009). Interestingly, the role of underlying visual processes in reading disability is gaining significant researcher interest once again (Stein & Kapoula, 2012).

Clearly, there are many children who struggle to learn to read for reasons other than poor teaching. For this reason, the fact that there are some who question the value of the term "dyslexia" may appear puzzling, particularly to those for whom the existence of such difficulties is all too real. However, the primary issue is not whether biologically based reading difficulties exist (the answer is an unequivocal "yes"), but rather how we should best understand and address literacy problems across clinical, educational, occupational, and social policy contexts. Essentially, the dyslexia debate centers on the extent to which the dyslexia construct operates as a rigorous scientific construct that adds to our capacity to help those who struggle to learn to read.

Definitions of dyslexia

Without an agreed-on definition that can be implemented reliably and validly, understanding the nature, causes, and best treatments for reading disability is unlikely. Similarly, an agreed-on definition is essential for practice. (Brown Waesche, Schatschneider, Maner, Ahmed, & Wagner, 2011, p. 296)

Somewhat paradoxically, defining dyslexia is seemingly both very easy and very difficult. It is easy, largely because most parties agree that the definition should principally concern the inherent and particular difficulties encountered by those who struggle to read text. It is difficult because the field has been unable to produce a universally accepted definition that is not imprecise, amorphous, or difficult to operationalize. As noted in the section-opening quotation, without a universally agreed-on operational definition, we cannot be sure that assessments are measuring the same thing, and as a result, there are likely to be serious doubts about any resultant diagnosis or classification (Siegel & Lipka, 2008).

One of the particular difficulties concerning definitions of dyslexia is that the term has variously been seen as different from, or synonymous to, several other labels that involve problems with literacy. These include specific reading retardation, reading difficulties, specific reading difficulties, reading disability, learning disability, unexpected reading difficulty, and specific learning difficulties. These overlap substantially and vary according to causal assumptions (Rice & Brooks, 2004). Thus, some (National Institute of Child Health and Development, 2007; Pennington & Bishop, 2009; Siegel & Mazabel, 2013; Wagner, 2008) do not differentiate between the terms "dyslexia" and "reading disability," and many (e.g., Swanson & Hsieh, 2009) use the term "reading disability" as synonymous with a number of terms: "dyslexia," "reading disorder," "learning disabilities in reading," and "specific reading disabilities." However, many other researchers, clinicians, and educators seek to reserve the term "dyslexia" to describe a smaller group within the larger pool of poor decoders. Determining the particular constellation of difficulties that marks out such a subgroup introduces a further set of contested definitions and understandings.

The U.S. National Research Council (Snow, Burns, & Griffin, 1998) identified three broad reasons for reading difficulty. These concern (1) difficulties of understanding and using the alphabetic principle in order to develop accurate and fluent reading; (2) poor acquisition of the verbal knowledge and strategies that are important to comprehend written material; and (3) a lack of motivation to read. In general, those who use the term "dyslexia" are concerned with the first of these, although poor reading comprehension and a lack of motivation to read are often associated by-products of word-reading difficulties (Morgan, Fuchs et al., 2008), and the motivational problems of some poor readers are likely to affect their response to intervention (Vaughn et al., 2009).

While there appears to be a bidirectional relationship between reading and motivation, it is not clear to what extent this latter variable serves to moderate the impact of a preexisting difficulty (Catts & Adlof, 2011) although there is some evidence that high engagement in reading-related activities can serve as a protective factor for young children at risk of future reading disability (Eklund, Torppa, & Lyytinen, 2013). There is also some evidence that students with reading disabilities tend to mix together in school peer groups, and this may result in lowered motivation and educational achievement, particularly for males (Kiuru et al., 2011).

Some believe that not all of those who struggle to decode text should be considered dyslexic, with the relative influence of nature and nurture often seen as a key factor. Herein lies a critical conceptual and diagnostic issue: In what ways is it meaningful and potentially valuable to conceive of a dyslexic subgroup within a larger pool of poor readers who all find reading accuracy (and, for some, fluency) problematic?

The critical question in dyslexia research is not whether dyslexic people in particular differ from 'normal' readers. It is *whether dyslexic people differ from other poor readers.* (Rice & Brooks, 2004, p. 33; emphasis in the original)

It is important to recognize that the value of a definition may be tempered by its purpose. Thus, as Stanovich (1992) has noted, there are definitions that are designed to serve scientific purposes, with fairly strict scientific criteria, and others that are employed for determining the allocation of additional educational resources for students with learning difficulties of various kinds. Some definitions are used by advocacy groups to highlight specific learning problems and to gain formal legislative support. For such groups, strict conceptual rigor may not be desirable, particularly where its use to guide resource planning might lead to the reduction of services to those deemed to be in need of these (Kavale & Forness, 2003):

The highly restrictive definitions of the research community are resisted by school personnel, who often want the broadest definition possible in order to allow themselves discretion in providing services for children with generic school learning problems. (Stanovich, 1992, p. 279)

Irrespective of the breadth of the definition, it is widely agreed that the core problem of dyslexia – a difficulty in decoding text – should be contrasted with the ultimate goal of reading – taking meaning from the written word. While these two processes are clearly related, they each involve a number of different skills, and strengths and weaknesses may be found in either one or both of these processes. Some can understand considerably more of a passage of text than one would expect on the basis of their reading skills; others may decode well but take little meaning from the print before them. The term "hyperlexia" is used to describe the phenomenon where an individual's word-reading skills are considerably higher than are their levels of reading comprehension, verbal functioning, or general cognitive functioning (Grigorenko, Klin, & Volkmar, 2003). Unsurprisingly, however, those who experience severe difficulties with decoding will usually experience associated problems of reading comprehension, in part because the effort that must be expended on decoding is likely to detract from the capacity to focus on deriving meaning. However the dependence of reading comprehension on word recognition appears to be lesser for older children (Hulslander, Olson, Willcut, & Wadsworth, 2010). In other words, there appears to be some age-based dynamics in the relationship between decoding and comprehension. They appear to be more closely related at the beginning of the process of reading acquisition but are more dissociated at the later stages when comprehension becomes increasingly dependent on skills of inferencing, capitalizing on general knowledge and vocabulary, deriving meaning from context, and so forth.

Fletcher (2009) notes a shift from a conception of general reading disorder to a description of more specific forms of reading difficulty. A differentiation can be made between dyslexia – which, he contends, describes a difficulty in decoding single words – and other forms of reading difficulty involving problems of reading fluency and comprehension. The child with dyslexia will most likely encounter problems in all three domains because of the decoding "bottleneck." For Fletcher, such individuals can be contrasted with a small number of nondyslexic poor readers who may demonstrate particular difficulties with fluency or comprehension but have few problems with single-word reading. Many people with reading difficulties succeed in overcoming the worst problems of decoding yet continue to struggle to read fluently (Biancarosa & Snow, 2006). (Note: The emphasis on single-word reading reflects the fact that, unlike for passages of continuous text, semantic and syntactic knowledge cannot be used to help decode the target words [Fletcher, 2009; Vellutino, Fletcher, Snowling, & Scanlon, 2004]).

Much of the literature on reading in international journals has had a strong Anglocentric focus, although this situation is being redressed with studies of reading difficulties in other languages now appearing more widely in prestigious international journals. Nevertheless, it has been argued that current knowledge has largely been derived from a highly idiosyncratic, "outlier" orthography (i.e., English) that has only limited relevance for a universal science of reading (Share, 2008). In transparent languages, the main reading difficulty tends to center on reading fluency rather than accurate word reading. In contrast, the complexities of letter-sound correspondence in the English language have resulted in a heavy focus on accuracy and a corresponding neglect, until relatively recently, of fluency in relation to both reading research and classroom instruction. Currently, the precise nature of reading fluency, its causal mechanisms, and whether the many features that are associated with it represent a single construct or a range of abilities are unclear. It remains to be seen whether greater interest in fluency, something that 'involves every process and subskill involved in reading' (Wolf & Katzir-Cohen, 2001, p. 220), will reduce the current emphasis on single-word reading in English-language speakers.

Recognition of the advantages of greater specification of different forms of reading difficulty would appear to be reflected in the recent psychiatric classification literature. The draft revision to the fifth version of the American Psychiatric Association's *Diagnostic and Statistical Manual* (DSM-5) originally suggested the replacement of the term "learning disorder" with that of "dyslexia" in order, it was stated, to render APA terminology consistent with international use. It was proposed that the term "dyslexia" should be employed to describe difficulties in reading accuracy or fluency that are not consistent with the person's chronological age, educational opportunities, or intellectual abilities.

In an update (May 2012), however, the draft proposals were amended. The diagnosis of *Learning Disorder* was now to be changed to *Specific Learning Disorder*, and the various named types of learning disorder (including dyslexia) were no longer recommended. The key reason for this was the variety of international conceptions and understandings of dyslexia (and other similar terms such as dyscalculia) that exist (Tannock, personal communication). Within the overarching category of *Specific Learning Disorder*, clinicians are required to specify for a given individual which particular domains of academic difficulty and their subskills are impaired. For *reading*, the particular skills identified are word reading accuracy, fluency, and reading comprehension. A second literacy-related domain, entitled *written expression*, includes spelling, grammar and punctuation, and clarity or organization of written expression.

One of the key difficulties of those who have tried to produce a definition of dyslexia concerns the extent of its inclusivity. Even relatively general definitions have been criticized as too inclusive by some groups and too exclusive by others. For example, a British Psychological Society (BPS) Working Party sought to provide what was described as a *working*, rather than an *operational*, definition (Reason, 2001). It is not immediately apparent exactly what this distinction means in practice, but it is likely that members of the Working Party were wary of producing a definitive account that might be subject to challenge in the courts or elsewhere in relation to specific cases. The BPS definition links accuracy and fluency together as follows: "Dyslexia is evident when accurate and fluent word reading and/or spelling develops very incompletely or with great difficulty. This focuses on literacy learning at the "word" level and implies that the problem is severe and persistent despite appropriate learning opportunities" (British Psychological Society, 1999, p. 64).

In the United Kingdom, the government-sponsored Rose Report (Rose, 2009) definition, geared primarily to a professional audience, took a similar stance: "Dyslexia is a learning difficulty that primarily affects the skills involved in accurate and fluent word reading and spelling" (p. 30). The highly general nature of this definition was subjected to criticism by the House of Commons, Science and Technology Select Committee (House of Commons, 2009) on the grounds that "[t]he Rose Report's definition of dyslexia is . . . so broad and blurred at the edges that it is difficult to see how it could be useful in any diagnostic sense" (paragraph 71, p. 26).

As previously noted, general definitions of this type can result in mutual dissatisfaction from otherwise opposing camps. On one side are those who think that such conceptions are too inclusive and spuriously include nondyslexic poor readers. On the other are those who believe that these are overly exclusive and rule out recognition of those "true" dyslexics who do not present with significant decoding problems but instead have other manifest forms of difficulty that stem from the condition. Situated within the former camp are those who believe that there are marked differences at the cognitive level between dyslexics and other poor readers. For such individuals, broad definitions fail to permit appropriate differentiation between these two groups (Herrington & Hunter-Carsch, 2001; Thomson, 2002, 2003). Thomson (2002) criticizes the BPS definition because, in his opinion, descriptive definitions of this kind downplay the importance of diagnosis, something he considers crucial for determining the most appropriate form of intervention.

In the latter camp are those who believe that descriptive definitions that focus on reading wrongly exclude from the diagnosis those who have other symptoms of dyslexia. Thus Cooke (2001, p. 49) was "in no doubt" that parents, teachers, and adult dyslexics would be concerned that the BPS definition could exclude those whose reading was no longer highly problematic but who nevertheless struggle with a range of problems such as being personally disorganized, experience difficulty filling in forms correctly, or find mathematical or musical notation problematic (a group, according to Cooke, that is sometimes misguidedly known as "compensated dyslexics"). In similar vein, she is also critical of the focus on reading at the word level on the grounds that this emphasis may exclude those whose primary difficulties concern reading fluency and comprehension.

If we wish to define dyslexia in a way that is more discriminating than that employed in the BPS or Rose solutions, the definition would need to be framed in a fashion that embodies either symptoms, causality or prognosis (Tønnessen, 1995). Symptoms refer to "observable and/or measurable signs of underlying conditions and processes. When we describe reading behaviour or reading achievement without reference to their underlying causes, then we are at the symptom level" (Tønnessen, 1997, p. 80). Symptom-based definitions of dyslexia may be inclusionary or exclusionary; the presence of the condition may be signaled by the absence of certain symptoms or by the presence of others.

Heaton and Winterton (1996) suggest that there are many reasons why a child may experience difficulties in learning to read. Key factors are:

- low intelligence
- socio-economic disadvantage
- inadequate schooling
- physical disability (e.g., visual or hearing difficulties)
- visible neurological impairment which goes beyond reading and writing
- emotional and behavioural factors which might affect attention, concentration and responsiveness to teacher direction
- dyslexia.

On such a basis, dyslexia could be defined and identified by the absence of the other six factors listed (Lyon, 1995). However, the field has tended to move away from identification on the base of exclusion (Lyon & Weiser, 2013) largely because when we seek to operationalize the construct on the basis of this conception, problems rapidly emerge.

As is discussed in some detail later in this chapter, the use of IQ for diagnostic purposes in dyslexia has been the subject of much debate and is now largely discredited. It would appear that for intellectual abilities to be considered as an exclusionary factor in a diagnosis, the individual would need to be functioning at a level sufficiently low to be considered to be "mentally retarded" – that is, scoring two or even three standard deviations below the mean on an IQ test. Such a perspective would imply that those with IQs no further than two standard deviations below the mean (typically, 70+) would not be automatically excluded from the possibility of a diagnosis of dyslexia. Such a view clearly differs from others (e.g., Nicolson & Fawcett, 2007), who consider dyslexic children to have average or above-average intelligence. Thus, these researchers are critical of a study by White et al. (2006), in which some children scoring below an IQ of 90 form part of the dyslexic sample, because this might lead to the inclusion of some with "no discrepancy between their reading and general performance" (Nicolson & Fawcett, 2006, p. 260).

Socioeconomic disadvantage is another highly problematic criterion, primarily because its use as an alternative explanation for reading difficulties could reduce the possibility of a diagnosis of dyslexia in poor readers from impoverished backgrounds (Rutter, 1978). Clearly, negative environmental circumstances, particularly disruptive early life experiences resulting from extreme poverty, and low levels of parental education will have a strong effect on the development of children's language and literacy (Hartas, 2011; Herbers et al., 2012). Wolf (2007), for example, cites a study of an impoverished Californian community (Hart & Risley, 2003) in which by the age of five, some of the children studied would have heard 32 million fewer words spoken to them than the average middle-class child. Socially disadvantaged children are less likely to have high levels of print exposure in the home, a resource that, while important for all children, appears to be particularly valuable for low-ability readers (Mol & Bus, 2011). There is also some evidence of a multiplicative relationship between socioeconomic status and phonological awareness (the latter often considered to be a key factor in dyslexia) whereby those from disadvantaged backgrounds may have reduced access to those experiences and resources that would help them overcome those reading problems that are underpinned by a phonological deficit (Noble, Farah, & McCandliss, 2006, although see Monzalvo et al., 2012, for a contrasting finding). From neuroscience, there is complementary evidence of socioeconomic status differences in brain structure (Jednoróg et al., 2012) and functioning that are arguably the product of environmental experience (Hackman & Farah, 2009; see also Hackman, Farah, & Meaney, 2010, for a discussion of possible causal factors).

It would surely be incongruous and unfair if distinctions between dyslexic and nondyslexic poor readers, and the differential expectations and perceptions and access to additional support that might result from these, were predicated on the basis of judgements about children's life experiences that reflected a strong social class component. All too easily a situation could emerge where either biological (dyslexic) or environmental (nondyslexic) explanations are ascribed to an individual on the grounds of their social circumstances. The reality is that, contrary to the picture that is often promoted by clinicians, it is impossible to distinguish between neurobiological and environmental etiologies when considering the needs of individual children who have scored poorly on reading-related measures (Fletcher, Lyons, Fuchs, & Barnes, 2007), and current biological evidence for a dyslexic subgroup does not yet permit diagnosis at the individual level (Rutter, Kim-Cohen, & Maughan, 2006).

Similarly, while the suggestion that inadequate schooling could rule out a diagnosis of dyslexia might at first appear to be relatively noncontentious (see, for example, Taylor, Roehrig, Soden Hensler, Connor, & Schatschneider, 2010), making a valid judgment in a clinical context would typically be very difficult. Should such a conclusion be based on the extent of the child's attendance at school? The nature of the reading (or wider) curriculum? The approaches to teaching and learning employed? The perceived skills of the teaching staff? The quality of the classroom learning environment? Or the extent to which parents actively support and reinforce the school's work? As noted in Chapter 4, when the whole-language approach to the teaching of reading held sway, and structured approaches to the teaching of reading were anathema to many, it may have been rather easier to offer a judgment that a child's difficulties were exacerbated by an inappropriate teaching approach. However, even here problems remain, for it is the interaction of underlying reading disability and an inappropriate, unstructured educational environment that together lead to the greatest likelihood of difficulty.

Equally difficult is any attempt to disentangle dyslexia from emotional and behavioral difficulties. Many children diagnosed as dyslexic show evidence of poor attention and concentration, and some present with a range of emotional or behavioral difficulties. Mugnaini, Lassi, La Malfa, and Albertini's (2009) review of the dyslexia literature found a significant association with internalizing disorders such anxiety and depression. Given the importance and significance of literacy activities in school and wider life, it is hardly surprising that a history of struggle often leads to a variety of emotional problems in adolescence (Eissa, 2010; Goldston et al., 2007).

Children encountering reading difficulties can sometimes present with externalising behavior. Thus, Morgan, Farkas, et al. (2008) found that reading problems in first grade increased the likelihood of problem behavior in third grade even after controlling for prior behavior and potential demographic-related confounds. Noting that early behavioral problems also predicted subsequent reading difficulties, the authors suggested a bidirectional causal model in which initial difficulties create a negative feedback cycle that results in disengagement from academic activity and increasingly problematic behaviour (see also McGee, Williams, Share, Anderson, & Silva, 1986). In a similar vein, there is some evidence that young children with decoding difficulties gradually become less concerned about getting things exactly right in class (Grills-Taquechel, Fletcher, Vaughn, & Stuebing, 2012).

Several commentators have pointed to a strong relationship between reading disability and juvenile offending (Grigorenko, 2006; Kirk & Reid, 2001), although the precise nature of the link between dyslexia and criminality is disputed (Rice, 1999; Samuelsson, Herkner, & Lundberg, 2003).

Attentional difficulties are common in struggling readers, and there is strong evidence of comorbidity for reading disability and attention deficit hyperactivity disorder (ADHD) in both clinical (Cheung et al., 2012 Mayes & Calhoun, 2006) and epidemiological samples (Gilger, Pennington, & DeFries, 1992). McGrath et al. (2011) note that while reading disability and ADHD occur in approximately 5% of the population, between 25% and 40% of children with one of these disorders also meet the criteria for the other. Indeed, it is claimed that ADHD is the most common developmental disorder that co-occurs with reading disability, although definitional difficulties, differences in methods of assessment, and limited epidemiological evidence render it difficult to achieve a clear picture of the prevalence (Sexton, Gellhorn, Bell, & Classi, 2012) or possible causal pathways of these conditions (Taylor, 2011).

It appears that correlations with reading achievement are higher for the inattentive than for the hyperactive dimension of ADHD (Chhabildas, Pennington, & Wilcutt, 2001; McGrath et al., 2011; Willcutt, Pennington, Olson, & DeFries, 2007; Willcutt et al., 2010). Evidence of inattention difficulties in those with reading disabilities has similarly been found in experimental studies. Thus,

Ben-Yehudah and Ahissar (2004) found inattention in a dyslexic sample to be greater than for controls but not within the range scored by an ADHD sample. However, within the dyslexic group, reading and attention scores were uncorrelated. A recent neuroscience study of kindergarten children at risk for reading disability, albeit involving only a very small sample, has pointed to a relationship between the neural mechanisms of selective attention and early reading skills (Stevens et al., 2013).

As with the criterion of intelligence, it is not clear whether exclusionary factors such as those previously discussed should concern only that very small proportion of children with the most profound difficulties – cases where a judgment may be made relatively easily – or a significantly larger group where determining a clear set of causal factors for the difficulties observed becomes highly complex. In practice, the major emphasis has historically been on discrepancies between reading achievement and IQ, and other exclusionary factors, especially those that concern the quality of the child's environmental and instructional experiences, have not proven to be influential (Tunmer, 2008).

Rutter and Maughan (2005) find the widespread use of exclusionary definitions to be surprising, a position shared by Fletcher (2009) who expresses dissatisfaction about the use of definitions that indicate what dyslexia is not. However, much may depend on the purpose that the definition is being employed to serve. Exclusionary definitions of dyslexia are often utilized by researchers (Rice & Brooks, 2004; Vellutino, 1979) so that meaningful comparisons between sound and poor readers can be undertaken. On some occasions, restrictions to a dyslexic sample may be made in order to isolate, for the purpose of research, certain underlying cognitive processes (Snowling, 2008), but in such cases it would be a mistake to consider the sample as being representative of all individuals with dyslexia.

In clinical practice, diagnosis is typically based on the presence of associated symptoms. While there is no shortage of these listed in the literature, using them to effect a meaningful judgment about the presence of dyslexia for a given individual is a problematic exercise. Lists of symptoms of dyslexia often include: difficulties in phonological awareness, poor short-term (or, working) verbal memory, poor ordering and sequencing, weak spelling, clumsiness, a poor sense of rhythm, difficulty with rapid information processing, poor concentration, inconsistent hand preference, impaired verbal fluency, poor phonic skills, frequent letter reversals, poor capacity for mental calculation, difficulties with speech and language, low self-image, and anxiety when being asked to read aloud. Critics of such lists (Elliott & Gibbs, 2008; Rice & Brooks, 2004) note that none of the symptoms is necessary or sufficient for a diagnosis. A further difficulty concerns the observation that many "signs of dyslexia" can be found in poor readers who may not universally considered to be dyslexic, and also in other individuals without reading problems. Some difficulties seen as typical of dyslexics – for example, letter reversals – are also commonly found in younger normal readers reading at the same age level (Cassar et al., 2005). To add to this complexity, similar characteristics are widely employed in the diagnosis of other developmental disorders such as ADHD, dyscalculia, or dyspraxia (Elliott & Place, 2012).

Drawing on the work of Bishop (1997), Frith (1997), and Snowling (2000), the Rose Report (2009) stated that, as a disorder of development, the difficulties experienced by the dyslexic child are likely to change as he or she passes through school and enters adulthood. According to the Report, at the preschool stage, signs of dyslexia are most likely to be delayed or problematic speech, poor expressive language, poor rhyming skills, and little interest and/or difficulty in learning letters. In the early school years, problems are most likely to include poor letter-sound knowledge, poor phoneme awareness, poor word attack skills, idiosyncratic spelling and difficulties in copying. In the middle school years, typical difficulties will include slow reading speed, poor decoding skills when confronted by new words, and difficulties with spelling. In adolescence and adulthood, principal difficulties will most likely be poor reading fluency, slow speed of writing, and poor organization and expression in work. Within the adult workplace, others have suggested that the processing difficulties of dyslexia are likely to affect organization, time management, social communication, writing (in particular, organizing ideas), spelling, reading (most likely comprehension rather than accuracy) and mathematics (McLoughlin & Leather, 2009).

The Rose Report identified three characteristic features of dyslexia: weakness in phonological awareness, weakness in verbal memory, and weakness in verbal processing speed. Each of these is examined in detail in Chapter 2. However, it should be noted at this point that none of these markers is deemed necessary for a diagnosis. Similarly, problems of language, mental calculation, motor coordination, concentration, and personal organization, while possibly comorbid, cannot by themselves be recognized as markers of dyslexia.

In respect of diagnosis, the Rose Report is somewhat confusing. In line with current thinking that reading disability/dyslexia reflects a dimension rather than a categorical diagnosis (Pennington & Bishop, 2009; Snowling, 2008), it is stated that

dyslexia is best thought of as a continuum, not a distinct category, and there are no clear cut-off points. . . . Until recently, a child was deemed to either have or not have dyslexia. It is now recognised that there is no sharp dividing line between having a learning difficulty such as dyslexia and not having it. (p. 33)

Despite this claim, the Report suggests that an accurate diagnosis can be made by specialists. Such a perspective reflects a belief that categorical labels such as dyslexia are more helpful than dimensional accounts are for communicating the nature of the difficulty (Hulme & Snowling, 2009), a position that has been criticized for glossing over the practical realities of identification and resourcing of children with special educational needs (Norwich, 2010). To be effective, such an approach requires consensual understandings as to the meaning of the categorical term concerned. However, a particular problem for dyslexia is that this is clearly not the case.

A focus on symptomatology or underlying causes differs from an alternative position in which the key criterion is the individual's place on a continuum ranging from poor to good readers (Swanson & Hsieh, 2009). Thus, those who might be described as reading disabled or dyslexic would be those who score at the left-hand tail of a normal distribution of readers. Mazzocco and Grimm (2013), for example, employ the 10th percentile as a cut-off point (on a nonword reading test) to differentiate between children deemed to have reading disability and other poor readers scoring in the 11th–25th percentile, who were described as being low achieving in reading. Similarly, in a longitudinal study of dyslexics, Pennington et al. (2012) take for their sample those scoring at the 10th percentile or below, although this time a reading fluency test was employed. In retesting the children the following year, they note that some other children in their study scored below the criterion level and, as a result, "became dyslexic" (p. 221).

The Rose Report appeared to conflate these differing understandings. It endorsed the construct of dyslexia, argued that it was at the more severe end of a reading performance continuum, and appeared to support a medical model in which experts retain a role in determining who is and who is not dyslexic. The Report set out a three-level model for assessment and diagnosis. At Level 1, class teachers "will be aware of the possibility that some children may have dyslexia. However, they will not declare that a particular child has dyslexia" (p. 53). By Level 3, appropriately qualified specialists "would make a decision on whether or not the child has dyslexia, and with what severity" (p. 53). How exactly such a determination might be arrived at was rendered rather less clear. Such phrasing seems inconsistent with the claims of a member of the Rose Expert Advisory Group that "it was not a question of dyslexia, yes or no" (Reason & Stothard, 2013, p. 12), and seems to strike a dissonant chord with the Report's other remarks about dividing lines. This apparent tension reinforces a perception that influential professional and other lobby groups had succeeded in ensuring the continuation of a model in which experts offer diagnostic pronouncements (see House of Commons, Science and Technology Committee, 2009, for criticism of the influence of dyslexia lobby groups on the UK government).

A further approach is to define dyslexia as *unexpected* poor performance in reading, writing, or spelling (e.g., World Federation of Neurology, 1968). However, this is not easy to operationalize:

Developmental dyslexia or reading disability refers to unexpected poor performance in reading. Poor performance in reading typically is defined as performance markedly below that of one's peers or expectations based on some form of standards. What constitutes an unexpected level of poor performance in reading has been more difficult to define. (Wagner, 2008, p. 174)

In practice, the markers used to indicate unexpected performance are likely to overlap closely with what might commonly be seen as key exclusionary factors, and, thus, in practice, these two approaches may not differ greatly in outcome. Shaywitz (2005), however, offers a rather different conceptualization by suggesting that unexpectedness is revealed by an uneven cognitive profile in which a decoding weakness is typically surrounded by a "sea of strengths" (p. 58), which may include high functioning in respect of reasoning, problem solving, critical thinking, vocabulary, comprehension, and general knowledge. Such a profile may, to some extent, be an artifact of studies of dyslexia clinic populations which, at least where fees are involved, are likely to involve families enjoying higher levels of cultural and linguistic capital.

The suggestion that sound general knowledge and vocabulary may be markers of dyslexia contradicts the position of others who have argued that poor scores on the Information subtest (a measure of general knowledge) of the Wechsler Intelligence Scales are an important component of a dyslexic profile (Vargo, Grossner, & Spafford, 1995). It also runs counter to the fact that poor vocabulary is an expected consequence of the reduced reading experience of those who struggle with literacy. A reduced vocabulary is also likely to impact the young child's capacity to decode unknown printed words, particularly where these are partially decoded or irregularly spelled. This, in turn, will hamper the further development of the child's phonological recoding skills (Tunmer & Greaney, 2010). A further difficulty resulting from the "sea of strengths" conception concerns how best to represent those children whose cognitive profiles are relatively flat (Fletcher, Stuebing, Morris, & Lyon, 2013). To avoid the use of the learning disabilities label (of which reading disability/dyslexia is but one component) for such children is quite rightly considered to be "absurd" (Fletcher, Morris, & Lyon, 2003, p. 52).

It is difficult to determine whether the additional presence of mathematical difficulties should reduce or increase a perception that poor reading is unexpected. Mathematical, particularly arithmetical, difficulties are frequently found in the dyslexia literature and often listed when symptoms of dyslexia are provided. However, it is possible to conclude that the presence of difficulties in other academic disciplines such as math would reduce the unexpected nature of the reading problem. One additional complexity results from limited consideration of the relationship between arithmetic/mathematics performance and differing types of reading difficulty. One recent study, for example, has found that children with word reading difficulties tend to demonstrate weaker mathematics performance than those who encounter problems with reading comprehension (Vukovic, Lesaux, & Siegel, 2010).

Inconsistent findings as to the comorbidity of reading and mathematical disabilities have added complexity to an issue that is currently receiving significant attention (Branum-Martin, Fletcher, & Steubing, 2013, Fuchs, Fuchs, & Compton, 2013). Willcutt et al. (2013) state that reading disability and math disability co-occur in 30% to 70% of those with either disorder. Landerl and Moll (2010) similarly report varying rates across studies, stating that between 11% and 56% of children with a reading disability also show arithmetic problems, and between 17% and 70% of those with arithmetic disorder also are having problems with reading. They suggest that these wide variations result from the use of different measures that tap different constructs (with some mathematics tests making significant demands upon reading) and the use of different cut-off points. Cut-off points would appear to be significant; Dirks, Spyer, van Lieshout, & de Sonneville (2008), for example, found that comorbidity between arithmetic and reading difficulties declined sharply as selection criteria became more stringent. Indeed, for those scoring below the 10th percentile, comorbidity was a mere 1% – a level that might be expected by chance. A similar finding was found in a large-population study (Landerl & Moll, 2010) when the cut-off was reduced from -1 SD to -1.5 SD. The authors suggest that this phenomenon may be explained by the fact that the less stringent the criteria, the higher the likelihood that children whose problems are primarily environmental will be included (Bishop, 2001). Environmental factors tend to depress academic performance across the board and thus inflate comorbidity rates. On the basis of existing findings and their study of a sample of 684 Grade 3–5 students, Compton, Fuchs, Fuchs, Lambert, & Hamlett (2012) conclude that most students with learning disabilities do not experience severe academic deficits in both reading and mathematics.

Unexpectedness is often seen to be present when there is a discrepancy between reading performance, as measured by a standardized test, and linguistic or cognitive skills, usually involving a standardized measure of intelligence. Indeed, Thomson (2003) goes so far as to argue that only measures of discrepancy can demonstrate that an unexpected problem exists. However, as is discussed in the following section, this approach is problematic.

Dyslexia as a discrepancy between reading and IQ

For the general public, and indeed for many education professionals (Machek & Nelson, 2007), understandings of dyslexia typically involve a picture of an able person whose abilities are masked by a specific problem with literacy. Indeed, the long-standing association between IQ and dyslexia has rendered it almost impossible to disconnect the two from social and political discourse

(Elbeheri & Everatt, 2009). In relation to dyslexia, much debate has focused on the value of the "two-group" hypothesis in which poor readers are divided on the basis of their IQ. Poor readers with high IQs (so-called dyslexics), it was believed, could be differentiated from non-dyslexics ("garden variety" poor readers) whose difficulties were deemed to be more likely the result of general cognitive weakness.

In order to have any direct utility for tackling reading difficulties, differences between IQ-discrepant groups and nondiscrepant groups may involve:

1. identification of valid differences on the basis of academic and/or cognitive factors that underlie reading performance (e.g., phonological processing);
2. differences in response to reading instruction;
3. differences in prognosis.

The reality is that IQ has been consistently unable to make meaningful differentiations on any of these bases. Meta-analyses and scorecard reviews (Fletcher et al., 2007; Hoskyn and Swanson, 2000; Stuebing et al., 2002, 2009) have yielded little evidence to support the suggestion that IQ-achievement discrepancy is an important predictor of decoding-related differences between those deemed to be low-achieving children and those considered to have dyslexia.

Importantly, studies have repeatedly shown that IQ scores cannot differentiate between poor readers who can be successfully remediated and those who are likely to be more resistant to intervention (Gresham & Vellutino, 2010). Neither do they yield valuable data that can be used for engineering differing forms of intervention to address decoding difficulties. On the basis of their meta-analysis, Stuebing and colleagues conclude that IQ predicted only 1% to 3% of the variance in the children's response to reading intervention. Noting that a small effect might still be relevant, particularly where any costs involved are minor, it was pointed out that in comparison with relatively expensive IQ procedures, baseline assessment of word reading skills proved to be a much stronger predictor. For this reason the authors queried why anyone would choose to use IQ rather than "a shorter task with a much stronger relation with outcome" (Vellutino et al., 2008, p. 45). Another indicator more effective than IQ would appear to be children's response to classroom intervention (Vellutino et al., 2008).

Finally, studies undertaken in which students were repeatedly tested over many years (Flowers et al., 2001; Francis et al., 1996) have shown that IQ discrepancy offers little prognostic information about future reading performance.

To date, there is no significant neurophysiological evidence of different aetiologies for discrepant and nondiscrepant groups (Fletcher et al., 2007; Tanaka et al., 2011). However, there is some evidence for a stronger genetic contribution to reading difficulty for those with high IQ (Wadsworth, Olson, & DeFries, 2010).

Stanovich and Stanovich (1997) argue that if there is no empirical evidence to support the suggestion that we should make separate classifications and treatments for discrepant and nondiscrepant groups, such a step would need to be based on a social policy decision arising from notions of social justice in relation to the fulfillment of the child's educational potential. Thus, the argument would run, children with high IQ scores have a greater severity of need (cf. Ashton, 1996, 1997) because the realisation of their higher potential is undermined by their reading difficulties. However, this position is highly problematic.

The notion that IQ tests provide a picture of fixed potential that places a limit on academic achievement has a long tradition. As Sir Cyril Burt, England's first school psychologist, noted, "Capacity must obviously limit content. It is impossible for a pint jug to hold more than a pint of milk and it is equally impossible for a child's educational attainment to rise higher than his educable capacity" (Burt, 1937, p. 477). Given that IQ was designed originally to predict subsequent educational achievement, a task in which it is relatively successful (Sternberg & Grigorenko, 2002), it seems plausible to argue that poor readers with high IQs are particularly likely to benefit from additional assistance. If this were true, identifying dyslexic children on this basis and providing them with additional assistance might seem to be a logical way of gaining most benefit from the distribution of limited resources. However, in addition to the ethical issues this raises, such a proposition can also be contested on scientific grounds; IQ was always meant to function as a general predictor across the curriculum, not as a means to make focused predictions in specific curriculum areas. Furthermore, reliance on such measures is problematic not only because IQ scores appear to be less stable in children than was once thought (Ramsden et al., 2011), but also because the use of the IQ test as a proxy for cognitive potential is itself highly contested (Lidz & Elliott, 2000; Sternberg & Grigorenko, 2002). In addition, there is some evidence that reading less (and less well) not only affects reading development but also undermines performance on IQ tests themselves (Ferrer et al., 2010), an example of the "Matthew effect" (Stanovich, 1986) that can lead to an underestimation of the cognitive potential of those with severe reading difficulties.

A further policy-related argument concerns the use of a discrepancy model to identify those children whose reading is poorer than their cognitive ability, but whose literacy difficulties are not sufficiently low to be deemed eligible for additional educational support. In a longitudinal study undertaken in Connecticut (Shaywitz, 2005; Shaywitz, Morris, & Shaywitz, 2008), it was found that 75% of children identified by discrepancy criteria also met low-achievement reading criteria. These researchers suggest that the remaining 25% may still be struggling with their reading but not to a level that is recognized on the basis of comparisons with peers using norm-referenced measures.

For some (e.g., Shaywitz et al., 2008; Thomson, 2009), such children merit additional assistance; others disagree on the grounds that finite resources should be targeted toward those whose absolute levels of literacy performance are weakest.

Some have argued that while global IQ scores appear to have little diagnostic or clinical utility in themselves, various combinations of subtests from these measures may yield useful diagnostic information. The use of subtest profile analysis for diagnosing dyslexia has proven attractive to some educational psychologists, although support for this approach has tended to come from clinical accounts rather than from rigorous empirical investigation (Watkins, Kush, & Glutting, 1997). Popular among clinicians during the 1980s and 1990s was the ACID profile in which low scores on arithmetic, coding, information, and digit span subtests from the Wechsler Intelligence Scales for Children were considered to be indicative of dyslexia (Vargo et al., 1995). The most common procedure is to compare an individual's scores on the ACID profile with their performance on the other subtests that together make up the full IQ score. If all the four ACID subtest scores are equal to, or lower than, the lowest score on the other subtests, the individual is considered to have a positive ACID profile. (Note: Kaufman [1994] suggested a rather different subtest cluster [SCAD] in which the Information measure was replaced by the Symbol Search subtest).

While children with reading difficulties often score poorly on these subtests, the incidence of the overall ACID profile is typically low, generally 4–5% in samples of learning-disabled children (Prifitera & Dersch, 1993; Ward et al., 1995; Watkins, Kush, & Glutting, 1997). Ward and colleagues also examined a subset of children with marked IQ-reading discrepancies but found the incidence even lower, at 3.9%. Such incidence levels do not result in useful clinical information for diagnosing and intervening with individuals. Somewhat puzzlingly, Thomson (2003), a long-standing advocate of psychometric testing for poor readers, found a much higher rate of 40% in a sample of children at a special school for dyslexic children where he was employed, although this finding, remarkably different to other major studies, may merely reflect local education authority diagnostic practices and referral patterns. In Thomson's (2003) study, particular weaknesses were found on Digit Span, Coding and Symbol Search although poor performance on Arithmetic and Information subtests was also noted. Subsequently, using a later version of the Wechsler Scales (WISC-IV), arithmetic was substituted by a new subtest, letter-number sequencing (Thomson, 2009). The subtests in both studies generally tap those cognitive processes (working memory, rapid naming) that are widely agreed to be problematic for poor readers (see Chapter 2), and so weaknesses in these areas are unsurprising. (Information seemingly taps a different set of skills. Low scores on this subtest, a measure of general knowledge, will, in part, reflect reduced opportunity to gain information from reading.)

Profiling on the basis of IQ subtests is now generally agreed to be of little diagnostic value for identifying dyslexic children (British Psychological Society, 1999; Frederickson, 1999; Ward, Ward, Hatt, Young, & Molner, 1995). Indeed, the weaknesses of this approach appear to range wider than just reading; Watkins et al. (1997) contend that all forms of WISC subtest analysis for learning difficulties have proven fruitless and should be abandoned. However, more recently it has been argued that subtest profiling on the WISC-IV may be valuable, largely because of the addition of working memory items (De Clercq-Quaegebeur et al., 2010). However, these authors accept that particular WISC-IV profiles cannot be employed to indicate the presence, or absence, of dyslexia. An alternative case for considering IQ subtests is that these may point to specific forms of intervention (Thomson, 2009). As noted elsewhere, this claim has little empirical support. Indeed, there appears to be little value in using profiles from IQ tests for any valid form of clinical classification or diagnosis (Canivez, 2013).

In pointing out the lack of utility of IQ for assessing the nature of reading difficulty, Stanovich (2005) outlines three key findings from research:

1. The primary subcomponent of reading that is problematic for children with severe reading problems is word recognition.
2. The primary psychological process underlying the word-recognition difficulties of reading disabled individuals is a problem in phonological coding due to weak segmental language skills.
3. Both the distal processing problem in the phonological domain and the proximal word-recognition problem can in part be remediated with intensive intervention.

The problem for the discrepancy assumption . . . is: *none of these facts correlate at all with IQ!* (p. 104) (emphasis as in original).

Given the wealth of research on the limited role of IQ in relation to dyslexia, with similar findings in other languages with a more regular orthography such as Finnish (Kortteinen, Närhi, & Ahonen, 2009) or Spanish (Jiménez & Garcia de la Cadena, 2007), it is unsurprising that the state-of-the-art review by Vellutino et al. (2004) concluded that "intelligence tests have little utility for diagnosing specific reading disability" (p. 29). Practitioners were advised to "shift the focus of their clinical activities away from emphasis on psychometric assessment to detect cognitive and biological causes of a child's reading difficulties for purposes of categorical labelling in favour of assessment that would eventuate in educational and remedial activities tailored to the child's individual needs" (p. 31). Such advice has been supported by several, more recent studies that show that a focus on identifying students' academic skills may offer the most helpful information for determining appropriate forms of instruction suited to the child's individual needs (see Connor, 2010, for a detailed discussion).

The demise of the IQ discrepancy model has done much to undermine the clinical utility of the dyslexia construct. From a position in which it was thought relatively easy to differentiate – from within a wider group of poor readers, a dyslexic subgroup with genuinely different abilities and needs – the finding that IQ had little to offer to diagnosis or intervention in respect of accurate and fluent reading resulted in a construct that now appeared to have little to offer that was additional or unique.

Despite the overwhelming scientific evidence against the utility of the IQ discrepancy model for diagnosis and intervention, there continues to be a significant proportion of teachers and school psychologists (Machek & Nelson, 2007; O'Donnell & Miller, 2011) and even some researchers (Warnke, Schulte-Körne, & Ise, 2012) who continue to advocate its use. While such resistance can seem puzzling (Stanovich, 2005), there are a number of reasons that help explain this phenomenon.

First, average or above-average intelligence has for so long been a defining feature of dyslexia (Catts & Kamhi, 1999), that this association, steeped in everyday understandings, has proven difficult to break.

Second, some prominent researchers have persisted with the argument that developmental dyslexia concerns an unexpected difficulty in learning to read for those with average or above-average intelligence (e.g., Nicolson & Fawcett, 2007). However, whether the lower endpoint of the "average" range is taken to be one or two standard deviations below the mean is not always made clear. Snowling (2008) appears to conceive of "normal" IQ as falling within one standard deviation from the mean in line with the majority of researchers who tend to select this point as the cut-off – that is, full-scale IQ >85 (Rice & Brooks, 2004, pp. 148–152). But this would mean that a child with an IQ in the low 80s could not be classified as dyslexic – for many this would represent an untenable position. A common practice is to set the cut-off at 1.5 standard deviations (Peterson and Pennington, 2012). Below two standard deviations (<70), children in the United States most likely would fit a classification of intellectual disability (formerly known as mental retardation), which is typically employed as an exclusionary factor.

Third, the association is perpetuated by the widespread use of IQ as a criterion in the selection of participants for research studies (Rice & Brooks, 2004). Some researchers appear to experience little dissonance between their acceptance that dyslexia/reading disability is a problem encountered by those at all levels of intellectual ability and their own continued employment of dyslexic samples where average or above-average IQs are a criterion for selection. In such instances, it would often appear that a distinction is made between clinical and research activity, and that while identifying groups on the basis of IQ does not serve a clinical or diagnostic function, studying poor readers with normal-range IQs may help shed light on underlying cognitive mechanisms that may not otherwise be easily revealed (Snowling, 2008).

Fourth, it has been argued that the continued use of IQ in the assessment of dyslexia reflects the absence of appropriate alternatives. In putting forward such a position, Elbeheri and Everatt (2009) argue that positive (inclusive) diagnostic indicators are still not sufficiently robust and until these "are fully explored and reliably measured, the arguments for using IQ tests as a basis of indication will be difficult to refute" (p. 30). However, there is strong evidence to suggest that this approach is gradually being supplanted by the use of a response to intervention (RTI) model (O'Donnell & Miller, 2011).

Fifth, IQ tests have long held an important role in many countries in determining eligibility for additional education services. A riposte to the challenge to the discrepancy model is that without measures of intelligence, some highly able children may not receive the additional services they require. Thus, following this line of reasoning, IQ tests may help identify intellectually able children whose reading levels, while depressed, are not so poor that they would typically be identified as requiring special services (Shaywitz, 2005). (As noted earlier, there are a number of problems with this argument.) Unfortunately, the converse would be true, and the application of an IQ-achievement model could serve to exclude less intellectually able children from specialized literacy-related intervention (Catts, Hogan, & Fey, 2003).

Sixth, it is clear that there is a relationship between IQ and higher-order reading skills. Cognitive tests may help shed light on the specific nature of a child's higher-order reading comprehension difficulties involving such processes as reasoning, inference, and logical deduction (Christopher et al., 2012; Vellutino et al., 2004) or assisting in the prediction of responsiveness to instruction when this is assessed by complex reading tasks (Frijjters et al., 2011).

Seventh, the IQ test is an instrument whose usage is restricted to those with appropriate qualifications and thus is a means of reserving and maintaining professional influence and status. Thus, with some evident frustration, Stanovich (2005) cites a comment in the house journal of the American Psychological Association that provides an analogy with an iconic tool of medicine: "[T]he intelligence test is our stethoscope, like it or not" (Kersting, 2004, p. 54). Despite powerful research evidence demonstrating the problems of the IQ-reading discrepancy model, the psychology profession is accused of continuing to resist reform from the inside (Stanovich, 2005). However, this does not merely reflect a lack of engagement with current scientific knowledge, for it would be a mistake to consider professional practice as a purely scientific pursuit devoid of political and personal concerns. To accept the admonitions of Vellutino et al. (2004) that practitioners should change the focus of assessment from cognitive testing to reading-related behaviors is to introduce a threat to many professionals schooled in the psychometric tradition who may lack high-level expertise in curricular and pedagogic practices.

Finally, for many poor readers there is a powerful desire to ensure that their reading difficulties are not perceived by others as indicative of low intelligence.

As Covington (1992) has shown, the desire to demonstrate underlying ability when the risk of low achievement is high can be very powerful, and this may result in the exercise of a range of self-protective behaviors. Personal accounts in the media and in the scientific and professional literatures (Riddick, 2010) often describe the hurt and humiliation that result from the widespread and pervasive misunderstanding that poor decoders are intellectually weak. The great attraction of a diagnostic label that not only decouples intelligence and reading ability but is also suggestive of higher-level intellectual functioning is understandable. The frequent references in the mass media to gifted dyslex- ics (e.g., Albert Einstein, Thomas Edison and Winston Churchill) merely feed this perception. It is not surprising, therefore, that academic challenges to the usefulness of the concept of dyslexia have been met by strong emotion and occasional hostility (Elliott, 2008). To add to this problem, a common parental concern is that teachers may incorrectly perceive their child as unin- telligent because of their literacy difficulties. Such perceptions are likely to result in lower teacher expectations, which may have a detrimental effect on the effort and support expended by classroom staff to help the child progress. In turn, teachers may convey negative messages to the child, which can serve to undermine their sense of competence and self-efficacy and further reduce academic motivation and engagement. Such pressures may equally exist in higher education contexts, where some academic staff may mistakenly find it difficult to accept that the intellectual abilities of those with reading disabilities may be little different from those of their peers (Callens, Tops, & Brysbaert, 2012).

A recent study by van Bergen et al. (in press) highlights the complexity of issues concerning IQ, dyslexia, and general reading difficulties. In this study it was found that four-year-olds who were later classified as dyslexic performed relatively poorly in both verbal and nonverbal IQ subtests. The authors conclude that this finding challenges the discrepancy model that assumes that dyslexic children should not demonstrate poor performance on cognitive (IQ) measures. However, the children in the study were identified as dyslexic on the basis of poor performance on a word reading fluency test (<10th percentile). As dis- cussed earlier, most advocates of the discrepancy model have argued that this should be used to differentiate between those who are "garden variety" poor decoders and others who are dyslexic. Perhaps what van Bergen and colleagues' work demonstrates is a gradual shift in the conception of dyslexia. This term is now less commonly employed by researchers to describe a particular, diag- nosable condition found in a subset of poor decoders, but instead is used as a more inclusive term to describe all those who struggle to decode. As previously noted, however, such a shift may be less evident among clinicians for whom the capacity to offer intragroup diagnostic classifications may continue to be more attractive.

Dyslexia and language disorders

Although early language skills are related to subsequent reading performance (Hayiou-Thomas, Harlaar, Dale, & Plomin, 2010), the relationship between speech and language disorders and dyslexia is complex, and the two conditions are not easily disentangled. Indeed, some prominent researchers have argued that dyslexia should be considered as a particular subtype of general language-processing difficulty (Bishop & Snowling, 2004; Catts, Fey, Tomblin, & Zhang, 2002). Specific language impairment (SLI, sometimes known as developmental dysphasia or developmental language disorder) concerns impaired receptive or expressive language. Children with SLI, it is argued, will typically share some similar features with those with dyslexia (particularly in the area of phonological processing and the consequent problems this will cause for the acquisition of literacy skills [McArthur & Castles, in press]), yet the individual with SLI would usually be expected to have broader language problems involving comprehension, vocabulary, and syntax (Stackhouse & Wells, 1997).

McArthur et al. (2000) examined 110 Australian middle school children diagnosed as having a specific reading disability, and 102 classified as having a specific language impairment. They found that just over half (53%) could have been diagnosed with either condition. Fifty-five percent of the children with an SRD had impaired oral language and 51% of those with an SLI had reading accuracy difficulties (reading comprehension was not assessed). The authors concluded that for those with both reading and language problems, the particular diagnostic label that had been provided reflected their current placement, a mainstream classroom or language center, rather than any particular features of their reading and language difficulties. Given these findings, the authors query whether the term "specific" should really apply to such cases.

It is possible to examine the potential overlap between SLI and reading difficulty even before children learn to read. Thus, Nash et al. (2013) compared the language skills of young children (aged 3.5 to 4.5 years) who were at family risk of dyslexia with those of children with SLI and typically developing controls. One-third of those in the at-risk group met the diagnostic criteria for SLI.

The presence of a broader language difficulty does not necessarily mean that reading will be problematic. Several studies have identified children with language impairment who are competent at single-word reading yet who do not display any significant phonological impairments (e.g., Bishop, Mcdonald, Bird, & Hayiou-Thomas, 2009; Catts, Adlof, Hogan, & Weismer, 2005; Ramus, Marshall, Rosen, & van der Lely, 2013). Thus, it would appear that specific language impairment and reading disability are best considered as distinct disorders that are often comorbid (Ramus et al., 2013).

In line with what has been termed the simple view of reading, which differentiates word recognition from language comprehension (Gough & Tunmer, 1986), it has been suggested that the individual with dyslexia is typically one who struggles with word recognition but has little difficulty in understanding its message when it is read aloud for them (Tunmer, 2008). Those who have problems in both decoding and comprehension of oral language are sometimes described as having a mixed reading disability (see also Catts & Kamhi, 2005). While there is support in the literature for the argument that word reading and language comprehension are relatively independent processes, there remains a degree of overlap, and their independence should not be overstated (Ricketts, 2011).

The changing demands of the reading process over time help explain why the composition of poor reader groups is often far from stable as children gravitate from elementary to high school (Adlof, Catts, & Lee, 2010), and why those with specific language impairment may not be identified as poor readers at a young age. In the early years of school, an ability to decode simple words may be sufficient for such children to cope with noncomplex narratives of commonly used words. In later years, as texts become more syntactically and semantically complex, language-based weaknesses are likely to become more problematic for reading, particularly in relation to comprehension (Hogan & Thomson, 2010).

Another form of language disorder, concerning the production of correct speech, is known as speech sound disorder (SSD). The defining characteristics of this condition are substitutions or omissions of sounds from words and poor intelligibility because of speech production errors (Pennington & Bishop, 2009). In a longitudinal study comparing SSD with control children, Peterson, Pennington, Shriberg, & Boada (2009) found that while reading appeared to be more problematic in the SSD group, many of these children did not develop reading disabilities. Furthermore, it was found that it was broad language function, rather than early speech production, that predicted reading disability. In general, it appears that children whose difficulties are limited to expressive phonology may develop unimpaired levels of literacy, and the risk to reading development posed by SSD in isolation is negligible (Pennington & Bishop, 2009). However, it would seem that reading difficulties are likely to be greatest when both SSD and SLI are both present (Bishop & Adams, 1990; Catts, 1993).

Definitions based on causal explanations

Tønnessen (1995) suggests that an alternative to focusing on symptoms is to seek a definition that can offer a causal explanation. Such definitions often retain the notion of "unexpectedness," with many emphasizing phonological factors.

The International Dyslexia Association cites the definition provided by the U.S. National Institutes of Child Health and Human Development:

Dyslexia is a specific learning disability that is neurological in origin. It is characterized by difficulties with accurate and/or fluent word recognition and by poor spelling and decoding abilities. These difficulties typically result from a deficit in the phonological component of language that is often unexpected in relation to other cognitive abilities and the provision of effective classroom instruction. Secondary consequences may include problems in reading comprehension and reduced reading experience that can impede growth of vocabulary and background knowledge. (Lyon, Shaywitz, & Shaywitz, 2003, p. 2)

In line with this definition, Torgesen, Foorman, and Wagner (undated) differentiate between dyslexics (whose problems are considered to stem largely from neurobiological factors) and other poor readers whose problems are seen largely as being a consequence of adverse environmental experiences. However, it is difficult to separate out individual poor readers into such categories. Some students from challenging backgrounds, or who have experienced poor teaching, may also have reading problems that have a neurobiological origin, and, to render matters more complex, environmental factors can have an impact on the child's neurological development. Moreover, there exists no assessment technique that can identify, for any given individual, a biological cause that can be used to confirm or deny that they have dyslexia. For this reason, the distinctions offered by such definitions are currently more valuable for guiding scientific research than for informing clinical or educational practice. Accordingly, most leading researchers (including Torgesen and his colleagues) do not routinely employ biological/nonbiological differentiations to help guide intervention program planning (Vellutino et al., 2004, pp. 28–30).

As is shown in subsequent chapters, there continues to be considerable debate as to the merits of underlying causal explanations, and none of the major existing theories provide a "clear-cut, definitive, and unequivocal set of diagnostic criteria that would pinpoint the ultimate (neurobiological) origin of the child's reading difficulties" (Vellutino et al., 2004, p. 28).

Response to intervention

An alternative approach, response to intervention (RTI), dispenses with a search for deficits in specific cognitive functions when difficulties are first presented and instead places the emphasis on gauging the individual's progress over time. Such an approach fits Tønnessen's (1995) suggestion that rather than delineating symptoms, or providing causal analyses, a third approach to defining dyslexia could be on the basis of the individual's progress.

In the United States, the use of RTI (both as an intervention tool and as a means of classifying or diagnosing children with special educational needs), in contrast to traditional psychometric assessment, has gained considerable support in recent years. However, because of legislation in relation to the resourcing of special education, discussion and debate have largely played out in relation to the diagnosis of learning disability (LD) rather than reading disability/dyslexia, its most common component.

Crucially, with this approach, any unexpected component is no longer related to variable levels of functioning in relation to an individual's strengths and weaknesses, but rather is determined on the basis of the child's failure to respond to standard and validated instruction (Fuchs & Fuchs, 2009). Here, a discrepancy is still emphasized but, instead of referring to ability-ability differences, the focus is now on within-individual discrepancies relative to age-based expectations and instruction (Fletcher & Vaughn, 2009). This conception is believed by its advocates to have more utility for determining the nature of intervention than do approaches based on the identification of uneven cognitive profiles (Reschly & Tilley, 1999).

Although there are varying models of RTI with differing numbers of tiers or levels (Fuchs, Fuchs, & Compton, 2012), they all share a similar basic structure. Initially (Tier 1 or T1) there is a universal process of screening in the relevant domains (e.g., reading and math). Those children deemed to be at risk of academic failure subsequently receive specialized intervention and regular monitoring (Tier 2 or T2). Should the child continue to fail to make sufficient progress, input becomes gradually more intense and more individualised (Tier 3 or T3). In the United Kingdom, similar stages are described as Waves, with Waves 1–3 approximating to those of Tiers 1–3 in the United States.

Despite the growing popularity of RTI, there remain a number of operational difficulties (Hale et al., 2010; VanDerHeyden, 2011). One major weakness is that there are several different RTI models with no agreed-on single method of determining how best to measure response to intervention. In general, the leading approaches vary on whether they emphasize rate of growth and/or a cut-off score of some kind, and the longitudinal stability of classification decisions appears to be rather poor (Brown Waesche et al., 2011). As a result, these approaches are not consistent in identifying poor responders (Fuchs & Deshler, 2007). Such differences, however determined, are likely to have significant implications for children who may require additional services (Berkeley et al., 2009), although differences between leading RTI models tend to be smaller than when compared with the traditional discrepancy approach (Brown Waesche et al., 2011).

The RTI approach has been heavily criticized by researchers with a strong allegiance to traditional psychometric approaches. Reynolds and Shaywitz (2009a, 2009b), for example, criticize the scientific evidence for RTI and suggest that there is much still to learn about appropriate procedures, which, they contend, are currently guided by "guesswork" (2009a, p. 47). For these writers, the RTI approach cuts at the central component of the traditional conception of learning disability – an unexpected difficulty in relation to ability (based on comparison of strengths and weaknesses within the individual). A further weakness, they argue, is that bright children performing below their potential but at a level commensurate with less able peers might fail to be identified where this approach is used in isolation. Similar criticisms are also offered by Kavale, Spaulding and Beam (2009) for whom RTI is conceptually flawed, inadequate for practice, and politically, rather than scientifically, motivated.

A core area of debate concerns the forms of intervention that may result from differing identification procedures. Reynolds and Shaywitz (2009a) have little doubt about the importance of assessment of cognitive processes:

One of the major purposes of a comprehensive assessment is to derive hypotheses emerging from a student's cognitive profile that would allow the derivation of different and more effective instruction. By eliminating an evaluation of cognitive abilities and psychological processes, we revert to a one-size-fits-all mentality where it is naively assumed that all children fail for the same reason.... At the current stage of scientific knowledge, it is only through a comprehensive evaluation of a student's cognitive and psychological abilities that we can gain insights into the underlying proximal and varied root causes of reading difficulties and then provide specific interventions that are targeted to each student's individual needs. (pp. 46–47)

This position has been strongly contested and cognitive profiling approaches have been criticized for questionable reliability leading to an inability to provide scientifically rigorous diagnoses (Kramer et al., 1987; Stuebing et al., 2012), and also because of their limited ability to relate findings obtained to subsequent intervention (see also Fletcher et al., 2013).

Fletcher and Vaughn (2009) are critical that Reynolds and Shaywitz (2009a) offer no data to support their claim of the value of cognitive profiling for intervention, adding that they have been unable to identify any such data themselves (Fletcher et al., 2007). Gresham (2009) argues along similar lines and in responding to Hale et al.'s (2006) call for traditional cognitive assessments to guide intervention, contends that it is beholden to those advocating the use of cognitive and neuropsychological data for the purpose of formulating differentiated interventions to provide empirical evidence to support the existence of aptitude × treatment interactions. Gresham adds that, to date, no data-based studies (other than individual case studies) have been cited to support such claims, whereas hundreds of studies in a variety of different areas of learning have failed to show such a phenomenon (Cronbach, 1975; Cronbach & Snow, 1977; Pashler, McDaniel, Rohrer, & Bjork, 2008). Fletcher (2009, p. 6) provides a powerful assertion that has yet to be convincingly challenged:

Despite claims to the contrary (Hale et al., 2008) there is little evidence of Aptitude ×
Treatment interactions for cognitive/neuropsychological skills at the level of treatment
or aptitude (Reschly & Tilley, 1999, pp. 28–29). The strongest evidence of Aptitude ×
Treatment interactions is when strengths and weaknesses in academic skills are used to
provide differential instruction. (Connor, Morrison, Fishman, Schatschneider, & Underwood, 2007)

Similarly, and despite their advocacy of cognitive profiling for studying the
nature of learning disabilities, Compton, Fuchs et al. (2012) assert that empirical support for interventions tied to the individual's unique cognitive strengths
and weaknesses is "equivocal at best" (p. 79). Interestingly, a white paper by
58 leading scholars in the United States (Hale et al., 2010), many of whom are
closely associated with the psychometric tradition, argues that evidence indicating the value of cognitive and neuropsychological assessment for determining
responsiveness to academic and behavioral intervention is only now beginning
to emerge, although it concedes that further research is needed. However, the
extent to which such knowledge will be able to inform the selection of different interventions for students with different cognitive profiles is still unclear.
Fletcher et al. (2011), for example, found that while cognitive processes were
able to differentiate subgroups defined on the basis of poor response and low
achievement after a tier 2 (T2) intervention (i.e., small group work), this seemed
to reflect the severity of impairment in reading skills rather than qualitatively
distinct differences in the cognitive profiles of these groups. As a result, it was
concluded that the assessment of cognitive processes failed to provide sufficient
value-added benefit to justify their use. One must be careful, however, to differentiate between the use of cognitive variables to inform appropriate forms of
targeted educational intervention and their use in informing predictions about
students' likely future progress – in other words, one should not confuse identification (for example, of learning disability status) with treatment (Fuchs et al.,
2012).

Finally, if a link between a classification based on some form of psychological
profiling and a corresponding instructional method were ever identified, such
a finding would only apply to that particular classification, and it would also
need to be shown that any additional benefits could justify the high costs of providing individual cognitive assessment and tailored instruction (Pashler et al.,
2008).

One of the complexities of the RTI model is determining how this ties
into conceptual understandings of dyslexia. In the case of reading, those in
the United States who fail to make significant progress, given high levels of
structured intervention, would, with this approach, be likely to be diagnosed
as learning disabled. However, the label would then be indicative of treatment

resistance rather than reflect any underlying cognitive processes or biological etiology. Given that there are many reasons why children may not respond adequately to interventions (McKenzie, 2009), some have argued that "inferring specific learning disabilities from failure to respond to intervention is not scientifically or clinically justifiable" (Hale et al., 2010, p. 227). On the other hand, there is little research to suggest that inadequate and adequate responders differ from one another other than in respect of their defining characteristics – poor initial reading-related skills and poor response to intervention (Fletcher et al., 2011). Which of these has the most predictive power continues to be subject to debate (Stuebing, Fletcher, & Hughes, 2012; Swanson, 2012; Tran et al., 2011).

The prevalence of dyslexia

Given the lack of current consensus about what exactly constitutes dyslexia, it is hardly surprising that estimates of its prevalence vary substantially. Such a problem is by no means new; almost a century ago, Hinshelwood (1917) disparagingly commented that some educationalists saw congenital word-blindness as very common, involving as many as one in a thousand. He noted that such estimates often included cases where there were "slight degrees of defect in the visual word center, while the early writers had reserved it for only those grave cases which could be regarded as pathological" (p. 82). Two decades later, Orton (1939) suggested that slightly more than 10% of the school-aged population had reading disabilities. He also introduced the notion of a continuum of disabilities, rather than clear pathological categories, arguing that experience of work with hundreds of cases indicated that clear divisions did not reflect the gradations of difficulty that he had encountered.

The prevalence of dyslexia (or reading disability) reported in the literature tends to vary according to the definition that is adopted, where cut-offs are made, and whether data from school, clinical, or large population samples are employed (Rose, 2009). Shaywitz's (2005) longitudinal study in Connecticut identified approximately 17.5% of the sample as having a reading disability, defined on the basis of reading performance that was below age, grade, or level of intellectual ability. In citing this figure it would appear that the term "reading disabled" was seen as synonymous with "dyslexic" given that the terms are employed interchangeably in the text:

The apparent large-scale underidentification of reading-disabled children is particularly worrisome because even when school identification takes place, it occurs relatively late – often past the optimal age for intervention. Dyslexic children are generally in the third grade or above when they are first identified by their schools; reading disabilities diagnosed after third grade are much more difficult to remediate. (p. 30)

Indeed, in an earlier, highly influential article, Shaywitz (1996) claimed that "dyslexia affects a full 20 percent of schoolchildren" (p. 100). Her position reflects the belief that reading difficulties lie along a continuum with no clear-cut distinction between good and poor readers. Citing the words of Kendell (1975) – "Classification is the art of carving nature at the joints; it should imply that there is indeed a joint there, that one is not sawing through bone" (p. 65) – Shaywitz argues that despite the fact that there is no natural joint separating dyslexic and good readers, or "a gap of nature" (p. 27), educational services have often been based on just such a belief.

A similar figure is provided by the U.S. National Institutes of Health. Here it was stated that reading disabilities, "synonymous with 'dyslexia'" (Coles, 1998, p. 190), affect at least 10 million American children, or approximately 20%. More recently, the National Institute of Child Health and Development (2007) has claimed that between 15% and 20% of the U.S. population have a language-based disability, and of these, most have dyslexia.

The prevalence rates for dyslexia provided by national support groups also vary widely. Thus, Crisfield (1996), writing on behalf of the British Dyslexia Association, suggests that as much as 10% of the population may have "mild" dyslexia with 4% having a more severe form. The Dyslexia Foundation of New Zealand (2008) also claims that 10% of children in that country are dyslexic. The International Dyslexia Association avoids specifying the precise figure, but in its fact sheet it is suggested that as many as 20% of the population as a whole have some of the symptoms of dyslexia (http://www.interdys.org/ewebeditpro5/upload/DyslexiaBasicsREVMay2012.pdf, retrieved 25 August 2012).

Working with a sample of Dutch children, van Bergen et al. (2012) identify as dyslexic those whose scores on a reading fluency test corresponded to the weakest 10% of the population. Fletcher et al. (2007) recognize the disparities that exist and suggest a prevalence of between 6% and 17% of the school age population depending on the criteria employed. Butterworth and Kovas (2013) report an estimated prevalence of 4–8% for dyslexia. The same estimate is provided by Snowling (2010), although in other publications by this author (Hulme & Snowling, 2009; Snowling, 2013), figures between 3–6% and 3–10% are suggested. As she has repeatedly pointed out, however, such cut-off points are wholly arbitrary, as dyslexia is not a clear-cut diagnostic category.

Clearly there are very significant differences in the ways in which this label is operationalized, even by leading scholars in the field. Additionally, estimates from clinical accounts often differ from the larger proportions typically identified in research studies where the cut-off using reading or spelling tests will often be one standard deviation below the mean (e.g., Gooch, Snowling, & Hulme, 2011). Snowling (2013) emphasizes the continuous nature of reading skill and suggests the deployment of cut-off points at 1.5 standard deviations and 2 SDs below the mean for representing moderate and severe reading difficulty.

An alternative use for the term (Elliott & Gibbs, 2008; Snowling et al., 2011) reflecting an RTI perspective might be to use the term to describe that proportion of poor readers that appears to be resistant to current evidence-based forms of remedial intervention. However, this suggestion does not reflect most contemporary understandings.

It has been found that in most school systems and cultural settings girls tend to be better readers (and, indeed, writers [Berninger et al., 2008]) than boys, with the gender gap greatest at the extremes of the distribution (Chiu & McBride-Chang, 2006; Machin & Pekkarinen, 2008). However, many studies of other orthographies appear to provide little evidence of gender differences in respect of reading disability – for example, Spanish (Jiménez et al., 2011), Chinese (Chan, Ho, Tsang, Lee, & Chung, 2007), and German (Landerl & Moll, 2010). Interestingly, a recent study in Finland suggests that reading disability appears to have a more deleterious impact on boys' attainment than that of girls with similar literacy difficulties (Rimkute et al., 2013).

There is some evidence to suggest that a greater proportion of boys than girls demonstrate phonological awareness difficulties in preschool (Lundberg, Larsman, & Strid, 2012). While there seems to be strong evidence that more males experience reading disability (Miles, Haslum, & Wheeler, 1998), the size of the gender ratio is disputed, partly because those figures that are reported often vary according to the differing definitions and measures employed. On the basis of clinically referred samples, Finnucci and Childs (1981) reported a ratio of 5.90:1, Katusic et al. (2001) reported a ratio between 2.00 to 3.00:1, and Wolff and Melngailis (1994) reported a ratio of 4.28:1. A review of four independent epidemiological studies in New Zealand and in Britain (Rutter et al., 2004) also indicated substantially higher rates of reading disability (taken as the bottom 15% of reading performance) for boys. Sex ratios in these studies varied from 3.19:1 to 1.39:1. Other epidemiological studies suggest a rate of approximately 1.5:1 (Flannery et al., 2000; Flynn & Rahbar, 1994).

Some of the confusion may result from a gender discrepancy between epidemiological and referred samples (Smith, Gilger, & Pennington, 2001), with a lower ratio of boys to girls in research-defined, compared with clinic, studies (Share & Silva, 2003). Analysis from Shaywitz's longitudinal Connecticut study indicated that school identification procedures resulted in three to four times as many boys as girls being identified as reading disabled. In contrast, her research team's own testing program indicated no significant gender differences. Shaywitz's primary explanation for the "myth" of male vulnerability to reading disability (Shaywitz, 1996, p. 98) was that girls, who tend to be less obtrusive and attention seeking, are more likely to be overlooked for further clinical evaluation. Boys with reading difficulties are more likely to present with comorbid externalizing disorders, whereas girls will often demonstrate internalizing problems (Pennington, 2009). As schools tend to refer to clinical services children with conduct rather than internalizing disorders (Bramlett et al., 2002), disproportionate referral rates of boys and girls for reading-related problems may be an inevitable outcome [although see Quinn and Wagner (in press) for a counter position]. Willcutt and Pennington (2000) found a male-to-female ratio of 1.3:1 in their reading-disabled population sample, but where an externalizing disorder was present, the male-female ratio was 2.6:1, a proportion that reflects the range typically found in referred samples (Pennington, 2009).

Although there continue to be marked differences of opinion, most commentators now appear to accept that there is a slightly higher proportion of males with reading disability. While one detailed review of the literature (Liederman, Kantrowitz, & Flannery, 2005) has estimated a ratio between 1.74 and 2.00:1, the middle ground would seem to suggest a rather lower figure of approximately between 1.3:1 and 1.6:1 (Fletcher et al., 2007) with the ratio increasing in line with the severity of reading disability under examination (Quinn & Wagner, in press).

The broader notion of learning disabilities and its relationship to dyslexia

A number of key issues concerning the dyslexia debate have played out by reference to the broader construct of learning disability (LD), a term that incorporates difficulties in a variety of achievement-related areas. The primary reason for the widespread use of this rather general term is perhaps because in many countries a diagnosis of learning disability can result in the provision of ring-fenced resources (Kavale & Forness, 1995).

The term "learning disabilities" has a long history (Hallahan & Mock, 2003), but its origins as a formal diagnostic category are linked to the work of Kirk who first introduced the term in print in 1962. He defined LD as referring to

a retardation, disorder or delayed development in one or more of the processes of speech, language, reading, writing, arithmetic, or other school subject resulting from a psychological handicap caused by a possible cerebral dysfunction and/or emotional or behavioral disturbances. It is not the result of mental retardation, sensory deprivation, or cultural and instructional factors. (Kirk, 1962, p. 263)

Since that time, there have been many revisions and "official" definitions, most recently stimulated by the proposals for DSM-5 (Scanlon, 2013). However, the one constant is that definitions have always been considered to be problematic (Kavale et al., 2009). In an exact parallel to the dyslexia debate, the lack of consensus about how to define LD has led to disputes about whether it really exists as a discrete entity (Kavale & Forness, 2003) and whether it is preferable to move away from attempts to make categorical decisions to intervening whenever a particular learning difficulty is observed (Fletcher et al., 2013).

The U.S. Individuals with Disabilities Education Improvement Act (IDEIA, 2004) defines the term "specific learning disability" as a

disorder in one or more of the basic psychological processes involved in understanding or in using language, spoken or written, which disorder may manifest itself in the imperfect ability to listen, think, speak, read, write, spell or do mathematical calculations.

Such disabilities should not be primarily the result of visual, hearing, or motor disabilities, of mental retardation, of emotional disturbance, or of environmental, cultural, or economic disadvantage.

In the United States, approximately 7% of school-aged children are classified as having a learning disability, with this group being seen as approximately half of all those identified as having disabilities of one form or another (U.S. Department of Education, 2007). However, the significant rise in the number of U.S. students identified with this label in the 1995–2005 period, although more recently declining (Zirkel, 2013), has led to the claim that such shifts weaken the amount of confidence one can have that a given student is "truly" LD (Kavale & Forness, 2003, p. 83). For some, definitional imprecision has led to a situation where "no one knows what an SLD (specific learning disability) is" and "operational definitions of SLD have . . . in essence, developed 'out of thin air'" (Kavale et al., 2009, p. 46).

Debates over the definition and operationalization of dyslexia are closely paralleled in respect of LD. For both constructs, there is disagreement as to whether there should be evidence of both strengths and weaknesses in order to differentiate these conditions from other conceptions, sometimes known as the specificity hypothesis (Fletcher et al., 2007). In both cases, there are strong political (advocacy) drivers that have "overwhelmed" scientific considerations and which have resulted in terminology that "is defined loosely and treated unsystematically, primarily on the basis of advocacy and expedience" (Kauffman, Hallahan, & Lloyd, 1998, p. 276). Diagnostic fuzziness may not sit well with those seeking scientific understanding, but it is not necessarily perceived as a problem for those whose primary goal is advocacy. As noted earlier, for such groups, ensuring that those who encounter difficulties in school receive special assistance is often deemed to be more important than obtaining conceptual clarity (Kavale & Forness, 2003). In the United States, for example, the desire to include as many as possible as LD, in order to ensure maximum funding, resulted in a gradual increase in the number of children being diagnosed with LDs, from 2% in 1976 to more than 6% in 2000 (Büttner & Hasselhorn, 2011). One difficulty that results from such enterprises is that students identified as LD by teachers and clinicians may often fail to fit the description provided by scientific accounts.

For both dyslexia and LD, it has proven easier to offer a general, somewhat anodyne conceptual definition than it has to provide a consistently applied operational definition. For Rice and Brooks (2004), dyslexia is not one clear thing but many, with the term serving as a conceptual clearinghouse for a variety of difficulties, deficits, and causes. As for dyslexia, the LD construct has been articulated by means of so many different operational definitions there is now little consensus about the nature of the condition (Kavale et al., 2009). In commenting on the lack of correspondence between the many differing operational definitions of LD, Siegel and Lipka (2008) observe that if the same variable is measured in different ways by different researchers, it is difficult to argue that they are all measuring the same concept:

In order to assess whether or not a student has LD, accepted common criteria must be established. Following that, a set of measuring tools must also be used to demonstrate some consistency among students. For academic and methodological purposes, one needs to define the criteria for a diagnosis of LD when collecting samples for research. If different investigators use different criteria, then the findings of research have limited generalizability and practical utility. (Siegel & Lipka, 2008, p. 294)

Such precision is of more than just theoretical interest, for whether we are considering the broader notion of learning disability or the more specific case of dyslexia, differing forms of operationalization, employing different cut-off levels, are likely to result in some children failing to receive the additional educational support that others with similar strengths and weaknesses might receive elsewhere (Macmillan & Siperstein, 2002).

Levels of analysis: the biological, the cognitive and the behavioural

One factor that has complicated our understanding of reading difficulties in general, and dyslexia in particular, is the tendency of researchers to operate at differing levels of analysis, depending on their particular perspectives, disciplines, and specialties. Frith (1997) points out that the examination of reading difficulties can take place at the level of the biological, the cognitive, and the behavioral. Each of these levels can shed light on the reading process, but the particular samples studied often differ and research findings from these levels are not easily integrated. Thus geneticists and neuroscientists tend to include all those with reading difficulties in their samples, rather than a subgroup that might be termed as dyslexic on some clearly and consistently defined basis. At the cognitive level, some researchers attempt to compare those with dyslexia, defined on the basis of certain cognitive features, with other, "garden variety" poor readers; most working at this level, however, do not make such a distinction. On some occasions, dyslexic and non-dyslexic poor reader samples are differentiated on the basis of certain cognitive features (e.g. IQ), to enable closer examination of underlying cognitive processes, even though such features

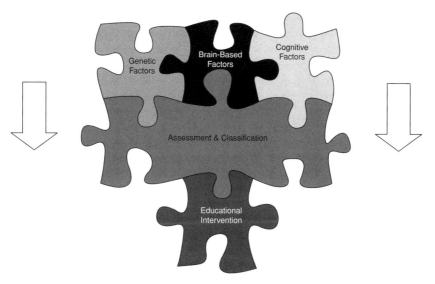

Figure 1.1 Assessment for intervention feeding directly from each level of analysis: genetic, neuroscientific, and cognitive

do not differentiate between dyslexics and typical readers (decoders). At the behavioral level, debate rages as to whether there are clear signs, or symptoms, of dyslexia as something other than reading disability, and whether such indicators serve to guide early detection and intervention.

Perusal of media or professional accounts might lead one to assume that the assessment of dyslexia for the purposes of intervention can be undertaken using data obtained at each of these levels. In such circumstances, assessment and classification/diagnosis would draw on data obtained from the direct assessment of an individual's genetic, neuropsychological, and/or cognitive profiles (see Figure 1.1). Others recognize that while, given the current state of knowledge, genetic and neuroscientific data cannot presently be used to directly inform assessment of specific individuals, biologically based reading problems can be indirectly assessed through the use of cognitive assessments (see Figure 1.2). Others consider that at the present time, assessment primarily at the level of educational performance represents a more valid, meaningful, and effective use of resources (e.g., Vellutino et al., 2004).

Irrespective of the current limitations of clinical assessment, in order to derive sophisticated understandings of reading disability/dyslexia, there is a clear need to derive complex models operating at biological, cognitive, and behavioral levels that interact with one another and with the environment (Hulme & Snowling, 2009). Such an enterprise will, perhaps, be the key task for the next

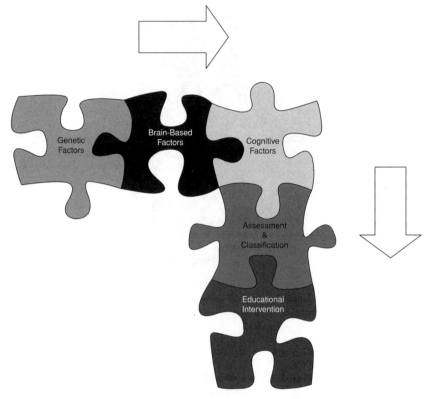

Figure 1.2 Assessment for intervention commencing from the cognitive

decade. In the following chapters we examine cognitive and biological (genetic and brain) factors in turn and consider the extent to which these help shed light on the dyslexia debate.

Summary

Despite claims to the contrary, it is incontrovertible that there are many people who struggle to learn to read (decode) for reasons other than poor teaching. While this condition is widely known as dyslexia, achieving a clear, scientific, and consensual understanding of this term has proven elusive.

Table 1.1 illustrates the diverse and often overlapping understandings of dyslexia that can be found in the literature. For some, the construct of dyslexia describes all those who struggle to decode (and is a term that can be used

Table 1.1. *Differing understandings of who may be considered to have dyslexia*

- Anyone who struggles with accurate single-word decoding.
- Anyone who struggles with accurate and/or fluent decoding.
- Those for whom decoding is merely one element of a more pervasive dyslexic condition marked by a range of comorbid features. This can include compensated dyslexics who no longer present with a severe reading difficulty.
- Those who score at the lower end of the normal distribution on an appropriate test of reading accuracy or fluency. Cut-off points vary but are typically 1, 1.5 or 2 standard deviations below the mean.
- Those whose decoding difficulties cannot be explained in alternative ways (e.g., because of severe intellectual or sensory impairment, socioeconomic disadvantage, poor schooling, or emotional/behavioral difficulty).
- Those for whom there is a significant discrepancy between decoding performance and IQ.
- Those whose decoding difficulty is deemed to be unexpected.
- Those whose poor decoding skills contrast with strengths in other intellectual and academic domains.
- Those whose decoding problems are biologically determined.
- Those whose decoding problems are marked by certain associated cognitive difficulties (in particular, phonological, rapid naming, and verbal short-term or working memory deficits).
- Those with a history of very poor spelling.
- Those poor decoders who also present with a range of symptoms commonly found in those with dyslexia (e.g., poor motor, arithmetical, or language skills, visual difficulties, and low self-esteem).
- Those who demonstrate a discrepancy between decoding and listening comprehension.
- Those who fail to make meaningful progress in decoding even when provided with high-quality, evidence-based forms of intervention.

interchangeably with constructs such as reading disability or specific learning disability); for others, poor reading is but only one aspect of a broader and highly complex dyslexic condition.

For many, particularly a significant proportion of professionals operating in clinical and educational settings, not all who struggle to decode text should be considered to have dyslexia. For many years the key criterion was evidence of a discrepancy between reading accuracy and IQ; however, the subsequent discrediting of this notion has resulted in significant conceptual difficulty and doubts as to the added value of the label. For some, the dyslexic reader is now merely an individual who scores at the tail of a normal distribution on a given measure of reading accuracy. For others, the predominant feature is the condition's biological basis (and thus some dyslexic individuals can potentially score higher on measures of reading accuracy than other poor readers deemed to be non-dyslexic). In practice, however, achieving meaningful differentiation between underpinning biological and environmental factors for an individual poor reader is usually an unrealistic goal.

Although a number of exclusionary features have been identified for the identification of dyslexia, these are highly problematic in relation to individual diagnosis. While adverse environmental factors will typically impair the development of children's literacy skills, the presence of a biologically based difficulty for a given individual can rarely be ruled out.

At the current time, it is unclear how any particular individual can be meaningfully identified as a member of a dyslexic subgroup within a wider pool of poor decoders. Given that not all conceive of dyslexia in this way, it is hardly surprising that prevalence estimates range from 3% to 20%.

An alternative to searching for underlying indicators of dyslexia involves identifying individuals with reading-related problems as early as possible and then monitoring their response to high-quality, evidence-based intervention. In such cases, a diagnostic label is no longer necessary for the purposes of undertaking remediation, and a "wait to fail" scenario can be avoided. While those who favor psychometrics have criticized the scientific basis of RTI, its advocates have challenged opponents to specify how profiles derived from psychometric tests can meaningfully inform diagnosis and aid reading intervention. To date, a convincing response has yet to be offered.

Our understanding of reading difficulties has been aided by developments in cognitive, neurological, and genetic sciences. It is often believed that these disciplines can be drawn on not only to gain greater understanding of the true nature of dyslexia, but also to facilitate differential diagnosis and subsequent intervention. It is to the contribution of each of these disciplines that the book now turns.

Note: The terminology employed in this book

As this chapter has demonstrated, the use of the terms "dyslexia," "reading disability," "reading difficulty," and other closely related constructs varies greatly, with these often being employed interchangeably. This discrepancy renders problematic the use of such terms in this book where a key aim is to achieve greater conceptual clarity. Our solution to this conundrum is, wherever possible, to use the particular constructs that are employed in the publications that are cited. In the case of more general discussion and reflection, the terms "dyslexia" and "reading disability" are used interchangeably to refer to decoding difficulties in relation to both single-word reading and the fluent reading of text. Where appropriate, however, the distinction between reading accuracy and fluency is highlighted and examined.

The important difference between decoding and reading comprehension is recognised in the text. Throughout, the term "reading difficulties" is employed where reference is made to a broad group of different types of reading problem, including accurate and fluent decoding and reading comprehension.

The concluding section of this book (Chapter 5) returns to the exploration of conceptual issues and provides recommendations with the aim of achieving more precise and rigorous use of terminology.

2   Explanations at the cognitive level

Introduction

In order to develop a causal model of RD (reading disability) that can inform intervention, it is necessary to develop a theory at the cognitive level of explanation. . . . Although some causes of RD have a genetic origin, and environmental factors play an important role, cognition mediates brain-behaviour relationships and at the present time, the cognitive level offers a necessary and sufficient level of explanation for the development of principled interventions. In short, we need to understand the cognitive difficulties that underpin reading problems, regardless of whether their origin is constitutional or environmental. (Snowling & Hulme, 2011, p. 4)

This chapter examines the evidence concerning the nature and role of a number of cognitive processes that have been proposed as influential in dyslexia/reading disability (i.e., phonological awareness, rapid naming, short-term/working memory, low-level sensory auditory and visual processing, scotopic sensitivity, attentional factors, and motor processing). In each case the implications of the available research evidence for clinical and educational intervention will be considered. As this chapter demonstrates, this highly complex field is rendered additionally problematic by often contrasting and inconsistent research findings that have resulted in much debate and little consensus, beyond widespread agreement that reading disability appears to be explained by multiple deficits.

The phonological deficit hypothesis

For most of the past four decades, the *phonological deficit hypothesis* (Stanovich, 1988; Stanovich & Siegel, 1994) has been the dominant cognitive explanation (Vellutino et al., 2004). Studies of cognitive functioning in children with reading problems have consistently found three processes – phonological processing, short-term/working memory, and processing speed – that appear particularly significant when comparisons are made with typically achieving readers (Johnson et al., 2010). For each of these processes there appears to be a phonological component that is particularly important for reading. According to some theorists, the phonological deficit incorporates elements that map onto these three major dimensions: phonological awareness, verbal short-term memory, and slow retrieval of phonological information stored in long-term memory, as exemplified in rapid automatic naming tasks (Wagner & Torgesen, 1987). However, this grouping is controversial, and others argue that it is not helpful to conceive of verbal short-term/working memory and naming speed as core elements of phonology (Nicolson & Fawcett, 2008).

Tunmer (2011) lists a number of aspects of phonological processing. These include:

encoding phonological information (phonetic perception), gaining access to and performing mental operations on phonological information (phonological awareness), retrieving phonological information from semantic memory (lexical retrieval), retaining phonological information in working memory (short-term verbal recall), and translating letters and letter patterns into phonological forms (phonological recoding). (p. x)

Confusingly, phonological awareness is sometimes employed as the superordinate construct. Thus, Duff, Hayiou-Thomas, and Hulme (2012) include measures of phoneme awareness, short-term memory, and rapid automatized naming as measures of phonological awareness. For the purposes of the following section, however, we have treated these as separate constructs.

An important distinction that has been drawn is that between implicit and explicit phonological processing (Melby-Lervåg, Lyster, & Hulme, 2012). Tasks involving verbal short-term memory or rapid automatized naming are deemed to involve implicit phonological processing because they do not involve any conscious awareness of, or reflection on, the sound structure of spoken words. In contrast, explicit phonological tasks are considered to be those that require reflection on and manipulation of such speech sounds (Melby-Lervåg, Lyster, & Hulme, 2012).

Phonological decoding is important because it enables the reader to map speech sounds onto orthographic patterns (letters) and thus decode unfamiliar words (Share, 1995, 1999, 2004). Phonological awareness – the ability to detect and manipulate the sounds of spoken language (Liberman & Shankweiler, 1985) – operates at both the phoneme (the most basic elements of speech) and syllable levels within words (Bryant et al., 1990). It appears to follow a developmental sequence with awareness of the larger segments, syllables and rimes, preceding that of smaller segments, phonemes (Carroll et al., 2003). Phonemic awareness – the ability to segment spoken words into phonemic elements – appears to be a particularly important factor for reading. To develop this ability, children must learn to attend to meaningless phonemes rather than the more recognizable morphemes and words. For most children, this skill is necessarily advanced by tuition in learning to read. Where phonemic awareness is poor, children are likely to struggle to acquire the ability to discover spelling to sound relationships and, as a consequence, fail to develop alphabetic coding skills (Ehri, Nunes, Stahl, & Willows, 2001; Shankweiler & Fowler, 2004).

According to the phonological deficit perspective, children with dyslexia are hindered by faulty representation of speech sounds, which leads to problems involving the precise processing of spoken words. These representations become degraded (more fuzzy, noisy, less specified, or with a lower resolution) and as a result, the child struggles to acquire a range of phonological skills such as phonological awareness, alphabetic mapping, letter-sound decoding, and associated skills such as orthographic awareness (Blachman, 2000; Vellutino, Scanlon, & Spearing, 1995; Vellutino et al., 1996). Weak phonological coding may render it difficult for the child to establish strong links between the visual and verbal counterparts of printed words. This is likely to impair the ability to store high-quality representations of word spellings, thus affecting rapid word identification and reading fluency. The theory gained prominence following studies of preschool children that sought to ascertain which pre-reading skills were the best predictors of later reading and writing ability. Phonological awareness emerged as an important factor (Bradley & Bryant, 1983). Poor performance on relevant measures led to the identification of children who were later to struggle with reading. Other studies comparing older poor readers with younger children without difficulties, reading at the same level, showed significant phonological deficits for the older groups (Olson, 1985; Rack, Snowling, & Olson, 1992).

Since the groundbreaking work of the 1980s, a vast number of studies have pointed to the importance of phonological awareness for reading development, although prediction appears to be strongest in the early years where an emphasis on sequential letter-to-sound decoding, rather than automatic word recognition, is likely to be greatest (Vaessen & Blomert, 2010). Phonological awareness appears to be a better predictor of reading ability in general than reading disability in particular (Scarborough, 1998).

Although awareness at the phonemic level has been considered to be more important than that of larger units (Snowling, 2000), it appears that both are important for early readers. A large-scale meta-analysis of studies reporting correlations between early skills and subsequent reading performance (National Early Literacy Panel, 2008) found that for decoding, the average correlation with phoneme awareness was somewhat higher than awareness at the subphonemic level (e.g., syllable awareness) (.42 and .36, respectively), but this difference was not significant. Composite measures of phonological awareness proved to be the best predictors (average correlation = .47). Phonological tasks that involved analysis of sounds (i.e., deleting, counting, substituting sound units) were better predictors of subsequent decoding and reading comprehension than those that involved judgments involving synthesis (i.e., combining sound units) or identification (i.e., matching initial sounds in words). Of the various phonological measures, rhyming tasks provided the weakest correlations with reading.

A meta-analytic review of the relationships between phonemic awareness, rime awareness, and verbal short-term memory and children's word reading skills (Melby-Lervåg et al., 2012) found phonemic awareness to be the strongest predictor. Where studies had compared poor readers with typically developing (younger) children reading at the same level, a large deficit in phonemic awareness was found for the struggling readers (an effect size of $d = -0.57$, compared with -0.37 for rime awareness and -0.09 for verbal short-term memory). It was further found that the relationship of these latter two elements to reading could be explained in terms of shared variance with phonemic skills. The authors concluded that these findings lend support to the "pivotal role of phonemic awareness as a predictor of individual differences in reading development" (Melby-Lervåg et al., 2012, p. 322). Further support for the argument that a deficit in phonemic awareness is the most powerful neuropsychological predictor of reading disability has more recently been provided by Willcutt et al. (2013).

While phonological/phonemic awareness seems to be a predictor in most alphabetic writing systems, it may be rather less important for the later stages of literacy development in the case of transparent languages (Arnoutse, van Leeuwe, & Verhoeven, 2005; Furnes & Samuelsson, 2010; Landerl & Wimmer, 2000; Ziegler, Bertrand, et al., 2010). Indeed, it has been argued that the preponderance of studies in the English language may have resulted in an overestimate of the importance of phonological/phonemic awareness in reading development (Share, 2008). However, it is important to note that not all findings support the suggestion of differences across orthographies (e.g., Furnes & Samuelsson, 2011).

Prediction can involve many different outcome criteria and vary across methods and contexts. The focus may be on predicting reading outcomes in all children, solely those struggling to learn to read, or the reading gains that will be made by those with difficulties once high-quality interventions are put into place. The predictive power of phonological awareness and other reading-related cognitive skills also appears to vary on the basis of what sorts of measures are employed (e.g., different tests of reading accuracy, fluency, or comprehension) and, as noted earlier, whether the relevant language is opaque (e.g., English) or transparent (e.g., German). A further complication concerns the theoretical complexities that have resulted from findings that cognitive processes sometimes predict reading outcomes when considered as univariates but fail to do so once more complex multivariate models are constructed (McGrath et al., 2011).

Studies in which phonological deficits have been linked to reading difficulties have generally been correlational or cross-sectional in nature (Melby-Lervåg et al., 2012) and thus have been unable to resolve issues of causality (Castles & Coultheart, 2004). Nevertheless, claims for a causal link have been given greater weight by studies that have demonstrated that phonological training for beginning readers, as part of an overall reading intervention, result in improved word identification, spelling, and general reading ability (Bryant & Bradley, 1985; Vellutino et al., 2004).

It is difficult to separate causes from consequences, and the relationship appears to be bidirectional: the development of reading skill can also improve phonemic awareness (Castles & Coultheart, 2004; Ehri, 1999). Bishop (2006) outlines three lines of research evidence that suggest that literacy skills can affect performance on phonological tasks. Firstly, orthographic knowledge about how a word is written can influence phonological judgments. Secondly, those who have significant literacy difficulties because of reduced opportunity to learn to read tend to perform more poorly on phonological tasks than do normal readers. Finally, children who have had no exposure to reading instruction also tend to perform poorly on such measures yet often make rapid progress once introduced to print, a finding that supports the argument that poor phonemic awareness may sometimes reflect children's early experiences at home and in preschool (Corriveau, Goswami, & Thomson, 2010).

The argument that children's phonemic awareness is not a cause but a consequence of their reading development has been partially undermined by longitudinal studies that suggest that measures of phonological competence, prior to the commencement of school, can predict future reading performance (Hulme & Snowling, 2009). In one research program, the Jyväskylä Longitudinal study of dyslexia (Lyytinen et al., 2006; Richardson et al., 2003), researchers interviewed pregnant women and identified an at-risk group on the basis of familial predisposition to dyslexia. Two groups of about 100 children each were constructed: one where children came from families with high relative risk, and a second group where there were no indicators of relative risk. Children in both groups were regularly tested and interviewed, every six months initially and subsequently with greater intervals. In their first year of school (aged seven years), some of the predicted children were found to be experiencing major difficulties in acquiring literacy. It was found that those at risk had proven to be less able, even from the age of six months, to discriminate subtle differences in speech sounds (phonetic durations – an important skill in the Finnish language). This difficulty was also found in many of the dyslexic parents. Another longitudinal study, this time involving Dutch dyslexic children (Boets, De Smedt, Cleuren, Vandewalle, Wouters, & Ghesquire, 2010), also found a general phonological deficit to be present prior to the onset of formal reading instruction, although the authors noted a reciprocal relationship with reading ability. However, it is necessary to be cautious about making causal claims on the basis of longitudinal studies of this kind as it is difficult to ensure the elimination of confounding factors, such as children's learning rate (Byrne, 2011; Olson, 2011) that might be the true underlying cause of any statistical associations (Melby-Lervåg et al., 2012).

Theoretical difficulties have resulted from findings that reading-disabled children can perform normally on tasks and in conditions where the phonological deficit theory would be expected to predict poor performance (Ramus & Ahissar, 2012). One possible explanation for this is that the underlying problem may not, in actuality, concern the quality of the phonological representations. On the basis of a series of experiments with young adult poor readers (Ramus & Szenkovits, 2008; Soroli, Szenkovits, & Ramus, 2010; Szenkovits & Ramus, 2005), it was suggested that rather than being degraded in some way, phonological representations generally appeared to be normal (although these may be problematic for a very small minority). However, the existence of a phonological deficit was not questioned; the participants in the studies showed clear weaknesses on phonological measures. Noting that the tasks that made significant demands on short-term memory and retrieval speed appeared to cause the greatest problems, Ramus and Szenkovits (2008) hypothesized that the core phonological deficit may involve not the quality of the phonological representations, but rather the ability to access these. Similar ideas, they point out, were earlier put forward by Shankweiler and Crain (1986) in their processing limitation hypothesis, and also have parallels with Hulme and Snowling's (1992) conception of an output deficit. Some further support for Ramus's hypothesis has been provided by a number of experimental studies (e.g., Berent, Vaknin-Nusbaum, Balaban, & Galaburda, 2012; Mundy & Carroll, 2012). However, Ramus acknowledges that his theory is still at a "sketchy and underspecified" stage (Ramus & Ahissar, 2012, p. 108).

Despite the popularity of phonological explanations for dyslexia, there continue to be a number of difficulties, with some researchers claiming that phonological factors may be less important than is generally accepted (Byrne, 2011). Not all children with reading disabilities demonstrate a phonological deficit (Castles & Coultheart, 1996; Frederickson & Frith, 1998; White et al., 2006), and children with poor phonological abilities can nevertheless develop good reading skills (Catts & Adlof, 2011; Howard & Best, 1996). In studies of children with speech and language difficulties, it has similarly been found that in many cases phonological awareness deficits do not lead to literacy problems (Bishop et al., 2009; Peterson et al., 2009). Further evidence challenging the phonological theory has been provided from studies of brain-damaged individuals (e.g., Tree & Kay, 2006).

As is discussed later in this chapter, it appears that for a small proportion of poor readers, reading problems can be traced to other cognitive deficits.

In addition, studies of adults with reading disabilities suggest that phonological awareness appears to be rather less important for older poor readers than it is for children, with other processes such as verbal memory, vocabulary, and naming speed playing an equally significant role in differentiating between those with and without reading disability (Swanson & Hsieh, 2009). However, as discussed later in this chapter, much depends on the breadth of the use of the term "phonological" and the extent to which it includes a variety of cognitive processes such as working memory and rapid naming. Ramus et al. (2013), for example, have found some support for his suggestion that many of those with dyslexia have difficulties in relation to the exercise of phonological skills, rather than poor phonological representations. For these authors, phonological skills are understood as the "things that one can do with one's phonological representations, but that require additional skill: awareness and meta-cognitive skills, short-term or working memory, rapid and serial retrieval" (p. 639).

To add to the complexity, some researchers (Nicolson & Fawcett, 2008) suggest that a weakness of the phonological theory stems from the observation that deficits in this area are not specific to those with dyslexia (as they understand this term) but appear to be characteristic of all poor readers. Of course, this argument does not sit easily with definitions of dyslexia in which phonological difficulties are presented as a major diagnostic criterion, or those where a dyslexic subgroup is not distinguished from other poor decoders (see Chapter 1 for a discussion of this definitional complexity).

Despite overwhelming evidence from both behavioral and neuroimaging (Diehl et al., 2011) studies pointing to the importance of phonological awareness in reading, theoretical understanding continues to be unclear:

> While it is almost universally agreed that a phonological deficit is a key factor for most children with reading disability, there continues to be significant debate as to its precise nature and role. Despite more than thirty years of research into the phonological deficit, " . . . we still don't know what it is." (Ramus & Szenkovits, 2008, p. 165)

Given that a single phonological deficit is not necessary or sufficient to cause reading disability (Catts & Adlof, 2011), current thinking sees this as one of multiple deficits that are likely to interact to cause reading disability (Peterson & Pennington, 2012), with some, as is discussed later in this chapter, giving greater weight to the role of visual factors (Valdois, Lassus-Sangosse, & Lobier, 2012; Vidyasagar, 2012).

Snowling (2008; Moll, Loff, & Snowling, 2013) has suggested that, rather than being conceived of as a direct marker of reading difficulties, various phonological (and other) deficits may be better conceptualized as *endopheno-types*, heritable processes that operate between the genotype and the behavioral phenotype. Endophenotypes are considered to be state-independent, that is, they are manifest in an individual, albeit often in a less pronounced fashion, whether or not the particular condition (e.g., reading disability) is present. The suggestion that phonological awareness deficits may be endophenotypes for reading disability has been strengthened by studies demonstrating that family members of those with reading difficulties, but who are typically developing readers themselves, tend to show lower performance on phonological tasks than do controls (Boets et al., 2010; Moll et al., 2013; van Bergen et al., 2012).

Research into phonological deficits has resulted in the development of a range of related interventions for struggling readers that have been shown to improve these skills and, consequently, reading performance (see Chapter 4). Nevertheless, doubts have been expressed about their long-term effectiveness (Olson, 2011), and there continues to be a significant proportion of struggling readers for whom phonological interventions are insufficiently effective.

Rapid naming and the double deficit

A long-standing finding in the dyslexia literature is that a significant proportion of children with reading difficulties are slower in naming quickly visual stimuli that are already well known to them (a process often termed *rapid automatized naming* [RAN]). Typically, measures of RAN (Denckla & Rudel, 1976a, 1976b) assess the speed in which the individual can name a series of familiar items (letters, numbers, colors, or objects) placed in front of them. Using such measures, Denckla and colleagues (Denckla, 1972; Denckla & Rudel, 1974) found correlations between naming speed and reading performance, and from this stemmed the influential work of Wolf, Bowers, and colleagues (Bowers & Wolf, 1993; Norton & Wolf, 2012; Wolf & Bowers, 1999). According to these researchers, fluent reading requires the ability to integrate a range of perceptual, attentional and naming mechanisms that enable the matching of visual representations to phonological codes, precisely, and at speed. Thus, problems of rapid naming do not concern a single isolated problem, but rather a number of difficulties involving several high and low-level processes.

Naming speed appears to be related to almost all aspects of the reading process (J. Kirby et al., 2010), and while a relationship between RAN and general reading ability has usually been found, its predictive power appears to vary (Savage, 2004) depending on whether the naming task involves letters and numbers or pictures and colors (Christopher et al., 2012; Mazzocco & Grimm, 2013; Poulsen, Juul, & Elbro, in press; Schatschneider et al., 2004), and whether the outcome of interest is reading accuracy or fluency (Savage & Frederickson, 2005). It appears that the link with reading fluency is strongest when the naming task requires serial rather than discrete processing (i.e., where stimuli are presented in a series of rows, rather than singly, one after the other on a computer screen) and oral production of the names of the stimuli is required, rather than a nonverbal paper-and-pencil response (Georgiou et al., 2013).

The role of rapid naming for predicting the progress of typical readers of English appears not to be large. In a large-scale meta-analysis of early skills that might predict later reading, writing, or spelling, rapid naming was shown to be only moderately correlated with reading (National Early Literacy Panel, 2008). Rapid naming of letters/digits demonstrated an average correlation of .40 for decoding and .43 for reading comprehension, with correlations of .32 and .42 in the case of objects and colors.

However, rapid naming appears to have greater predictive power for poorer readers (Lervåg, Bråten, & Hulme, 2009; Meyer et al., 1998; Scarborough, 1998), although this has not been found in all studies (Koponen et al., 2013). J. Kirby et al. (2010) speculate that the relationship may be curvilinear, with a steep rise at the lower levels of ability and a flattening out at higher levels. Certainly naming speed has been repeatedly shown to be deficient in many children who struggle with reading difficulties (Wolf, Bowers, & Biddle, 2000), with the problem often persisting into adulthood (Pennington et al., 1990; Vukovic, Wilson, & Nash, 2004). It appears to be most predictive when related to younger children, and its effects tend to be reduced after Grade 3 (Wolf, Bowers, & Biddle, 2000). Hulslander et al. (2010), for example, found that rapid naming failed to predict word reading performance for children of varying reading ability aged between 8 and 13 years when they were retested approximately 5 years later.

While the rapid-naming effect appears to be "universal" (Wolf et al., 2009, p. 85), its predictive importance appears to be greater in transparent (Furnes & Samuelsson, 2010; Torppa et al., 2010; Wimmer, Mayringer, & Landerl, 2000) and logosyllabic (Liao, Georgiou, & Parrila, 2008; Tan et al., 2005), rather than more opaque, languages (Compton, 2003; Compton, DeFries, & Olson, 2001). Somewhat surprisingly, Ziegler, Bertand, et al. (2010) found limited influence for RAN across five languages lying at different positions along a transparency continuum (Finnish, Hungarian, Dutch, Portuguese, and French). This finding appears not to fit with other studies (e.g., Landerl, Ramus et al., 2013), possibly because of the use of different age groupings. However, Ziegler, Bertrand et al.'s study (op. cit) assessed object, rather than alphanumeric RAN, which, while considered to be a purer measure of naming-speed deficits (on the grounds that it is not confounded by letter recognition), tends to be more weakly correlated with reading scores.

The apparently greater importance for RAN in transparent languages is unsurprising as for such orthographies the primary difficulty after the first two years at school is typically slow, laborious reading rather than specific decoding errors (Klicpera & Schabmann, 1993). Studies of reading in transparent languages often employ measures of reading fluency rather than reading accuracy, although this is not always made explicit in published research abstracts. There is also a tendency for children to score highly on phonological awareness tests in transparent languages, resulting in reduced range and, potentially, an underestimate of its contribution to reading (Vaessen et al., 2009).

According to Wolf's double deficit hypothesis model (Wolf & Bowers, 1999), dyslexics can be subdivided into three groups: those with phonological difficulties but with average naming speed ability, those with a rapid naming deficit but average phonological skills, and those with both phonological and rapid naming difficulties. According to her model, those with the double deficit would be likely to have the most severe form of reading difficulties – a suggestion that has been largely confirmed by empirical studies in both opaque (Wolf, Bowers, & Biddle, 2000) and transparent (Torppa et al., 2013) languages, although contrasting findings showing no differences between children with a double or single deficit have also been reported (Ackerman et al., 2001; Vaessen et al., 2009).

Evidence to support the suggestion that there exists a subgroup of poor readers with naming speed deficits but no phonological deficits (a single naming speed deficit) has been described as "mixed" (Vaessen et al., 2009, p. 204). Whereas Wolf, Bowers and Biddle (2000) have reported a number of studies in which a significant number of poor readers exhibited a single naming speed deficit, other studies have not found this. In their review of three cross-sectional studies undertaken by Badian (1997), Morris et al. (1998), and Pennington et al. (2001), the reviewers (Vukovic and Siegel, 2006) conclude that most of the children who had naming speed difficulties also demonstrated phonological processing deficits. While it appeared that those with both naming speed and phonological problems tended to have the most severe reading difficulties, there were relatively few who had rapid naming problems but intact phonological skills. Vaessen, Gerretsen, and Blomert (2009) found that 10.5% of their sample of dyslexic primary school children demonstrated a single naming speed deficit, but noted that there was little difference on literacy performance between these children and the other groups.

A detailed review of naming speed by Kirby, Georgiou, et al. (2010) concludes by calling for a cautious response to the mixed findings that have been reported for the double deficit hypothesis. While the majority of these indicate that the greatest difficulties are experienced by those with both phonological and naming speed deficits, any definite claims should be treated with caution. Contradictory findings across research studies may stem from differences in orthographies and in the nature of study samples (see also Georgiou & Parrila, 2013). Some studies use typically developing readers; others, those with reading disabilities. Arbitrary cut-off points and age groupings vary substantially. The authors suggest that given significant difficulties of group stability over even short periods, a "purer test" of the hypothesis might involve adolescents or adults (Kirby, Georgiou, et al., 2010, p. 350), although there appear to be no longitudinal studies involving the former and conflicting evidence from the latter.

As noted earlier, rapid naming has been more closely associated with reading fluency than single-word identification and letter-sound decoding (Manis, Doi, & Bhadha, 2000; Sunseth & Bowers, 2002), although Fletcher et al. (2011) did not find this to be the case when comparing good and poor responders to a small-group reading intervention. Whereas some researchers have considered fluency to be primarily a by-product of successful decoding, Wolf and her colleagues believe it to be a developmental process related to all key aspects of reading, from basic phonological and decoding skills to semantic and morphological knowledge (Wolf, Gottwald, Galante, Norton, & Miller, 2009). As much of the dyslexia research in English has placed an emphasis on word recognition, the importance of naming speed in the development of skilled, fluent reading has arguably been overlooked. Those who understand dyslexia as primarily a problem of word reading accuracy (e.g., Fletcher et al., 2007) do not consider rapid naming to be a core deficit, and poor readers who demonstrate difficulties solely in relation to reading speed (rather than accuracy) would not necessarily be labeled as suffering from dyslexia.

As is the case for much of the research work in dyslexia, it has proven more difficult to arrive at a widely agreed-on theoretical explanation for the nature and role of rapid naming than it has been to demonstrate an association between this process and reading disability (Georgiou & Parrila, 2013), and the double deficit hypothesis has been criticized for lacking sufficient specification to enable its theoretical underpinnings to be evaluated experimentally (Vellutino et al., 2004). Neither a clear consensus on an operational definition of rapid naming nor a clear account of how exactly this relates to reading has been achieved (Lervåg et al., 2009; Vukovic & Siegel, 2006). Achieving such understandings has been rendered particularly complex because naming speed appears to serve as an indicator of an underlying problem that impacts reading speed (Wolf, 2007). For Wolf, et al. (2000), "[n]aming speed is conceptualized as a complex ensemble of attentional, perceptual, conceptual, memory, phonological, semantic, and motoric subprocesses that places heavy emphasis upon precise timing requirements within each component and across all components" (p. 395).

Some researchers contend that rapid naming deficits are best conceived as reflecting an underlying deficit in phonological representations (Snowling & Hulme, 1994; Wagner & Torgesen, 1987). Within such an account, naming speed tasks tap rapid access to, and retrieval of, phonological information from long-term memory. Wolf and her colleagues (Wolf et al., 2002; Wolf & Bowers, 1999) have criticized this conception, arguing that these processes are more related to underlying timing problems and should therefore be considered as independent (see also Nicolson & Fawcett, 2006, p. 260, for criticism of the "ad hoc" lumping together of different processes under the phonology category). For some, "naming speed is phonological, but not only phonological" (J. Kirby et al., 2010, p. 356). An alternative theory is that poor naming speed disrupts skilled orthographic processing, the mechanism by which words seen frequently come to be speedily recognized as sight words (Bowers, Sunseth, & Golden, 1999; Bowers & Wolf, 1993; Georgiou, Parrila, & Kirby, 2009). A potential weakness with this account is that naming speed has been found to be equally strongly related to the speed of reading pseudowords as real words (Moll et al., 2009). As pseudowords cannot have been stored already, and thus cannot be familiar to the reader, this would appear to rule out the orthographic hypothesis. However, as pseudowords often contain familiar clusters of letters, some form of orthographic processing may still be operating, albeit not at the word level (J. Kirby et al., 2010).

A case for inclusion within a phonological account stems from the argument that if phonological representations of words are degraded or not easily accessible, they are unlikely to be easily retrieved, and as a result, naming speed would be reduced. In their detailed examination, Vukovic and Siegel (2006) are unable to provide an authoritative conclusion regarding this issue but support the argument that RAN might best be classified as a phonological task. They suggest that while rapid naming may indeed represent the ability to retrieve information from long-term memory and indicate global processing speed, as far as reading is concerned, difficulties may center on the ability to rapidly retrieve phonological codes.

Studies indicate that measures of naming speed and phonological processing are modestly correlated; Swanson et al. (2003) reported a correlation of .38 in their meta-analysis of correlational studies of phonological awareness and naming speed. However, Torppa et al. (2013) found only a weak correlation between these two variables for a large group of Finnish kindergarten children. In a study of Danish readers, Poulsen, Juul, & Elbro (in press) found that phonological awareness was an important mediator for RAN-reading correlations for measures of both accuracy and fluency. These authors concluded that while the degree of mediation was modest, RAN appears to measure phonological processing to some limited extent.

RAN measures have been found to be independent predictors of reading skill (Bowers & Wolf, 1993; Powell et al., 2007), with the relationship being stronger for measures of orthographic choice and exception word reading than nonword reading, this latter measure being closely linked to phonological ability. Powell and colleagues surveyed a sample of British children aged 7–9 years and found a pattern that supported the double deficit theory. Factor analysis and structural equation modeling of the data led to the conclusion that while phonological processes played a part in RAN performance, other processes, beyond generalized processing speed, also seemed to be important. Moreover, in a large Russian family study of reading skills (Naples, Chang, Katz, & Grigorenko, 2009), phonemic awareness and RAN were found to be distinct constructs that could not be substituted by each other. Each appeared to be heritable; there were indicators of genetic forces operating in both shared (i.e., contributing to both indicators) and unique (i.e., contributing to each indicator separately) fashion. Also, it was shown that, for each indicator, a number of genes were involved, revealing that there were pleiotropic (i.e., contributing to both indicators) and unique (i.e., contributing to each indicator separately) genes.

Taking an opposing position, Ziegler, Bertrand, et al. (2010) consider it "probably misleading" (p. 557) to conceive of RAN as an independent nonphonological component. They point to a study by Chiappe, Stringer, Siegel, & Stanovich (2002) showing that while 25% of unique variance in reading was explained by naming speed, 75% was shared with phonological awareness. Ziegler et al. (2010) suggest that while RAN tasks may incorporate only a relatively minor phonological component, it is this particular element that appears to be the best predictor of reading performance (Vaessen et al., 2009). Where measures of phonological awareness are insufficiently sensitive or reach the ceiling (as may often be the case in studies of transparent languages), most of the shared variance will be left to RAN and this will become the key predictor.

There remains considerable uncertainty about the exact nature of the cognitive processes that underpin naming speed, and its relationship to the reading process. Some have suggested that these are tied by the operation of a range of various executive processes including attention, working memory, and inhibition (Amtmann, Abbott, & Berninger, 2007) that together ensure skilled performance. For others, naming speed reflects a general processing speed deficit (Kail & Hall, 1994) that may disrupt the temporal integration of visual and phonological information and also timing-related deficits outside of the language domain (Bowers, Sunseth, & Golden, 1999; Farmer & Klein, 1995).

The notion of rapid naming as a subcomponent of general processing speed (Johnson et al., 2010) has been challenged by findings that RAN accounts for variance even after global processing has been controlled for (Cutting & Denckla, 2001; Powell et al., 2007, although see Catts et al., 2002, for a contradictory finding). Christopher et al. (2012) found that for a large sample of children, 26% of whom had a history of reading disability, naming speed for digits and letters independently predicted word reading after processing speed was controlled for, but this was not similarly the case for nonalphanumeric stimuli. In the light of their finding that speed of processing correlated with RAN but not with reading, Poulsen, Juul, & Elbro (in press) tentatively concluded that speed of processing was unlikely to be an explanation for the relationship between RAN and reading.

The term "global processing" may be somewhat misleading as it can conceal important distinctions between global and more specific forms of rapid processing (Bonifacci & Snowling, 2008; De Clercq-Quaegebeur et al., 2010; Naples, Katz, & Grigorenko, 2012; Shanahan et al., 2006). Vaessen, Gerretsen and Blomert (2009), for example, found no evidence of impaired visual matching speed in their sample of dyslexic children, and nonalphabetic processing accounted for only a small proportion of variance in reading speed (Wimmer & Mayringer, 2001). McGrath et al. (2011), however, found that symbolic processing speed was associated with single-word reading performance. To render this issue more complex, Savage (2004) has queried whether, given existing evidence, it is possible to conclude that rapid naming reflects automatic processing, and has called for more sophisticated studies that can go beyond questions about speed of processing to examine the automaticity of naming.

Stainthorp et al. (2010) found that children with slow RAN performance appeared to have difficulties on visual (but not auditory) discrimination tasks that could not be explained by general processing speed or by word reading ability. Although there was no significant difference between slow and normal RAN groups on accuracy, the former group took longer to make the discriminations, even after controlling for simple reaction times. The authors suggest that a general focus on accuracy, rather than on speed, may help explain the widely held view (Vellutino, 1979) that visuo-perceptual difficulties are not significant in dyslexia. Despite the fact that their low RAN group did not have significant reading problems, Stainthorp et al. (2010) offer a number of possible explanations for the relationship between RAN and reading difficulty involving an underlying visual discrimination problem. However, they accept that without detailed longitudinal studies, causal explanations are merely speculative.

While it is widely agreed that assessments of naming speed in young children can help identify those who may subsequently develop reading difficulties, its value for informing effective educational intervention programs is far from clear. To date, it has proven difficult to provide a detailed and full account of the cognitive components that underpin the RAN-reading relationship, and this has hindered attempts to provide targeted interventions (Poulsen, Juul, & Elbro, in press).

Unlike phonological processing deficits, where there is evidence supporting the value of targeted interventions, there remains significant doubt as to whether it is possible to increase naming speed and, even if this were possible, whether such gains would result in improved reading performance (Norton & Wolf, 2012). J. Kirby et al. (2010) outline two alternative scenarios. In one, naming speed operates as a distal predictor of reading; it is seen as relatively stable and not easily improved by intervention. Given this situation, it is probably wiser to follow the lead of Wolf et al. (2009) and introduce multi-component reading skill interventions. An alternative scenario is to conceive of naming speed as having more proximal effects on reading. Here, interventions would be geared to improving speed directly, and reading performance would be expected to improve as a consequence. The evidence in support of this latter approach is minimal, however, van der Leij (2013) and there continues to be insufficient knowledge as to what aspects of any such program would be important for the achievement of such an end.

Short-term and working memory

When considering the nature of reading, it is unsurprising that memory deficits are seen as having a causal effect on reading difficulties (Kipp & Mohr, 2008; Vellutino et al., 2004). Key processes in learning to read involve coding, storage, and retrieval of stable associations between speech and written language. Crucially important is the lexical retrieval process that requires visual recognition of an array of letters as forming a particular word and subsequent retrieval of its name and meaning from memory.

While there is some evidence that both verbal and visual long-term memory capacities tend to be weaker in poor readers (Menghini et al., 2010; Swanson, 1999), findings have tended to be inconsistent (e.g., Bell, 1990; Watson & Willows, 1995). One explanation for such discrepancies is that behavioral outcomes can be influenced by different systems within long-term memory (Nicolson & Fawcett, 2007), and research tasks have often been insufficient to enable differentiation between these (Menghini et al., 2010).

In relation to dyslexia, most studies of memory processes have focused on short-term or working memory, both of which involve limited capacity to hold information for a brief period of time. Whereas short-term memory merely involves the passive storage of information, working memory involves both storage and processing and thus draws on a central executive system in which controlled attentional processes are significant. These difficulties appear not to be related to IQ (Swanson, Zheng, & Jerman, 2009). Both types of memory have been shown to be associated with poor progress in reading (Gathercole, Pickering, Knight, & Stegmann, 2004; Kibby et al., 2004; Swanson, Ashbaker, & Lee, 1996), across a wide range of orthographies (although their role, similar across these, was relatively minor [Landerl et al., 2013]). There is also some support from neuroscientific studies using functional magnetic resonance imaging (fMRI) (Beneventi et al., 2010; Berninger et al., 2008). The relative importance of short-term versus working memory for reading disability is somewhat contentious. In their meta-analytic review, however, Swanson et al. (2009) reported that measures of short-term memory and working memory both made independent contribution to effect size differences between children with and without reading disability.

As is the case for rapid naming processes, there is disagreement as to whether short-term verbal memory difficulties should be incorporated within the phonological deficit model or considered separately within a broader conception of poor working memory. The phonological deficit case is prompted by findings that problems appear to be particularly related to the storage of verbal input (Siegel & Ryan, 1989; Swanson et al., 2009). As illustrated later in the chapter, however, working memory difficulties in poor readers can also be found in the visuo-spatial domain, although here too verbal processes may also play a role. Further doubts about the relationship of memory difficulties to the phonological model have been raised by findings that working memory problems can persist even in cases where nonverbal stimuli are used and phonology is seemingly not involved (Banai & Ahissar, 2004, 2010).

It is possible that working memory may have a disruptive role in the acquisition of literacy, only where problems are of a certain severity, with a particular performance threshold proving important for attaining an appropriate reading level (Nevo & Breznitz, 2011). Children with significant working memory difficulties tend to perform poorly on a variety of cognitive, academic, and behavioral measures (Alloway et al., 2009; Banai & Ahissar, 2004, 2010), including reading (Alloway, Gathercole, Kirkwood, & Elliott, 2009; Johnson et al., 2010). Similarly, a large proportion of those identified as having learning difficulties show working memory problems even when intelligence is controlled for (Gathercole et al., 2006). Working memory appears to be particularly impaired in children who present with a combination of academic difficulties such as reading, spelling, and mathematics (Maehler & Schuchardt, 2009, 2011, although see De Weerdt, Desoete, & Roeyers [2013]). Indications are that the memory problems of struggling readers do not improve with age (Cohen-Mimran & Sapir, 2007; Rose & Rouhani, 2012; Swanson & Hsieh, 2009; Swanson et al., 2009).

Many studies have demonstrated the importance of working memory in relation to reading comprehension (Carretti et al., 2009; Swanson, 1999; Swanson, Howard, & Sáez, 2006; Swanson & O'Connor, 2009), although its precise role continues to be controversial (Ricketts, 2011). Its influence may be less for accurate word reading, although Christopher et al. (2012) found that working memory predicted word reading and reading comprehension at similar levels. Memory difficulties may play a more powerful role when poor readers are required to decode complex, multisyllabic words. Here, there is a requirement for the reader to hold associations between sounds and letters while subsequently building these up into new associations in order to read the word (Compton, Fuchs et al., 2012; Conners et al., 2001). Problems on working memory tests tend to be greater for children who experience both decoding and reading comprehension difficulties in combination than for those with reading comprehension problems alone (Swanson et al., 2006) – hardly surprising given the processing demands that will ensue.

A sound and consensual understanding of the precise nature of the relationship between short-term and working memory and reading disability has proven difficult to achieve, in part because of the use of different terms, models, measures, and sampling (Cowan & Alloway, 2008). Indeed, this state of affairs has led researchers in some studies to seek to assess elements of working memory in ways that can be considered to be "theoretically neutral" (Gathercole et al., 2006, p. 267). Thus phonological and visuo-spatial short-term memory tasks involving storage can be contrasted with more complex memory tasks that are designed to tap working memory.

While several models of working memory feature in the literature (Baddeley, 2012) perhaps the most influential in studies of reading disability is that originally conceived by Baddeley and Hitch (1974). According to this, a modality-free central executive is responsible for controlling and regulating the cognitive processes in two domain-specific stores: the phonological loop and the visuo-spatial sketchpad. The central executive is also seen as responsible for the control of attention and processing involving a range of regulatory functions including the retrieval of information from long-term memory (Baddeley, 1996). The revised model (Baddeley, 2000) introduced a fourth component, the episodic buffer, which was held to be responsible for binding information across informational domains and memory subsystems into integrated chunks. However, there appears to be no published research considering this element in relation to learning disabilities (De Weerdt et al., 2013).

Verbal short-term memory and verbal working memory

Verbal short-term memory and working memory are typically assessed using recall of digits or word sequences. A widely employed measure involves repeating digits both forward and backward (e.g., the Digit Span subtest from the Wechsler Scales). Repetition of digits in the same order is often used as a measure of short-term memory, whereas tasks that require the participant to reverse the series of numbers are considered to test working memory. There are some doubts, however, as to the value of digit span tasks as the particular strategies involved may not generalize well to tasks such as reading (Swanson et al., 2009), and some consider that these may not be a true measure of working memory (Rosen & Engle, 1997). In experimental work, another favored memory task involves the use of nonwords, although the two main types of measure – nonword repetition and nonword matching – appear not to share common processing demands (Savage, Lavers, & Pillay, 2007).

The phonological loop is considered to be the site for verbal short-term memory (Baddeley, 1986) because of two key characteristics: it serves as a phonological input store and also utilizes an articulatory rehearsal process. Some have claimed that, in practice, verbal short-term memory and verbal working memory are synonymous constructs, at least when applied to children (Hutton & Towse, 2001). Swanson (2006) disagrees with this suggestion on the grounds that working memory tasks require participants to transform material in some way, rather than merely recall a sequence of items in the order in which they were presented. As this involves regulation processes, it can be seen to be tapping both the phonological loop and the central executive (see Bacon, Parmentier, & Barr, 2013; Smith-Spark & Fisk, 2007; Wang & Gathercole, 2013, for experimental support for this position). In relation to reading, working memory appears to have two important roles: it holds information that has been recently processed in order to make connections to the most recent input and it "maintains the gist of information for the construction of an overall representation of a text" (Swanson & O'Connor, 2009, p. 548).

Despite the presence of verbal short-term and working memory problems in many individuals with reading difficulties, there is some uncertainty as to their unique contribution. A five-year longitudinal study of children from kindergarten to fourth grade (Wagner et al., 1997), for example, found that while individual differences in phonological awareness exerted a causal influence on word-level reading, there were no independent causal influences for phonological memory. Wagner later noted (Wagner & Muse, 2006) that the apparent irrelevance of phonological memory in this study may have been a statistical artifact resulting from a strong correlation between measures of phonological memory and phonological awareness. In a wide-ranging review of the relationship between working memory and reading difficulties, Savage et al. (2007) examined the unique contribution of phonological memory (and other working memory) measures for later reading acquisition. When these were entered into regression equations with other accepted predictors of word reading, little evidence was found that the memory measures added to prediction for word reading. As suggested earlier, however, it is possible that working memory only becomes important when multisyllabic words are being tackled (Gilbert, Compton, & Kearns, 2011).

A more recent meta-analysis of studies of those with dyslexia and controls, where differences between phonemic awareness, rime awareness, and verbal short-term memory were examined (Melby-Lervåg et al., 2012), also found only a limited role for verbal short-term memory, with most of the variance apparently explained by phonemic awareness. It seems that the apparently greater predictive power of measures of phonological awareness may have resulted in reduced interest in working memory as a direct determinant of reading disability (Wagner & Muse, 2006).

It is difficult to conceive of any measure of phonological awareness that does not involve some component of verbal working memory, and this probably explains why phonological memory tasks often fail to contribute independent variability in multivariate studies (Fletcher et al., 2007). The difficulty of treating these two processes as separate elements is succinctly made by Wagner and Muse (2006):

[L]arge-scale studies indicate that measures of phonological memory and phonological awareness measure nearly the same thing at the preschool level, and very highly related things thereafter. . . . Simply treating them as two completely distinct constructs flies in the face of compelling data. (p. 53)

Visuo-spatial short-term memory and visuo-spatial working memory

According to Baddeley (2012), the visuo-spatial sketchpad is responsible for the short-term storage and manipulation of visual and spatial information. It includes linguistic information that can be recoded into a form that can be visualised. This system is typically assessed by measures that involve the recall of visually presented material such as sequences of tapped blocks, or of filled cells in a visual matrix.

Studies concerning the relationship of visuo-spatial short-term or working memory to reading disability are fewer in number than those examining verbal working memory (Johnson et al., 2010), and their findings have proven to be inconsistent (Jeffries & Everatt, 2004; Kibby, Marks, Morgan, & Long, 2004; Menghini et al., 2011; Olson & Datta, 2002; Smith-Spark et al., 2003; Smith-Spark & Fisk, 2007; Wang & Gathercole, 2013).

Two meta-analytic reviews of children with dyslexia have found effects for visual memory. In one of these (Swanson, Zheng, & Herman, 2009), moderate to high effect sizes were found for both visual short-term memory and visual working memory. However, hierarchical linear modeling indicated that overall memory problems were primarily moderated by difficulties in relation to verbal processes that tapped the phonological loop and the executive system. A second meta-analysis of studies comparing reading-disabled and typically achieving students (Johnson et al., 2010) reported effect sizes of −.64 for visual working memory in comparison with −.92 for verbal working memory.

Contrasting findings in studies utilising visuo-spatial tasks may, in part, be explained by differences in the nature of the samples, methods, and tasks employed (Menghini, Finzi, Carlesimo, & Vicari, 2011). It has been suggested that performance will be affected by the extent to which the visual stimuli can be phonologically recoded (Macaruso et al., 1995). Thus, Swanson (1978) found that poor readers performed worse than controls when names could be given to the stimuli and thus stored as phonological codes.

The central executive

More complex memory tasks have been designed to assess the central executive/attentional control aspect of working memory, typically in combination with verbal memory. For these, the individual is typically required to process and store increasing amounts of information until reaching the point at which recall errors are made. It is important to note, however, that despite burgeoning interest, there are many unresolved conceptual and methodological issues in relation to the measurement of executive functions (Friso-van den Bos et al., 2013).

The importance of the central executive likely depends on the nature of the task and the materials utilized. Compared with tests of single-word decoding, more complex measures of reading are likely to require greater capacity to hold onto task-relevant information in the face of competing distractions, and children with a range of learning disabilities (including reading) appear to struggle on tasks that place high demands on processing, in particular controlled attention (Swanson & Zheng, 2013). Swanson and colleagues (Swanson, 2003; Swanson & Howell, 2001) have shown that complex memory tasks predict reading ability independent of phonological short-term memory. These findings were further supported by their subsequent meta-analytic review of studies comparing working memory in poor and normal readers. Here, short-term memory and working memory each contributed unique variance (Swanson et al., 2009, although see Schuchardt, Maehler, & Hasselhorn, 2008, for a contrasting position).

However, there is some disagreement in the literature about the operationalization, validity, and reliability of working memory measures, and it is somewhat ironic that measures with the strongest empirical association with reading also have the greatest problems of construct validity (Savage et al., 2007). These can be contrasted with

other verbal STM tasks, whose empirical base as associates of reading is fairly weak but whose construct validity has rarely been questioned. . . . Together they add up to a knowledge base where claims of a clear and unambiguous association between reading disability and WM can still currently be questioned. (Savage et al., 2007, p. 214)

The central executive appears to have an important role in relation to reading comprehension, in part by regulating attentional control (Carretti, Borella, Cornoldi, & De Beni, 2009). In a review of relevant studies, Swanson (2006, p. 83) notes:

[I]n situations that place high demands on processing, which in turn place demands on controlled attentional processing (such as monitoring limited resources, suppressing conflicting information, and updating information) children with RD (reading disabilities) are at a clear disadvantage. . . . This impaired capability for controlled processing appears to manifest itself across visuospatial and verbal WM (working memory) tasks, and therefore reflects a domain-general deficit.

As appears to be the case for most underlying cognitive processes in dyslexia, memory deficits are not found in all struggling readers. In a study of French dyslexics, for example, a sizeable proportion of the sample (30%) did not present with such problems (De Clercq-Quaegebeur et al., 2010). An additional complexity is that the proportion of poor readers with working memory difficulties can vary significantly across studies (Swanson, Zheng, & Jerman, 2009). To some extent, such inconsistencies may reflect the complexity of the memory tasks involved (Ramus & Ahissar, 2012).

Despite the frequent presence of short-term and working memory difficulties in children with dyslexia, prediction is typically less powerful than for phonological processing or rapid naming (Savage et al., 2007). The National Early Literacy Panel's (2008) meta-analysis of studies involving early skills and subsequent reading reported average correlations for phonological short-term memory that were weak for decoding (.26) and moderate for reading comprehension (.39). Measures of visual memory produced weak correlations for both decoding (.22) and comprehension (.17). Melby-Lervåg et al.'s (2012) meta-analysis found only a very small effect size (–.09) for verbal short-term memory when dyslexics were compared with controls reading at the same level. Further evidence for the somewhat weaker predictive power of short-term and working memory, in comparison with phonemic awareness and rapid naming, has also been found in a large cross-cultural study involving orthographies of varying complexity (Landerl, Ramus, et al., 2013).

Working memory and educational intervention

Studies of short-term and working memory in those with dyslexia have not proven particularly helpful for guiding intervention. Perhaps this is because there may not be a simple causal relationship between short-term or working memory and word reading, but rather a complex number of factors, operating at many levels that interact to produce reading disability (Laasonen et al., 2012).

This more complex picture raises significant questions about how research into memory can be used to help reading-disabled children. As is the case for rapid naming, there are conflicting views as to whether particular underlying (memory) processes can be improved directly, and if so, whether this will subsequently lead to improved reading performance.

Rather than seeking to improve the underlying cognitive deficit, another option is to focus directly on teaching the relevant academic skills, in this case those concerning reading and spelling. However, whether the focus is on improving memory processes or focusing directly on academic content, it would seem to be valuable also to sensitize teachers to the need to modify their classroom practice when working with those with memory difficulties. Teachers need to understand reasons for not overloading working memory demands, and be advised on how best to help such children devise helpful memorization strategies (Gathercole & Alloway, 2008). While such advice would intuitively seem to be beneficial, it should be noted that a classroom working memory intervention involving close collaboration with teachers produced discouraging results (Elliott, Gathercole, Alloway, Kirkwood, & Holmes, 2010).

An alternative approach to tackling memory problems is to provide direct training sessions using specially designed computer programs. Despite positive findings from laboratory and field studies suggesting that children's performance on working memory tasks (almost always for those with ADHD) can be improved after such exercises (Alloway, Bibile, & Lau, 2013; Gray et al., 2012; Holmes & Gathercole, in press; Holmes, Gathercole, & Dunning, 2009; Klingberg, 2010; Loosli et al., 2012; Shiran & Breznitz, 2011), there remain significant concerns that gains reported may be largely short-term and fail to generalize (Melby-Lervåg & Hulme, 2013; Redick et al., 2013; Shipstead, Redick, & Engle, 2012). Interestingly, one training study (Dunning, Holmes, & Gathercole, 2013) demonstrated improvement in untrained working memory tasks, yet this had no impact on either classroom analogues of activities that tax working memory or academic skills, either immediately after the training, or one year later. A randomized clinical trial with children aged 7–11 with ADHD (Chacko et al., 2013) similarly found some near-transfer gains in memory storage but no treatment generalization to other aspects of working memory, academic performance, or changes in children's attentional difficulties. Such findings support claims that widespread methodological weaknesses in studies that have produced more promising results render their conclusions problematic (Shipstead, Hicks, & Engle, 2012; Chacko et al., 2013; von Bastian & Oberaver, in press). Despite the occasional positive finding, such as that reported by Egeland, Aarlien, and Saunes (2013) for word reading and Dahlin (2011) in respect of reading comprehension, there is little convincing evidence to support claims that working memory interventions can meaningfully impact academic performance in school. Certainly there is a significant need for longitudinal studies examining the long-term effects of experimental manipulations of this kind on children with various learning difficulties.

Low-level sensory processing

During the past decade, there has been a resurgence of interest in underlying auditory and visual factors in reading disability. Rather than directly competing with phonological accounts, these have often been integrated within explanations whereby phonological processing operates at "a layer above" more basic processes (Plante, 2012, p. 259). Thus, several theories suggest that phonological and other proximal reading-related difficulties can be traced back to more basic lower-level deficits involving auditory, visual, and/or motor processing (Ramus, 2003; Tallal & Gaab, 2006; Vidyasagar & Pammer, 2010a), with some suggesting that 20–30% of those with dyslexia have a sensory processing deficit that may contribute to their reading difficulties (Wright & Conlon, 2009). However, whether such processes exert a causal influence on phonological processing and reading, or instead serve merely as a marker for an underlying neurological abnormality (Heath et al., 2006; Pugh et al., 2013), is still subject to debate.

Auditory processing

The quality of the child's phonological awareness is likely to depend on their auditory processing; if this is impaired in some way, they are unlikely to be able to reflect appropriately on the sounds in words they hear. Such an assumption reflects a bottom-up perspective in which basic auditory processing problems are considered to be causally responsible for phonological deficits (Farmer & Klein, 1995; Klein & Farmer, 1995; Tallal & Gaab, 2006). In contrast, top-down explanations (Ramus et al., 2003; White et al., 2006) emphasize the role of higher-level linguistic processes. According to such accounts, auditory processing difficulties may be present but these do not impact phonological processing and, thus, would not play a causal role in reading disability (for a discussion, see Hämäläinen, Salminen, & Leppänen, 2013).

On the basis of earlier work showing that children with specific language impairment experienced greater difficulty in tasks of auditory sensitivity, Tallal (1980) examined whether these problems might also be a feature of those with reading disability. This proved to be case, with a positive correlation being found between auditory processing and reading. Tallal hypothesized that deficits in auditory processing affected speech perception, which in turn affected the development of phonological awareness and, ultimately, the acquisition of reading skills.

A variety of different auditory tasks have been employed in reading research, many focusing on the processing of short sounds and fast transitions involving a "rapid" or "temporal" deficit (Tallal, 1980; Tallal & Gaab, 2006). One measure (a time order judgment "repetition test") involves familiarizing participants with two distinct sounds and then asking them to state the order in which these are presented. The time interval between the two sounds indicates whether the task assesses rapid or slow auditory processing. Tallal's conclusions that difficulties centered on the perception of rapid tones were subsequently challenged on the grounds that she failed to check adequately that the problems she studied were specific to the temporal domain. In addition, studies by Ahissar, Protopapas, Reid, and Merzenich (2000) and McArthur and Bishop (2004) indicated that the deficient auditory problems of those with language and reading difficulties did not appear to be limited to stimuli that were presented in a rapid fashion, but also included tasks involving frequency modulation and longer inter-stimulus intervals (Mody, Studdert-Kennedy, & Brady, 1997; Share et al., 2002; Studdert-Kennedy & Mody, 1995).

An alternative, and increasingly influential, auditory theory has been proposed by Goswami and her colleagues (Corriveau, Goswami, & Thomson, 2010; Goswami et al., 2002). These researchers argue that the rapid processing hypothesis offers an insufficient account of the auditory difficulties encountered by those with reading disabilities. Instead, it may be more appropriate to focus on the perception of auditory signals underpinning speech rhythm, tempo, and stress. Impairments in this respect are likely to lead to difficulties in drawing on prosodic cues (involving the grouping, rhythm, and prominence of the elements of speech, ranging from subparts of the syllable to the phrase [Pierrehumbert, 2003]) that appear to be valuable in helping the child develop phonological awareness and early reading skills (Beattie and Manis, in press; Goodman, Libenson, & Wade-Woolley, 2010; Holliman, Wood, & Sheehy, 2010; Wood, 2006). One important element of rhythmic sensitivity is *rise time*, which refers to the rate of change of the amplitude of sounds (corresponding to the beats of syllables in the speech stream). In speech, rise time incorporates changes in frequency, duration, and intensity, factors that are important for prosodic prominence. Perhaps, therefore, it is unsurprising that rise time sensitivity appears to be a predictor of phonological awareness in young children (Corriveau et al., 2010), although the route and nature of its influence may be somewhat different in the case of older readers (see Beattie & Manis, 2012 for a discussion).

Poor performance on auditory measures has been repeatedly found for groups of reading-disabled children (Goswami et al., 2013) and adults, with correlations found between auditory processing, phonological, and language skills (Goswami, Gerson, & Astruc, 2010; Goswami et al., 2002; Stein, 2008; Talcott et al., 1999; Walker et al., 2006), although it should be noted that other studies have failed to detect a relationship (Halliday & Bishop, 2006; Nittrouer, 1999; White et al., 2006). Beattie and Manis (2012) compared rise time perception in three groups of children: those with reading difficulties, those with combined reading and language difficulties, and chronological age-matched typical readers. The age-matched controls performed significantly better on the rise time measures than the two groups of children with reading difficulties, with no difference on this measure between the latter groups. However, the majority of the children with reading problems did not perform poorly on these measures and, for each of the two poor reader groups, no significant correlations were found between the rise time tasks and reading or phonological awareness measures.

The auditory processing hypothesis in relation to reading disability has been criticized on both methodological and substantive grounds (Studdert-Kennedy, 2002; Vellutino et al., 2004). One common criticism concerns the lack of universality of this problem in reading-disabled children (McArthur & Bishop, 2001). Ramus (2003) suggests an overall aggregate from samples of those with reading disabilities of 39%. Roughly similar figures of "about a third" are provided by Boets, Wouters, van Wieringer, and Ghesquière (2007, p. 1614) and between 22% and 36% by Wright and Conlon (2009), although this latter estimate relates to single measures of either auditory or visual sensory processes. However, such an approximation can serve to mask large variations across studies (e.g., Griffiths et al., 2003; Van Ingelghem et al., 2001). McArthur and Hogben (2012) note findings in the 20–50% range, and Stein (2012a) states that estimates range from 10% to 70%. There appears to be some evidence that auditory processing deficits are less prevalent in some languages other than English (Georgiou, Protopapas, Padadopoulos, Skaloumbakas, & Parilla, 2010; Georgiou, Papadopoulos, Zarouna, & Parrila, 2012; Goswami et al., 2011; Surányi et al., 2009).

Recognition that auditory processing deficits cannot explain all cases should not directly lead to the conclusion that it cannot explain any of them (Stein, 2008). Indeed, a similar criticism can equally be applied to the phonological deficit hypothesis (Boets, Ghesquière, et al., 2007). Certainly, if one accepts a multiple risk factor account of reading disability, the fact that a risk factor affects some but not others should not be seen as theoretically problematic (Plakas et al., 2013), although the large variations between different samples does pose an empirical challenge (McArthur et al., 2008).

Another challenge to the hypothesis stems from the finding that some normal readers also demonstrate significant auditory and speech perception problems (Halliday & Bishop, 2006; Landerl & Willburger, 2010). It is unclear, however, whether this suggests a limited role for lower-level sensory processing in the acquisition of reading skills or, alternatively, that some children find ways to compensate for such difficulties (Boets, Ghesquière, et al., 2007).

The nature of the data obtained from studies is often such that it is difficult to claim that poor performance on auditory tasks is necessarily caused by a perceptual deficit rather than inattention, short-term memory, or other nonperceptual difficulties (Gooch, Snowling, & Hulme, 2011; Marshall, Snowling, & Bailey, 2001; Roach, Edwards, & Hogben, 2004). The picture may have been further complicated by the possible inclusion of children with comorbid ADHD within various study samples (Snowling, 2011). It appears likely that there is not one unitary perceptual deficit, but rather several contrasting reasons for poor performance on auditory tasks, with some being potentially more modifiable than others by training (McArthur & Hogben, 2012).

Methodological difficulties such as the use of correlational designs and the lack of statistical power that results from small sample sizes have rendered it difficult to establish causality (Studdert-Kennedy, 2002). Given that many poor readers do not experience auditory problems, it is possible that these serve as a marker of reading disability rather than play a causal role (Beattie & Manis, 2012). If, however, this is not the case and there is a causal relationship, this may be reciprocal rather than unidirectional (Studdert-Kennedy & Mody, 1995), or the effect may run in the opposite direction (Pennington, 2009). The few longitudinal studies that have been undertaken have generally failed to support any causal claims (Pennington, 2009), and there is little evidence of a direct connection between earlier auditory deficits and the emergence of subsequent reading difficulties (Heath & Hogben, 2004; Share, Jorm, Maclean, & Matthews, 2002, although see Boets et al., 2011, for an alternative view). Neither have intervention studies been able to demonstrate that enhancing the auditory processing of children with reading difficulties results in improved reading performance (McArthur et al., 2008; Pokorni, Worthington, & Jamison, 2004). Although a recent study has suggested that auditory training interventions can lead to gains in phonological awareness at both the rhyme and phoneme levels (Thomson, Leong, & Goswami, 2013), there is insufficient evidence to conclude that this will ultimately result in significantly improved reading performance.

It is conceivable that skilled readers might develop superior auditory skills as a result of their phonological prowess (Talcott et al., 2002). One study (Johnson et al., 2009), for example, tested children (most of whom had a speech disorder) at age five and eight years and found that phonological awareness at age five appeared to be a stronger predictor of auditory processing at age eight than the reverse. However, findings from a study of babies using brain event-related potentials, with follow-up tests during the following nine years (Leppänen et al., 2010), suggest that a proportion of struggling readers are affected by auditory-processing deficits from birth (see also, van Zuijen et al., 2013). Although these are unlikely, in themselves, to be the cause of dyslexia, they may act as risk factors that aggravate phonological processing difficulties (see also Boets, Ghesquière, et al., 2007; Plakas et al., 2013; for similar conclusions, and Raschle et al., in press, for fMRI evidence that supports the argument that auditory processing difficulties predate reading experience and instruction).

Noting that children with reading disabilities appear to have problems processing simple speech sounds but not analogous non-speech sounds, some have suggested that the auditory deficit is specific to speech (Mody, Studdert-Kennedy, & Brady, 1997; Schulte-Körne et al., 1998). However, inconsistencies in findings have proven to be a problem across different speech-processing studies (McArthur et al., 2008), and debate continues as to whether phonological problems typically found in poor readers are a product of a general auditory problem or of more specific speech perception deficits (Schulte-Körne & Bruder, 2010; Vandermosten et al., 2010; Zhang & McBride-Chang, 2010).

One study (Bruder et al., 2011) has indicated that children with dyslexia appear to be less attuned to native language speech representations. Interestingly, in another experiment (Perrachione, Del Tufo, & Gabrieli, 2011), it was found that a sample of those with reading disability experienced greater difficulty than did controls in identifying voices speaking their own language (English), although this difference disappeared when they were asked to differentiate between Chinese speakers. Given that it was not the meaning of the words that was important in this task, this finding may point to a problem in perceiving allophonic variation, that is, the different ways that a particular phoneme may be sounded (Peterson & Pennington, 2012) (see Bogliotti et al., 2008, for further discussion).

According to some speech scientists, studies of reading have often placed too great an emphasis on only one unit of speech – the "tyranny of the phoneme" (Peterson & Pennington, 2012, p. 1997) – and indeed, even determining in linguistics exactly what is meant by the term "phoneme" is not straightforward (Dresher, 2011). In reality, discrete elements of speech do not map directly onto phonemes, and accumulated evidence now suggests that auditory deficits in poor readers operate across the broader speech stream (Johnson et al., 2011). The long-term implications of this finding are that clinical interventions may need to focus on helping children recognize auditory structure at all levels rather than just that of the phoneme (Johnson et al., 2011).

Evidence for the greater presence of various auditory processing deficits in children and adults with reading disability is persuasive, with neural inconsistency in response to sound a possible contributory factor (Hornickel & Kraus, 2013). However, there is doubt as to the proportion of poor readers who encounter such problems, ignorance about the developmental trajectory of auditory processing skills during infancy and childhood (although see Boets et al., 2011), and uncertainty as to the extent to which there is a causal relationship between auditory problems and reading disability (Hämäläinen et al., 2013). Rather than being single cause predictors of dyslexia, auditory processing difficulties may represent risk factors that contribute cumulatively with other processes to the development of reading disability (Plakas et al., 2013). Finally, while it appears that training programs can help improve the auditory task performance of children with deficits, there is, to date, little evidence that gains resulting from these subsequently improve reading (McArthur, 2009). A suggestion that poor readers may benefit from wearing assistive listening devices in classrooms (Hornickel et al., 2012) is intriguing but results from a study of one school in isolation.

Visual processing

Given that reading requires precise visual recognition of letter strings prior to conversion to their sounds via grapheme-phoneme mapping (Share, 1995), it is unsurprising that visual deficits have long been held to be causes of dyslexia by researchers, the teaching profession, and the lay public (Stein & Kapoula, 2012;

Washburn, Joshi, & Cantrell, 2011). Although some visual problems have been shown to have greater presence in those with reading disability, the difficulty has been to establish causality. For example, oculomotor problems, sometimes associated with dyslexia (Jainta & Kapoula, 2011; Kapoula et al., 2008; but see Zeri, De Luca, Spinelli, & Zoccolotti, 2011, for an opposing finding), have been adjudged to be a consequence of reading difficulty, rather than a cause (Hutzler et al., 2006; Prado, Dubois, & Valdois, 2007).

The perceived role of visual factors in dyslexia was significantly undermined by Vellutino, who provided a detailed critique of flawed methodologies in the existing literature, alongside findings from his own carefully controlled experimental studies (Vellutino, 1979, 1987; Vellutino et al., 2004). This showed that deficits in a range of visual processes such as visualization, visual perception, visual memory, and visual sequencing did not appear to be causally responsible for reading disability.

More recently, there has been a resurgence of interest in the role of visual processing in reading disability, with increasing confidence being expressed in the light of new approaches and hypotheses that have yielded more supportive findings (Bellocchi et al., 2013; Heim & Grande, 2012; Quercia, Feiss, & Michel, 2013; Vidyasagar, 2012; van der Leij et al., 2013). Stainthorp et al. (2010) argue that Vellutino's critique should be treated with caution as the tasks employed in his experimental studies were complex and involved much more than just visual perception. Differences in testing formats, materials, and scoring methods may help explain inconsistent findings (Zeri et al., 2011), and the failure to identify visual processing deficits in those with dyslexia may be a consequence of the use of measures that are not always sufficiently sensitive to detect anomalies (Lachmann & van Leeuwen, 2007).

Visual processing and the role of the magnocellular system

A number of different forms of visual processing deficit in reading disability have been proposed. One influential theory suggests that the origin of the difficulty can be traced to the magnocellular system (Livingstone et al., 1991; Stein & Walsh, 1997). Magnocellular neurons (essentially those with a large cell body) are found in all areas of the brain and are instrumental in visual, auditory, and motor functioning (Stein, 2008). While temporal processing difficulties involving auditory, motor, and visual information have been associated with the magnocellular theory of dyslexia (Livingstone et al., 1991; Stein, 2012a; Stein, Talcott, & Walsh, 2000), it is visual processing that arguably has been of greatest interest. The magnocellular visual pathway comprises large cells that are responsible for detecting contrast, motion, and rapid changes in the visual field. In contrast, the parvocellular pathway consists of small cells that are sensitive to fine spatial detail. According to Stein and his colleagues, reduced sensitivity in the magnocellular system creates difficulties in suppressing visual information. As a result, retinal images persist longer than appropriate, and this results in an excess of visual information that creates a masking effect and some reduction in visual acuity, which then impedes the reading process.

As is the case for auditory processing, it has been suggested that those with dyslexia may have a rapid sensory processing deficiency (i.e., reduced sensitivity to stimuli that are presented very rapidly) via the dorsal pathway that is largely made up of magnocellular cells (Pammer, 2012; Vidyasagar, 2012). Such a deficit has been put forward as an explanation for poorer performance on a range of visual tasks, and a number of studies have found supportive evidence for a link between difficulties in this area and reading disability (Conlon, Sanders, & Wright, 2009; Cornelissen et al., 1995; Wright & Conlon, 2009).

Obtaining a clear picture has been complicated somewhat by overlap in the various terms employed in research studies. Skottun and Skoyles (2008, p. 666) list these as:

"rate processing problems" (Habib, 2000), problems in "temporal processing" (Au & Lovegrove, 2001; Farmer & Klein, 1995; Habib, 2000; Stein & Walsh, 1997), deficits in "temporal perception (temporal acuity)" (Talcott, Hansen, Willis-Owen, McKinnell, Richardson, & Stein, 1998), "transient processing defects" (Stein & Walsh, 1997), or reduced sensitivity to "dynamic stimuli" (Stein & Talcott, 1999).

Further complication has resulted from the different tests employed to investigate such deficits. These include measures of temporal contrast sensitivity, visual persistence, discrimination of stimulus sequences, temporal acuity, and coherent motion perception. Temporal contrast sensitivity concerns the ability to detect particular stimuli that change over time. Visual persistence refers to the brief continuation of neural activity after a given stimulus has been suddenly terminated. Discrimination of stimulus sequences involves identifying differences in the order of (rapid) presentation of the same stimuli. Temporal acuity involves making judgments about the gaps of time between stimuli presented consecutively (or sometimes simultaneously). Finally, coherent motion perception tests typically involve perception of the direction of movement of a series of dots. Some of the dots move around the computer screen at the same speed in the same direction; others move in a random fashion. The coherent motion threshold can be determined by varying the proportion of coherently moving dots until the direction in which they are moving is identified (see Skottun & Skoyles, 2008, pp. 667–670, for a more detailed description of each of these tests). A meta-analysis of 35 studies of motion perception in dyslexia (Benassi et al., 2010) found a moderate mean effect size ($d = 0.68$, n = 2334) for between-group differences (dyslexic versus normal readers) but a small effect size ($d = 0.18$) for correlational studies. The reason for this apparent discrepancy is unclear but may reflect the use of continuous measures that may reduce the effect size.

Skottun and Skoyles (2006a, 2006b) argue that some tests (visual persistence, coherent motion) are poorly suited for assessing magnocellular sensitivity, and the more sound measures (temporal contrast sensitivity, temporal acuity) have not consistently supported the theory. While some comparative studies of normal and poor readers have shown that a proportion of those with reading disability tend to demonstrate poor contrast sensitivity (Laycock, Crewther, & Crewther, 2012; Pellicano & Gibson, 2008; Wang et al., 2010), several others have failed to substantiate such findings (Gross-Glenn et al., 1995; Johannes et al., 1996; Skottun, 2000; Spinelli et al., 2002). Schulte-Körne and Bruder's (2010) review of relevant studies of those with dyslexia reported an inconsistent role for contrast sensitivity (deemed by Skottun & Skoyles, 2010a to be the most direct and reliable means of differentiating between magnocellular and parvocellular sensitivities), although noted stronger evidence for rapid motion deficits. Conlon et al. (2012) found that slightly more than a third of their sample of adults with dyslexia demonstrated a motion-processing deficit, a figure consistent with several previous studies (Conlon, Sanders, & Wright, 2009; Johnson et al., 2008; Ramus, Pidgeon, & Frith, 2003; Wright & Conlon, 2009).

Skottun and Skoyles (2010b) suggest that the key issue is not whether dyslexics require more time to complete visual tasks, or that they do more poorly on temporal order tasks than controls. Rather, the question is whether such differences reflect a true temporal processing disorder. It is conceivable that slower visual processing may be a consequence of a situation in which dyslexic samples simply find the tasks more difficult.

A number of studies have examined the influence of auditory and visual temporal processing in combination. Talcott et al. (2002) studied 350 randomly selected primary school children. They found that even though visual and auditory processing appeared to be related to literacy skills, once age and nonverbal IQ were controlled for, this accounted for only a small proportion of the variance (approximately 4%). In a study of a large sample of elementary school children, Landerl and Willburger (2010) found that temporal processing accounted for 3% of the variance in reading fluency (note the use of this variable rather than that of single-word decoding) once attentional differences had been controlled for. Correlations between auditory and visual temporal processing were moderate, suggesting that these tap into different aspects of temporal processing. Hierarchical regression analyses showed that measures of phonology and rapid naming, introduced after the temporal tasks, accounted for a much greater amount of variance. It would appear that suggestions that dyslexic individuals are often confronted by a cross-modal, or pansensory, temporal deficit (e.g., Laasonen, Service, & Virsu, 2001) have little empirical basis, and findings that are available offer minimal support for this (Skottun & Skoyles, 2010b).

The current picture is one of contrasting and confusing findings. A small proportion of poor readers show evidence of visual deficits, but these do not appear to be specific to magnocellular dysfunction (Amitay et al., 2002; Ramus, Rosen et al., 2003). Furthermore, a significant number of those who appear to have magnocellular deficits are able to develop adequate reading skills (Skoyles & Skottun, 2004). Vidyasagar and Pammer (2010a) support the argument that dyslexia is caused fundamentally by a visual deficit but argue that the visual problem should not be seen as being wholly restricted to the magnocellular pathway (see Conlon et al., 2012, for a similar suggestion). However, in a study of children with dyslexia, McLean et al. (2011) found significant deficits in magnocellular but not parvocellular temporal resolution, compared with controls, although the association with reading ability was relatively weak. Adding to this complex picture, Wright, Conlon, and Dyck (2012) found that differences between children with dyslexia and controls on a visual search task did not appear to be explained by a magnocellular deficit. Perhaps the most apposite conclusion is that provided by Skottun and Skoyles (2010b) for whom the evidence for magnocellular deficits in dyslexia is "modest" (p. 2229). Another set of criticisms has focused on methodological concerns, in particular the difficulty of generating appropriate behavioral assessments that can isolate magnocellular from other forms of functioning (Amitay et al., 2003; Skottun, 2011; see also Conlon et al., 2011, and a response by Skottun and Skoyles, 2011). Variability across experimental methods and the use of small and oftentimes very different samples that might potentially include other comorbid conditions have also rendered synthesis across research studies problematic (Schulte-Körne & Bruder, 2010).

Others have raised the problem of relating the hypothesized problems of the magnocellular system to reading difficulties (Skottun & Skoyles, 2008, 2010a). The theory seeks to explain how confusion may occur when scanning arrays of words but does not provide a satisfactory account of failure to decode single words in isolation, a task widely seen as the core problem of dyslexia. Several hypotheses as to how magnocellular deficits may lead to impaired reading have been proposed (Boden & Giaschi, 2007), but there is still insufficient evidence to justify any causal assertions. On the basis of their fMRI study, Olulade, Napoliello, and Eden (2013) found that while dyslexic children showed evidence of visual magnocellular dysfunction, there was no evidence to support a causal role for this in the development of reading disability. Indeed, as these children gained from an intensive reading intervention, visual system activity also increased. In light of this finding, it was suggested that any causal path that may exist is more likely to operate in the opposite direction, with reading experience influencing the development of the magnocellular system.

Stein (2008) has responded to some of these criticisms by arguing that opposition to the magnocellular theory is fueled in part by the mistaken belief that it challenges the view that dyslexics' main difficulties are phonological rather than visual. He disputes such a suggestion arguing that the theory offers a partial explanation for the existence of phonological difficulties. Visual input leads to recognition of the structure of words and the understanding that these can be broken down into separate phonemes. Where magnocellular difficulties are present, it is not surprising, he contends, that phonemic awareness may be impaired as a result.

The magnocellular theory remains highly controversial. According to Stein (2012a), a search through Pubmed (a database of the biomedical literature) showed that 90% of studies since 2000 examining magnocellular impairments in dyslexia have found some evidence of these. However, many argue that the theory has insufficient empirical support. Given the strong differences within the research literature and the uncertain implications for intervention, it is perhaps unsurprising that the magnocellular theory has yet to be widely accepted by professional groups. Thus a joint report provided by several U.S. medical associations (American Academy of Pediatrics, 2009) concluded that, given the contrasting findings in the literature, any "possible (magnocellular) deficit" (p. 839) has insufficient evidence on which to base treatment.

Visual stress/scotopic sensitivity

Some poor readers report that they find the visual aspects of reading physically unpleasant because of glare caused by light reflected from reading materials. This can result in a variety of symptoms such as physical discomfort (e.g., sore eyes, headaches) or visual-perceptual distortions and illusions and difficulties in seeing text clearly (Singleton, 2009a). As a result, they struggle with text and may avoid reading. This condition is variously known as visual discomfort (Conlon et al., 1999, 2012), scotopic sensitivity, or Meares-Irlen syndrome (Irlen, 1991), with claims that its incidence may apply to approximately 20% of the general population (Jeanes et al., 1997; Kriss & Evans, 2005). More strikingly, the Irlen Institute has estimated that visual stress may cause problems in as many as 46% of those with reading and learning problems (Perceptual Development Corporation, 1998).

It is generally accepted by researchers that while sensitivity of this kind may lead to poor reading fluency, it cannot explain the problems of those who present with complex decoding difficulties (Wilkins, 1995). Although visual stress has been associated with magnocellular dysfunction, there is little empirical support for this (Simmers et al., 2001; White et al., 2006), and it is misleading to describe it as a form of visual dyslexia. Nevertheless, visual stress difficulties may prove to be more of a hindrance for those with pre-existing reading disability. Such individuals, who often struggle with automatic recognition of words, may need to focus their attention more on the physical characteristics of letters, and this may exacerbate visual stress (Singleton, 2009a). In turn, this is likely to reduce their willingness to practice reading, and as a result, the gap with other readers may increase (the well-known Matthew Effect). However, as is noted in Chapter 4, there is little evidence that the standard tools used to address the problem of visual stress – colored lenses or overlays – are effective means of tackling complex reading difficulties.

In its *Joint Statement – Learning Disabilities, Dyslexia, and Vision*, the American Academy of Pediatrics stated:

[T]here is inadequate scientific evidence to support the view that subtle eye or visual problems, including abnormal focusing, jerky eye movements, misaligned or crossed eyes, binocular dysfunction, visual-motor dysfunction, visual perceptual difficulties, or hypothetical difficulties with laterality . . . cause learning disabilities. Statistically, children with dyslexia or related learning disabilities have the same visual function and ocular health as children without such conditions. (American Academy of Pediatrics, Section on Ophthalmology & Council on Children with Disabilities et al., 2009, p. 842)

While most researchers examining the role of visual processes in dyslexia are unlikely to disagree with the conclusions concerning some of the particular visual processes listed in this statement, it does appear that that the Academy's perspective may not do full justice to an increasing body of research pointing to a greater role for visual factors in dyslexia than was formerly appreciated (Bellocchi et al., 2013; Dehaene, 2009; Szwed et al., 2012). In relation to the origins of reading disability, "The weakness itself probably rests somewhere at the crossroads between invariant visual recognition and phonemic processing" (Dehaene, 2009, p. 243).

Attentional factors

Some researchers have argued that rather than focusing on low-level perceptual factors (as measured, for example, by motion or frequency detection tasks), it might be more helpful to explore the role of higher-level mechanisms of perceptual attention and memory (Amitay et al., 2003). Visual attention, which concerns the ability to select rapidly the most relevant visual information, ranges across various aspects of the reading process and is seen to be important at all levels of letter string processing, involving both top-down (goal-directed) and bottom-up (stimulus-driven) mechanisms (Ruffino et al., 2010; Vidyasagar & Pammer, 2010b; although see Whitney, 2010, for an opposing view). Some researchers have sought to link impaired attentional orienting to underlying magnocellular deficits (Franceschini et al., 2012).

One explanation for the auditory and visual temporal deficits observed by dyslexia researchers is that these may be partially explained by sluggish attentional shifting (SAS) (Hari & Renvall, 2001; Lallier, Donnadieu, Berger, & Valdois, 2010). According to this theory, some individuals suffering from dyslexia struggle to disengage from auditory or visual stimuli when these are presented in rapid sequence – a phenomenon sometimes known as an abnormal attentional blink. In relation to auditory processing, Hari and Renvall (2001) suggest that SAS could have the effect of distorting the perception of rapid speech streams, which in turn could hamper the development of phonological representations. While there is significant evidence that attentional blink and reading are related, suggestions of a causal relationship have been subject to challenge (Badcock, Hogben, & Fletcher, 2008; McLean et al., 2010).

Friedmann, Kerbel, and Shvimer (2010) outline three main functions of visual analysis. Firstly, it involves ascertaining the identity of each of the letters; secondly, it encodes their position within the relevant word; and finally, when a string of words is to be read, it establishes an "attentional window" that focuses attention on a single word (Coltheart, 1981; Ellis, Flude, & Young, 1987). Deficits in each of these functions can lead to different types of difficulty (see two detailed case examples in Friedmann, Biran, & Gvion, 2012). Thus, visual letter identification weaknesses may result in letter substitutions or omissions; problems involving letter positions within words can result in transposition of the letters such that a different word with a combination of the same letters is read, for example, fired/fried (Friedmann & Gvion, 2001; Friedmann & Rahamim, 2007). Such errors are more likely to happen in migratable words, that is, where the migration outcome is also a word formed from the same letters (Friedmann et al., 2010). Finally, difficulties in binding letters to words can result in "attentional dyslexia" involving the migration of letters between words. In reading strings of words, the process of attentional shifting involves recognition of those letters that are required for letter-sound mapping while filtering out others nearby that are redundant. In some cases, where problems emerge, letters in words are correctly identified but appear to be perceived as belonging to words that are nearby. Although appearing in an adjacent word, the identity of the letters concerned and their relative position within the word that is read are often unchanged (Shallice & Warrington, 1977); however, in a significant number of cases, a specific letter may be omitted where it appears in the same position in both words (Friedmann, et al., 2010).

There are some suggestions in the literature that relatively simple modifications to the ways in which text is presented can help those who struggle with visual attention. For example, Friedman et al. (2010) describe the case of a child with attentional dyslexia whose reading was severely disrupted by this type of migration of letters between words. When the child was provided with a cardboard overlay with a cut-out window, it was found that her difficulties appeared to be almost wholly eliminated (see also Friedmann and Rahamim, in press, for the potential value of finger tracking). Such anecdotes help explain the widely held view of the lay public that many dyslexics suffer from letters or words "jumping around the page."

Further support for the sluggish attention hypothesis is provided by findings from a 3-year longitudinal study in which 96 pre-reading children received a battery of measures in kindergarten and were subsequently followed up in Grades 1 and 2 (Franceschini et al., 2012). In addition to tests of phonemic awareness and rapid naming, the children were given two visual-spatial tasks: one a serial search (marking every occurrence of a given symbol across five rows), the other involving a spatial cueing task in which the children had to select the correct orientation of a shape briefly presented (100 ms) to the left or right of a central fixation point. In a subsequent condition, the children's attention was either drawn to that side of a computer screen where the target symbol was subsequently to be presented or, alternatively to the opposite side. In such a task, performance is typically improved where the child's attention is drawn to the side where the image will appear, and rendered poorer in cases where their attention is pulled away to the wrong side. Those who scored poorly on the visual-spatial tasks subsequently became the weakest readers. On the visual search task, those who were to become poorer readers made twice as many errors as those with normal reading ability. Interestingly, on the cueing task, those who were to become poorer readers only performed worse in cases where the cues were valid. Where there were no cues, or the cues prompted attention to the wrong side of the screen, a cueing effect was not significant. The researchers concluded that visual-spatial skills were independent predictors of future reading difficulty, and problems were a consequence of a deficit in attentional orientation rather than an impairment in peripheral vision. Their findings support claims that visual spatial attention may be a key factor in dyslexia (Vidyasagar, 1999), although there continue to be competing hypotheses about the mechanisms concerned (Gabrieli & Norton, 2012).

Most studies of visual deficits in poor readers examine children after literacy problems have emerged, and thus it is conceivable that any observed poor performance on visual measures is a consequence of their reading difficulties. The strength of Franceschini et al.'s (2012) investigation was that the assessments were undertaken before the children learned to read. However, we should not conclude that a causal link was demonstrated (Catts, 2012). The data were correlational, of modest size, and 40% of those with visual difficulties did not develop reading problems over the three-year period. Moreover, visual problems were also demonstrated by some children who later became sound readers.

Another form of visual attention problem, the visual attention span deficit hypothesis (Bosse, Tainturier, & Valdois, 2007), has also been implicated in reading disability. According to this position, the dyslexic individual is often limited in the number of letter string elements that can be processed simultaneously, This attentional rather than perceptual impairment may be unrelated to that of sluggish attentional processing (Lallier, Donnadieu et al., 2010; Lallier, Tainturier et al., 2010). Essentially one can distinguish between the visual attention span deficit hypothesis that focuses on potential "deficits in the allocation of attention across letter or symbol strings, limiting the number of elements that can be processed in parallel during reading" (Bosse et al., 2007, p. 200) and the sluggish attentional processing hypothesis according to which some poor readers have difficulty in shifting their attention from one location to the next in an array.

Interestingly, the proponents of the visual attention span theory have been more resolute than others working in the field of visual processing/attention in attesting that such difficulty may be unrelated to phonological problems and that this implies that there are likely to be different dyslexic subtypes (Valdois, Lassus-Sangosse, & Lobier, 2012a). Several studies have indicated that visual attention span difficulties are independent of phonological problems for a significant number of poor readers (Bosse et al., 2007; Prado, Dubois, & Valdois, 2007), although some may struggle with a double deficit that involves a combination of both phonological and visual attention span difficulties (Bosse et al., 2007). Visual attention span appears not to be solely relevant for those with dyslexia as this has also been found to contribute to reading performance in typically developing children (Bosse & Valdois, 2009). Proponents of the phonological hypothesis, however, have offered a challenge on the grounds that deficits appear to be more significant for verbal (letters and digits) than nonverbal (symbols) material when these modalities are employed in exactly the same experimental conditions (Ziegler, Pech-Georgel, Dufau, & Grainger, 2010; see also a similar finding from a study with adults [Collis, Kohnen, & Kinoshita, 2013]). Ziegler, Pech-Georgel et al. (2010) suggest that while their finding may be explained by visual recognition processes, it is more likely that the underlying problem stems from the fact that digits and letters, but not symbols, map onto phonological codes, and it is the link between visual and phonological codes that is, for them, the key problem of dyslexia. They conclude that what appears at first to be a visual impairment in processing letters and digits may not be one, in actuality, and if visual impairments are only obtained for verbal material, phonology can be put "back in the front row" (p. F12). However, countering this position, Romani, Tsouknida, di Betta, and Olson (2011) subsequently found a difference between dyslexic and normal readers on a task of symbol matching that did not require naming. It appears that evidence is accumulating against the notion that there is a phonological basis for the visual attention problems found in those with dyslexia, with support for this independence emerging from experiments (Lobier, Zoubrinetzky, & Valdois, 2012; Valdois, Lassus-Sangosse, & Lobier, 2012b), case studies (Dubois et al., 2010; Valdois et al., 2011), and brain function studies (Peyrin et al., 2011, 2012). Neither does it appear that reduced performance on visual span tasks can be ascribed to a short-term/working memory deficit (Romani et al., 2011; Stenneken et al., 2011).

Another explanation for apparent visual problems affecting reading is that of abnormal crowding (Aleci et al., 2012; Collis et al., 2013; Martelli et al., 2009; Schneps et al., 2013). Crowding here refers to the negative influence of nearby letter contours on visual discrimination. Thus, features unrelated to the target may be integrated in error, thus rendering letter discrimination more problematic. In support of this idea, several studies have demonstrated that artificially increasing the space between letters and words can result in improvement in reading performance. In two studies, the effects were found for half (Spinelli et al., 2002) and two-thirds (Martelli et al., 2009) of their respective dyslexic samples, a finding that led these authors to conclude that the causal role of crowding applied to some but not all of those suffering from dyslexia. Zorzi et al. (2012) similarly found that increasing letter spacing improved both reading accuracy and speed for their dyslexic sample, all of whom had normal, or corrected-to-normal, visual acuity. In addition, increasing letter spacing did not improve the performance of younger, reading-level controls, a finding that suggests that the deficits observed could not be held to be a consequence of a lack of reading experience. Perea et al. (2012) found gains in word and text reading for both normal and dyslexic readers when the gap between letters was widened, but these were substantially larger for the poor readers' group. This finding applied to words of six letters but not to those comprised of four letters. The crowding effect has also been found when differently oriented geometric shapes have been used. Here, Moores, Cassim, and Talcott (2011) found that crowding led to far greater deterioration in visual discrimination performance for a dyslexic group than for controls. However, while consistent with an attentional explanation, these authors concluded that existing theoretical accounts of visual attention in dyslexia were insufficient to explain all of their findings.

A further controversial theory used to explain poor performance on sensory tasks has been proposed by Ahissar and colleagues (Ahissar, 2007; Banai & Ahissar, 2010). According to their account, some dyslexics have unimpaired top-down attentional mechanisms, but are susceptible to deficient bottom-up processing and as a result struggle to reduce attentional load. Puzzled by their observations that dyslexics seemed to perform more poorly than controls in auditory processing tasks, such as two-tone frequency discrimination, only when the same stimuli were used repeatedly, they suggested that individuals with dyslexia may experience particular difficulty in drawing on regularities to help them in these tasks. Their experimental studies led them to hypothesize that when participants are repeatedly presented with the same stimulus (e.g., an auditory tone) alongside others that differ, the former operates as a perceptual anchor providing an internal reference point that facilitates future processing. When asked to make discriminations, participants implicitly draw on this stored information, thus reducing the requirement to undertake explicit computations on each occasion. Ahissar (2007) found that the performance of a dyslexic sample on an auditory discrimination task was highly correlated with phonological memory scores when the same reference tone was utilized, but this was not the case when different tones were used. In this latter variant of the procedure, creating an internal reference would have been of no value in reducing task demands. Following this reasoning, Ahissar and colleagues have argued that those with reading disability are more likely to encounter a domain general difficulty in anchoring, which underpins difficulties of perception, verbal memory, and reading. However, to date the anchoring hypothesis has been shown to apply only to the auditory modality, and no such deficit has been found in the visual modality (Ramus & Ahissar, 2012).

The anchoring deficit hypothesis of dyslexia can be challenged on the same grounds as other theories discussed in this chapter. In outlining the rationale behind the theory, Ahissar (2007) noted that many of those with attentional difficulties do not encounter problems with reading and suggested that a specific attentional deficit (i.e., in relation to perceptual anchoring) might be responsible. However, when studied experimentally, it appears that a perceptual anchoring problem can be found in both good and poor readers as well as those who score high or low on a measure of attention (Willburger & Landerl, 2010). However, Oganian and Ahissar (2012) found that, contrary to the findings of Willburger and Landerl (2010), anchoring task deficits could not be explained by poor sustained attention. In seeking to explain the discrepancy between the outcomes of these two studies, Oganian and Ahissar suggest that this may result from differences in the task, in the measures, or to the particular demands of a study of German participants (Willburger & Landerl, 2010) in comparison with their own Hebrew and English samples. A further criticism of the anchoring hypothesis (Ziegler, 2008) stems from the observation that those with dyslexia appear more able to form perceptual anchors in some auditory tasks than in others. In response to this, Ahissar and Oganian (2008) contend that the ability to anchor repeated stimuli varies across dimensions, and therefore such findings are not inconsistent with their theory.

While much recent research in attention focuses on either auditory or visual processing, it is possible that difficulties apply to both of these in combination. A multisensory deficit of attention would be problematic for the segmentation of both auditory and visual inputs in the form of speech and letter strings, respectively. However, only a few studies (Facoetti et al., 2005; Facoetti, et al., 2009; Lallier, Tainturier et al., 2010; Lallier et al., 2009) have examined this in the same dyslexic samples. In a study of Italian children comparing those with decoding difficulties with controls, and subsequently with another group containing slow but accurate decoders, Facoetti et al. (2009) found that only those with poor phonological decoding skills demonstrated a temporal multi-sensory deficit of attention. Individual case analysis confirmed that this finding was not attributable to the presence of a small number of atypical cases in the poor-decoder group. Individual differences in multisensory attention accounted for 31% of unique variance in nonword reading performance of all the poor readers in the study (both the poor decoders and the slow readers) after control-ling for age, IQ, and phonological skills. In their study of young dyslexic adults with phonological awareness deficits, Lallier, Tainturier et al. (2010) found correlations in visual and auditory processing, which appeared to support the suggestion that attentional shifting speed has to be synchronized between visual and auditory modalities in order to develop fluent reading (Breznitz & Misra, 2003).

In arguing that a multisensory attentional deficit is a crucial component of impaired phonological decoding in dyslexia, Facoetti et al. (2009) discount suggestions that this problem is merely a consequence of the reading difficulties themselves. To support their assertion, they point to their finding that younger children with the same IQ, and reading at the same level as the dyslexic sample, failed to show the same attentional difficulties. They also cite visuo-spatial attention training studies that appear to have resulted in improved reading performance (Facoetti et al., 2003). The possibility that attentional deficits are a consequence of temporal processing problems is also discounted by Facoetti et al. (2009) primarily because these deficits were present even when time intervals were relatively lengthy (see Ruffino et al., 2010, for similar reasoning). Indeed, it is possible to speculate that the relationship operates in the alternative direction such that auditory processing deficits may be a consequence of sluggish attention (see also Facoetti et al., 2005; Renvall & Hari, 2002).

In attempting to reconcile, in a unifying explanation, the differing positions of those who variously emphasize phonological, auditory, or visual processing in dyslexia, one may find the problems of access to phonological representations described by Ramus and Szenkovits (2008) to be helpful. Certainly, their theory helps explain why performance on phonological, auditory, and visual tasks appears to vary according to task requirements. Thus, while representations will usually be intact whichever form they take, for dyslexics, accessing these will often be problematic particularly under certain demanding task conditions such as those involving storage in short-term memory, speeded or repeated retrievals, and extraction from noisy stimuli.

Concluding remarks: the role of auditory and visual factor

The case for low-level sensory deficits as causal in reading disability is the subject of much ongoing debate, with research studies examining causality still "in their infancy" (Vidyasagar & Pammer, 2010a, p. 61). While such difficulties are a feature of some children with reading disability, these are clearly not universal, and the possibility has been raised that they may co-occur with reading disability rather than play a causal role (Pennington, 2009).

Beyond stating that a burgeoning number of research studies are showing that a number of perceptual and attentional auditory and visual processes seem to be important in reading disability, it is difficult to provide many firm conclusions from this literature. At the current time, the field is subject to a proliferation of competing theories and research tools with little consensus as to what can be considered to be secure knowledge of relevance for those working with struggling readers. Certainly, this emerging body of new work has yet to result in significant practical implications for clinical assessment and educational intervention (although see Franceschini et al., 2013, for somewhat optimistic claims concerning the potential of action video games to improve reading). Further work is needed, particularly as most studies have been conducted at a stage in children's development when any low-level processing deficits may already have been compensated (Snowling, 2010).

For some researchers in the field of visual attention, such processes are seen as independent of phonological factors in causing reading disability. For others, poor attentional sampling of the visual input may affect reading ability and phonological skills. Perhaps the most significant contribution of this work for practitioners at the current time is to demonstrate the need for caution against too great an adherence to an overly simplistic phonological model.

Psycho-motor processing

That there is a statistical relationship between motor skills and cognitive devel-opment is largely undisputed, with poor gross motor skills often proving com-mon for those with learning disabilities (Westendorp et al., 2011). However, the prevalence of motor impairments in dyslexic samples has varied greatly across studies, with the majority reporting such difficulties in 30% to 65% of cases (Chaix et al., 2007; Kaplan et al., 1998; Ramus et al., 2003). These differences are likely, in part, to reflect different methods of assessment and cut-off points.

Given this statistical association, it is not surprising that there has been a search for possible causal factors in dyslexia. Several theories have been put forward to explain the prevalence of tactile (Laasonen, Service, & Virsu, 2001) and motor (Ramus, 2003) difficulties in dyslexic groups, with the most influential theory being that of cerebellar dysfunction (Nicolson & Fawcett, 2006; Nicolson, Fawcett, & Dean, 2001a; Stoodley & Stein, 2011). According to this theory, cerebellar dysfunction results in a failure to achieve sound automaticity of various skills (e.g., rapid naming or information processing) that are important for reading acquisition. A core component of the theory is that for those with dyslexia, automaticity difficulties are present across a broad range of domains, including motor skills (Nicolson & Fawcett, 1990). Nicolson & Fawcett's argument is not that motor problems act as causal factors in reading disability, but rather that these signify underlying cerebellar impairments. It is important to note that the cerebellar theory operates at a neural systems, rather than cognitive, level. Thus, rather than competing with theories such as that of a phonological deficit, the theory seeks to explain reasons why these cognitive-level difficulties arise. This explanation is highly controversial (Bishop, 2002), however, and while it is accepted by some that cerebellar dysfunction may be implicated for a proportion of poor readers, there continues to be a lack of clarity about the mechanisms involved and a belief that impaired cerebellar function is unlikely to be the primary cause of dyslexia (Stoodley & Stein, 2011, 2013).

The role and relationship of motor difficulties for dyslexia is highly contested, with some reporting group differences between dyslexic and typical readers (Fawcett, Nicolson, & Maclagan, 2001; Ramus, Pidgeon, & Frith, 2003; Wolff et al., 1995) and others failing to find these (Kronbichler, Hutzler, & Wimmer, 2002; Savage et al., 2005; White et al., 2006). Chaix et al. (2007), for example, found no direct causal relationship between reading performance and motor scores in a large sample of children who had attended a clinic for language and learning disabilities.

Several studies have examined balance/postural stability and found that poor readers have greater difficulty in maintaining stability than controls (Fawcett & Nicolson, 1999; Getchell et al., 2007), although this appears to be less evident in the case of adults (Stoodley et al., 2006). It has been suggested that this problem may have a basis in the relationship between sensory (visual) and motor (postural) control systems (Barela et al., 2011; Sela, 2012), perhaps because of difficulties in integrating proprioceptive signals (Quercia et al., 2011). However, the overall picture concerning balance/stability is far from clear; particularly, as asimilar problems are found for a number of developmental disorders. A meta-analysis of 15 studies examining balance in dyslexic and control samples (Rochelle & Talcott, 2006) produced an overall effect of $d = .64$, but there were very large differences between the various studies. Furthermore, the differences in reading scores between the dyslexic and control groups did not appear to be significantly associated with the effect sizes. The authors concluded that the relationship between dyslexia and poor balance was most likely influenced by variables other than reading skill.

Despite apparent comorbidity, the evidence for a causal relationship between motor impairment and reading skills is generally regarded as weak (Rochelle & Talcott, 2006). In a detailed review, Savage (2004) concluded that the evidence base for the significance of motor deficits in general, and Nicolson and Fawcett's automaticity model in particular, was mixed, adding that improved research designs with better sampling and measurement were required. Particularly valuable would be longitudinal studies that could consider associations between automaticity in pre-readers and subsequent literacy and cognitive performance.

At the current time, there is little evidence that research findings in these areas can meaningfully guide intervention, and programs designed to improve cerebellar functioning continue to be highly controversial (see also Chapter 4).

The multifactorial nature of dyslexia

While the history of research involving children with dyslexia has long involved a search for factors that differ between groups of normal and poor readers, the simplistic notion that one can identify a single cause of dyslexia is now obsolete (Fletcher et al., 2007). It appears that isolated cognitive processes each seem to play only a modest role in predicting word reading, with correlations being considerably weaker for poor readers than for those with sound reading skills (Swanson, 2013).

Determining which particular processes have a causal role, rather than merely act as correlates (see Snowling, 2011), has proven difficult, and while the central role of phonological deficits for a large proportion of poor readers is widely accepted, there continues to be much debate as to the nature and role of underlying elements. Recent research has once more begun to place greater emphasis on the role of a combination of underlying auditory, visual, and attentional factors in reading (Blau et al., 2009; Wallace, 2009).

Ramus and Ahissar (2012) suggest that the "profusion" (p. 105) of diverse theories is a consequence of the fact that the vast body of research data on cognitive deficits in dyslexia cannot be incorporated within a single theory. As they note, it is indeed astonishing that dyslexic samples tend to perform more poorly than controls on so many different tasks. Theory formulation is rendered difficult because the general understanding of human cognition is limited, many constructs (such as anchoring) are insufficiently defined and integrated into key areas of cognitive functioning, and the heterogeneous nature of reading disability is such that particular theories may apply only to certain subgroups. Nevertheless, strong evidence for the existence of subtypes with clear cognitive or biological profiles has yet to be produced.

Although phonological processing difficulties appear to explain more variance in reading difficulty in the English language than any other cognitive deficits, several processes appear to be important elements of a multiple-deficit cognitive model (Pennington, 2006; Willcutt et al., 2008). Too often, the use of univariate analyses has precluded examination of the relationship between individuals' performance across several neurocognitive measures. To address this, Menghini et al. (2010) examined the role of a range of neurocognitive deficits in a comparative study of dyslexic and nondyslexic children. Using measures of phonological ability, visual processing, selective and sustained attention, implicit learning, and executive functioning, they found that the dyslexic children demonstrated deficits in both the phonological and the nonphonological tasks. The proportion of those with dyslexia who demonstrated a phonological deficit only was 18.3%, whereas more than three-quarters (76.6%) showed phonological deficits together with other problems. Forty-one percent of the dyslexic sample demonstrated impairments in four or five of the tasks. Hierarchical regression analysis showed that the nonphonological tasks were good predictors, accounting for 23.3% of the unique variance of word reading and 19.3% of nonword reading.

A similar picture is provided by Willcutt et al. (2010), who found in a large twin study that while phonemic awareness was the strongest predictor of reading disability, reading difficulties were independently predicted by naming speed, working memory, verbal reasoning, and processing speed. On this basis, it was concluded that reading disorder should be considered as a complex disorder, "with a multifactorial etiology that leads to multiple correlated cognitive weaknesses" (p. 1356).

Pennington's (2009) account serves as a sound summary of much current thinking:

(1) The etiology of complex behavioral disorders is multifactorial and involves the interaction of multiple risk and protective factors which can be either genetic or environmental; (2) these risk and protective factors alter the development of the neural systems that mediate cognitive functions necessary for normal development, thus producing the behavioral symptoms that define these disorders; (3) no single etiological factor is sufficient for a disorder and few may be necessary; (4) consequently, comorbidity among complex behavioral disorders is expected because of shared etiological

and cognitive risk factors; and (5) the liability distribution for a given disease is often continuous and quantitative rather than discrete and categorical. (p. 6).

Cognitive level explanation and educational intervention

In the opening section of this chapter, a quotation from two leading dyslexia researchers pointed to the important role of the cognitive level of explanation for developing theory and practice. As this chapter has demonstrated, there continues to be considerable disagreement about the nature, role, and relevance of underlying cognitive processes in dyslexia. It is unsurprising, therefore, that the elaboration of a widely accepted causal model that can meaningfully inform educational intervention has proven to be elusive.

Such a gap can in no way be seen as a consequence of a lack of research activity that has sought to achieve this end. However, while the difficulty of arriving at an overarching theory is understandable, and an adequately integrated model of cognitive and instructional factors eludes us (Swanson, 2013), lay observers – and indeed, many educationalists and clinicians – may be surprised to learn of the tenuous relationship between the vast body of accumulated research findings about underlying cognitive processes and our current knowledge of how best to help those who struggle to learn to read.

Doubtless, some researchers in these areas will point to individual studies where one or more of these processes – and in a few rare cases, particular aspects of reading – have been briefly improved as a result of experimental manipulation. Nevertheless, the reality is that, other than phonological awareness training for very young children (and even here significant doubts continue as to the long-term benefits of interventions that address a phonological deficit [Olson, 2011]), there is no substantial evidence that identifying and directly addressing any of the specific cognitive processes that are highlighted in the dyslexia literature lead to significant and sustained gains in the decoding abilities of those who struggle to learn to read. While it is possible to find isolated experimental studies where an intervention has produced a promising finding, we must be cautious of any overly ambitious claims that may result from this. Specifically, studies of rapid naming, short-term and working memory, magnocellular functioning, motor processing, auditory processing, visual processing, and attention have yet to meaningfully inform the design of targeted reading-related interventions that have proven to be effective for significant numbers of poor readers over time. Indeed, a recent review of intervention studies designed to improve low-achieving students' academic performance by strengthening underlying cognitive processes concluded that there was currently insufficient evidence to support their use (Kearns & Fuchs, 2013).

These observations, of course, should not be perceived as representing a criticism or demeaning of this important work. Increasing our understandings of the influence of key processes underlying all forms of reading difficulty, and ultimately deriving sound causal models, are outcomes that may well assist our efforts to develop more powerful forms of intervention, particularly for that small group of "treatment resisters" for whom our current best evidence-based practices continue to fail. At the current time, many leading researchers in each of these fields are actively turning their attention to the production of training studies that can improve deficient processes and, as a consequence, help overcome reading disability. However, despite these laudable intentions, it needs to be clearly communicated to education practitioners, clinicians, students and their families, and the lay public that research in these domains offers promise for the future rather than secure knowledge with immediate application for practice.

Summary

The phonological deficit hypothesis continues to be dominant in the reading disabilities/dyslexia literature, although there is a difference of opinion as to whether rapid naming and verbal short-term/working memory should be incorporated within this account. Problems of phonological/phonemic awareness have been repeatedly shown to be associated with poor decoding, although it is now recognized that these cannot account for all those with a reading disability. A significant proportion of poor readers do not present with phonological difficulties, and others with such a deficit do not encounter problems in learning to read. Difficulties in rapid naming are also frequently found, particularly in relation to reading fluency, although it is considered that this problem reflects other underlying problems. A significant proportion of poor readers manifest short-term/working memory difficulties, particularly in relation to verbal memory, although the centrality of these for an understanding of reading disability is controversial.

There is increasing evidence that underlying auditory and visual processing deficits play a role in reading disability, although (1) our understanding of these is still rudimentary, (2) there are abundant methodological difficulties for research studies, and (3) conceptual understandings and causal explanations are subject to significant debate. The possible role of attentional factors has gained in prominence in recent years, although, as for all the processes examined in this chapter, there exists a wide variety of hypotheses that require further investigation and refinement.

It is perhaps surprising that such a vast raft of studies has resulted in only limited understanding of how various cognitive processes underpin dyslexia/reading disability. Recognition of the complex, multifactorial nature of reading problems has resulted in greater acceptance that a simple causal account or model will not prove sufficient. Nevertheless, it is a sad fact that, with the exception of phonological/phonemic awareness, this voluminous literature has had relatively little impact on the development of widely employed, and empirically supported, classroom- or clinic-based educational interventions geared to address reading disability.

3   The neurobiological bases of reading and
       reading disability

Introduction

Typically, arguments for the neurobiological basis of reading disability/dyslexia
are drawn from two large bodies of research – one on the brain and the other
on the genome. This chapter first presents a discussion of the literature on the
so-called reading brain – the brain as it is engaged in reading and reading-
related processes (Wolf, 2007). After this, it turns to the genome, as variability
in its structure and function is thought to form the substrate, through the brain
and, perhaps, other organs of the human organism (e.g., the liver by means of
metabolizing Omega 3 fish oil, as discussed in Lindmark & Clough, 2007), of
the neurobiological foundation of reading.

The chapter necessarily makes reference to many technical terms (e.g., specific regions of the brain, biological processes) that are likely to be unfamiliar
to the nonspecialist. In order to conform to space restrictions and to maintain
narrative coherence and flow, descriptions and definitions of many of these
have not been provided. Helpful information about these terms should be readily available both from Internet sources and publications referenced in this
chapter.

The reading brain

The first part of this chapter is structured around a discussion of morphological
(both postmortem and in vivo) and functional (in vivo) investigations of the
brain. In setting out current knowledge about the brain machinery behind reading, it draws on studies aimed at understanding (1) the brain at the pre-reading
and reading stages (i.e., prior to the mastery of reading, and/or upon completion
of the acquisition of reading); (2) the brains of typical readers compared with
those who experience difficulties; and (3) the brains of poor readers both
before and after attempts have been made to remediate their difficulties.

The utilization of a variety of imaging tools such as magnetic resonance
imaging (MRI), functional magnetic resonance imaging (fMRI), structural T1
MRI, diffusion tensor imaging (DTI), magnetic resonance spectroscopy (MRS),

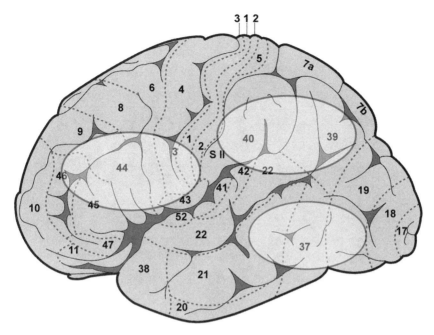

Figure 3.1 The consensual view of the neuronal network of reading: left inferior frontal (anterior component region, recruiting, partially, Brodmann areas, BA, 44, 45, and 6), posterior dorsal (temporoparietal region, recruiting, partially, BA 39 and 40), and posterior ventral (ventral occipitotemporal, recruiting, partially, BA 19, 21, and 37) brain areas. Adapted from Démonet, Taylor, and Chaix (2004). (See color plate.)

positron emission tomography (PET), magnetoencephalography (MEG), near-infrared spectroscopy (NIRS), and electroencephalography (EEG), has permitted researchers to build on the early brain anatomy findings that were obtained from postmortem studies of brains of individuals with reading difficulties. This technology has also permitted investigations of:

1. the functional peculiarities of the "reading brain" (i.e., what the brain does when a person reads);
2. the age and developmental aspects of the "reading brain," sampling it before, during, and after the acquisition of reading skills;
3. the brain functioning of individuals with reading difficulties compared to normal readers; and
4. the impact of remedial interventions aimed at improving the function of the "reading brain" for those experiencing difficulties.

Today's consensual view of reading avers that it takes place in a neuronal network that includes the following brain areas (see Figure 3.1):

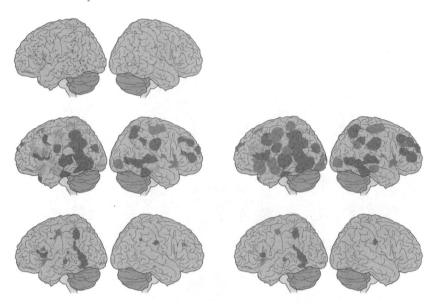

Figure 3.2 **(Top left)** Surface rendering of all input foci with underactivation (69) in red and overactivation (59) in green meta-analyzed by Richlan, Kronbichler, and wimmer (2009). **(Middle left)** Overlays of the separate maps for under- and overactivation, respectively; regions displayed in both maps are shown in yellow. **(Middle right)** Surface rendering of the difference map (after subtracting underactivation indicators from overactivation indicators). The blurred coloring results from discrepant activations at surface and deeper regions. **(Bottom left)** Surface rendering of the unthresholded difference map. **(Bottom right)** Surface rendering of the thresholded difference map. Adapted from Richlan, Kronbichler, and Wimmer (2009). (See color plate.)

- left inferior frontal (anterior component region, recruiting, partially, Brodmann areas, BA, 44, 45, and 6);
- posterior dorsal (temporoparietal [or parietotemporal] region incorporating the angular and supramarginal gyri and the posterior superior temporal gyrus);
- posterior ventral (ventral occipitotemporal or posterior inferior temporal regions incorporating fusiform and inferior temporal gyri).

There is broad agreement (see Figure 3.2) that there is a general pattern of activation of the network that differentiates skilled and poor readers, such that the former engage areas of the left side of the brain more than the latter, and the latter activate right-side regions more than the former (Maisog et al., 2008; Richlan, Kronbichler, & Wimmer, 2009), although it should be noted that the right-sided findings are less robust in meta-analyses (Richlan, Kronbichler, & Wimmer, 2011). There is uncertainty about the possible mechanisms of this disruption, and it is possible that these areas are affected in their functionality or, alternatively, that they endure deranged information transfer. For example, with regard to the first mechanism, it has been hypothesized that the insula, as a possible binding element between the posterior and frontal language areas, does not function properly in individuals with dyslexia (Paulesu et al., 1996). In relation to the second mechanism, it has been suggested that dyslexia may result from a "functional disruption" of the two (dorsal and ventral) posterior network areas (Horwitz, Rumsey, & Donohue, 1998; Ligges & Blanz, 2007; Pugh et al., 2000; Shaywitz et al., 2007).

As noted in Chapter 2, reading is now widely understood as a complex componential process. In line with this understanding, there is growing evidence that a variety of brain areas, individually and in combination, differentially support distinct components of reading (Katzir, Misra, & Poldrack, 2005; Vigneau et al., 2006). For example, phonological processing is thought to be carried out by superior temporal regions serving grapheme-phoneme mapping processes and inferior frontal regions serving as phonological rehearsal systems (Fiez et al., 2006; Jobard, Crivello, & Tzourio-Mazoyer, 2003). As studies accumulate, even greater differentiation appears to be warranted. For example, it has been shown that the left temporoparietal areas, including the supramarginal gyrus, are involved predominantly in sensorimotor transformation and phonological and semantic processing (Shalom & Poeppel, 2008), and that the middle-superior temporal cortex is principally important for speech-sound analysis (Aylward et al., 2003; Brambati et al., 2004; Brown et al., 2001; Eckert, 2004; Paulesu et al., 2001). The left inferior temporo-occipital gyrus/fusiform gyrus has been associated with rapid visual word recognition (Brambati et al., 2004; Brown et al., 2001; Kronbichler et al., 2008; Shaywitz et al., 2002; Silani et al., 2005; Simos et al., 2002; Turkeltaub et al., 2002), although its specificity to real words has been challenged as it also seems to be involved with the decoding of pseudowords (Jobard et al., 2003). However, it is possible that its functional significance might differ for typical and atypical readers (Wimmer et al., 2010).

So, to summarize, more than thirty years of research into the brain machinery underpinning reading have led to a widely accepted multicomponential reading pathway. This is characterized by partial specificity to various psychological aspects of reading (i.e., routing specific components of reading, such as phonological processing and word identification, through different anatomical structures in the brain). It also highlights dominant activation in the left hemisphere in typically developing individuals. In comparison, poor readers tend to hypoactivate the pathway in the left hemisphere when reading and hyperactivate it in the right hemisphere.

Postmortem studies

As noted in Chapter 1, ideas connecting severe reading difficulty to brain functioning (or, more specifically, to unknown brain lesions) were expressed in the late 19th century (Berlin, 1887; Hinshelwood, 1895). Berlin (1887) was the first to hypothesize that dyslexia originated from some kind of brain lesion. Hinshelwood (1895) suggested that the localization of this lesion was in the left occipital and parietal lobes. Morgan (1896), more specifically, proposed the involvement of the angular gyrus – a hypothesis that was substantiated by Hinshelwood (1902) in the light of findings from an autopsy completed on a patient he had followed for many years. These early ideas were further developed by Samuel Orton (Orton, 1937), who argued that, given the complexity of reading, researchers should think beyond the angular gyrus or even the parietal and occipital lobes, to other areas of the brain's left hemisphere. Orton (1937) accordingly posited the poor cerebral dominance hypothesis. Although, in general, Orton's specific theory was not confirmed, he certainly offered many insightful ideas that have proven to be relevant to the growing understanding of reading in general and reading disability in particular.

Yet, the views of these early clinicians remained mostly just ideas for many decades until the first systematic bits of evidence started to accumulate. Thus, Drake (1968) presented an autopsy case of a boy with reading disability who died from a brain hemorrhage caused by a vascular malformation, and whose brain contained a series of deviant brain formations in the cortical gyri of the left inferior parietal lobe. These malformations included ectopias – small areas of abnormally placed neurons originating from cortical dysgenesis – in the subcortical white matter of the brain. Capitalizing on Orton's idea and observations from other autopsies of poor readers, Geschwind and colleagues (Geschwind & Levitsky, 1968) proposed that the presence of small brain abnormalities caused the delayed lateralization of language, which, in turn, resulted in impaired acquisition of reading. Geschwind's disciples (Galaburda et al., 1985) continued with postmortem studies of individuals with dyslexia and have reported the presence of ectopias in the auditory cortex (Galaburda & Kemper, 1979), the lateral (Livingstone et al., 1991), and medial geniculate nuclei (Galaburda, Menard, & Rosen, 1994), the primary visual cortex (Jenner, Rosen, & Galaburda, 1999), and the cerebellum (Finch, Nicolson, & Fawcett, 2002). Moreover, researchers have reported qualitative differences in some neurons seen in individuals with reading difficulties as compared to those of normal readers. For example, in various structures of the thalamus, neurons of poor readers have been reported to be smaller, more variable in size and shape, and more disorganized (Galaburda, Schrott, & Sherman, 1996; Livingstone et al., 1991). Of interest is that there have been reports of gender differences in the distributions of ectopias, so that the brains of female poor readers were reported to have fewer and differently located microcortical malformations (Humphreys, Kaufmann, & Galaburda, 1990).

These observations, and the presence of concordant evidence from genetic studies of reading disability, substantiated the hypothesis that this disability is, at least partially, related to prenatal dysgeneses of the brain caused by deviations in the process of neuronal migration, resulting in the failure of neurons to reach their normal targets. Such dysgeneses, in turn, could be caused by a variety of events such as ischemic injuries triggered by autoimmune damage of vessel walls, which result in microinjuries of the cortex, scars, and disrupted blood flow (Galaburda et al., 1996).

Another line of research originating from postmortem studies of individuals with severe reading disability is based on the hypothesis of deviation from the typical asymmetry that is characteristic of average human brains (65%) (Geschwind & Levitsky, 1968) but which is thought to be less characteristic of a dyslexic brain (Galaburda et al., 1985; Humphreys et al., 1990). The focus of these investigations has been the planum temporal (especially the left planum), which is considered to be important for the formation of language lateralization (Galaburda, 1993; Shapleske, Rossell, & Woodruff, 1999). Proponents of this idea suggest that dyslexia is a disorder of language laterality whose biological substrate is a challenged planum temporale (and, correspondingly, altered asymmetry of the left and the right plana). However, some researchers have challenged the lack of asymmetry hypothesis (Livingstone et al., 1991) and, in contrast, have provided evidence of an exaggerated leftward asymmetry (Leonard & Eckert, 2008).

In summary, the field of neuroscience of the "reading brain" started with a handful of postmortem brain studies and over a period of more than a century has blossomed into a number of sophisticated, busy, and engaging subfields. Early postmortem studies were characterized by many methodological weaknesses (e.g., participants were not well characterized behaviorally; they and their brains were quite heterogeneous, and the sample sizes were small – typically from one to only a few), so that none of these early reports would be published in prestigious scientific journals today and their findings would be difficult to replicate and almost impossible to generalize. Yet, these studies were revolutionary in their main presumption – all hypothesizing that the root of reading in general, and reading disability in particular, is in the brain.

Studies of anatomical structure

Findings from early postmortem studies were a helpful platform to launch the neuroscience of reading when proper in vivo techniques such as MRI became available. These new techniques were able to visualize brain structure by examining measures such as gross as well as voxel-by-voxel regional volumes (voxel-based morphometry [VBM]), cortical surface area and thickness, and diffusion tensor imaging (DTI) of white matter structure. The main questions that were asked by this family of studies centered on *what structures* in the brain are engaged in the task of reading and *the degree* of their engagement.

The use of imaging studies of the "reading brain" in vivo has confirmed the results of early postmortem studies; they indicated the presence of a number of abnormalities in various brain structures in individuals with reading disability. A summary of these (Leonard et al., 2001) highlights the presence of a marked rightward cerebral asymmetry, marked leftward asymmetry of the anterior lobe of the cerebellum, combined leftward asymmetry of the planum and posterior ascending ramus of the Sylvian fissure, and a large duplication of Heschl's gyrus. More specifically, however, the abnormalities have been reported in the planum temporale, corpus callosum, and cerebellum.

Magnetic Resonance Imaging (MRI)   Planum temporale. A substantial body of research has extended findings from postmortem studies of the planum temporale. It has been reported that 60–70% of the general population have leftward asymmetry; it has also been noted that the lack of leftward asymmetry or the presence of rightward asymmetry is associated with a variety of language-related deficits (Dorsaint-Pierre et al., 2006; Foster et al., 2002). Concordantly, individuals with reading disability, as a group, tend to demonstrate less leftward and more rightward asymmetry (Hynd et al., 1990; Larsen et al., 1990; Rumsey, Donohue et al., 1997). Yet, not all studies indicate the presence of symmetry or divergent asymmetry (Heiervang et al., 2000). Moreover, there are reports that whereas the right planum temporale may be similar, the left one can be smaller in individuals with reading disability compared to typical individuals (Hugdahl et al., 2003). Furthermore, there have been reports of extreme leftward asymmetry of the planum temporale (Chiarello et al., 2006). Of interest also is that deviations from the patterns of symmetry and asymmetry have been observed in samples of individuals with reading disability not only for the planum temporale but for a variety of brain structures and areas (Duara et al., 1991; Habib et al., 1995; Kushch et al., 1993).

Corpus callosum. Only a few MRI studies have compared the size and shape/structure of the corpus callosum between individuals with and without reading disability. These studies are, at least in part, driven by the assumption that the processing of phonological stimuli requires the transfer of information across this brain structure (Badzakova-Trajkov, Hamm, & Waldie, 2005). While defective callosal transfer has been reported in poor readers (Fabbro et al., 2001), findings from studies have proven to be contradictory (Beaton, 1997). Specifically, some researchers have reported a larger corpus callosum in poor readers (Duara et al., 1991; Rumsey et al., 1996), whereas others have found it to be smaller (Hynd et al., 1995; Larsen, Hoien, & Odegaard, 1992; von Plessen et al., 2002), or have found no differences (Casanova et al., 2004).

Cerebellum. Similar types of comparison between poor and typical readers have focused on differences in the cerebellum. Here, results appear to be convergent (Casanova et al., 2004; Eckert et al., 2003; Leonard et al., 2001; Middleton & Strick, 1997; Schmahmann & Pandya, 1997). The consensus is that for those with reading disability, the right anterior lobes of the cerebellum, the bilateral pars triangularis, and total brain volume are often smaller (Eckert et al., 2003). Moreover, children with reading disability can demonstrate smaller rightward cerebellar hemisphere asymmetry (Kibby et al., 2008).

Voxel-based morphometry   *Voxel-based morphometry* (VBM) is an approach that permits an examination of the gray matter and cerebrospinal fluid areas, in the context of the entire brain, and also on a voxel-by-voxel basis (Mechelli et al., 2005). Decreased gray matter may reflect a regional decrease in neuronal number or neuropil (Selemon & Goldman-Rakic, 1999). Increased gray matter may reflect the classification of dyslaminations and ectopias of gray matter (Barkovich & Kuzniecky, 2000).

Studies have compared the amount of gray matter (i.e., the amount of the brain mass generated by the neuronal bodies, neuropil, glial cells, and capillaries) in individuals with reading disability and controls in samples from various countries including Australia, France, Germany, Italy, Norway, and the United States (Peterson & Pennington, 2012). Although the results found are quite divergent, they have consistently shown some alterations of gray matter in poor readers. Specifically, poor readers appear to have less gray matter in:

- the left semilunar lobule of the cerebellum (Eckert et al., 2003);
- the right cerebellar anterior lobe, right and left pars triangularis, the left and right lingual gyri, left inferior parietal lobule, and cerebellum (Eckert et al., 2005);
- left temporal lobe and the frontal area; left parietal region (Hoeft et al., 2007);
- bilateral fusiform gyrus, the bilateral anterior cerebellum, and the right supra-marginal gyrus (Kronbichler et al., 2008);
- both temporal lobes, specifically in the left temporal lobe, in the middle and inferior temporal gyri (Steinbrink et al., 2008; Vinckenbosch, Robichon, & Eliez, 2005);
- bilaterally in the planum temporale, inferior temporal cortex, and cerebellar nuclei (Brambati et al., 2004);
- the left temporal lobe and bilaterally in the temporoparietooccipital juncture, but also in the frontal lobe, the caudate, the thalamus, and the cerebellum (Brown et al., 2001); and
- the right posterior superior parietal lobule, the precuneus, and the right supplementary motor area (Menghini et al., 2008).

Moreover, altered ratios of gray to white matter have been reportedly found in the left hemisphere (Sandu et al., 2008) although this was not found to be the case by Casanova et al. (2004). Finally, there are also reports that for those with reading disability, some areas of the brain have increased gray matter density, specifically in the precentral gyri bilaterally (Frye et al., 2010; Silani et al., 2005; Vinckenbosch et al., 2005).

Diffusion tensor imaging   Diffusion tensor imaging (DTI) is a magnetic resonance imaging technique that permits the visualization and characterization of the white matter (i.e., axons in the brain). DTI can provide unique information about the integrity of white matter formations (anisotropy) and connectivity (fiber tracking) in the human brain (Feldman et al., 2010). Moreover, using DTI, it is possible to obtain quantitative measures (i.e., mean diffusivity and fractional anisotropy) reflecting underlying tissue properties that can be used to establish both milestones for typical and characteristics of atypical brain maturation (Lim & Helpern, 2002).

Being a relatively recent methodological development, DTI has not been widely used in the field of reading disability, although relevant studies are now increasingly being reported (Hasan et al., 2012; Lebel et al., 2013; Vandermosten et al., 2012; Yeatman et al., 2012). DTI has been utilized to both establish and quantify the connection between individual differences in the microstructure of white matter and individual differences in various reading indicators. In general, such studies have shown an association between lower anisotropy coherence and lower performance scores on various reading-related tasks both in typical and disabled readers (Beaulieu et al., 2005; Deutsch et al., 2005; Klingberg et al., 1999; Niogi & McCandliss, 2006).

DTI studies have delineated major white matter pathways that appear to be important in the acquisition of reading skill – the superior corona radiata, the corpus callosum (Hasan et al., 2012), and the superior longitudinal fasciculus, SLF (Ben-Shachar, Dougherty, & Wandell, 2007). In addition, compared with controls, lower fractional anisotropy values have been found in bilateral white matter tracts within the frontal, temporal, occipital, and parietal lobes (i.e., arguably, the whole brain) of poor readers (Richards et al., 2008; Steinbrink et al., 2008). There have also been attempts to combine tractography (a visual modeling technique) with region-of-interest analyses to identify specific hot spots in the brain that might drive the correlations between fractional anisotropy and specific reading skills. For example, one study has associated single-word identification scores with indicators of fractional anisotropy of the superior corona radiate (Beaulieu et al., 2005). Although interesting, this finding has been challenged by two case studies (Keller & Just, 2009; Yeatman et al., 2009), and further research is needed to clarify this contradiction.

As noted earlier, there have been relatively few DTI research studies of reading disability, and findings have proven somewhat inconsistent (e.g., in one study [Andrews et al., 2010], a positive association was found between fractional anisotropy of the corpus callosum and reading and reading-related scores, but in another study [Dougherty et al., 2007], the relationship proved negative).

However the emerging picture from this area of work suggests that reading disability is a neurodevelopmental condition that involves the detachment of brain structure and function. Yet, it appears that this process is malleable, as white matter development and myelination appear to be experience-sensitive; they can change as specific tracks are used at high(er) frequencies and intensity (Fields, 2008; Mattson, 2002). In this context, of particular interest is a study in which micro changes in the white matter (specifically significantly increased fractional anisotropy in a region of the left anterior centrum semiovale) were documented in poor readers, aged between 8 and 10 years, whose phonological decoding skills had improved after 100 hours of intensive remedial instruction (Keller & Just, 2009).

In brief, DTI studies generally demonstrate lower fractional anisotropy values in left temporoparietal and frontal areas in poor readers. The localization of these regions is being debated, with most studies pointing to the left SLF and corona radiata and rather fewer to the posterior part of the corpus callosum or to more ventral tracts such as the inferior longitudinal fasciculus or the inferior fronto-occipital fasciculus (Vandermosten et al., 2012). Interpreting DTI findings, Gabrieli (2009) has suggested that in the case of reading disability, there is a lack of balance in the white-matter pathways supporting reading; in fact, they appear to project too weakly within the primary reading network (thus hypoactivation of the left hemisphere components of the network) and too strongly between hemispheres (thus hyperactivation of the right hemisphere components of the network).

Studies of brain function

Functional imaging is a type of brain imaging aimed at detecting or registering changes in metabolism, blood flow, or regional chemical composition. In contrast to structural imaging, as discussed earlier, functional imaging reveals in vivo changes in the brain caused by specific experimental manipulations (e.g., introducing a chain of cognitive tasks), modeling changes exerted by the brain as it engages in specific cognitive activities (e.g., when reading) in the real world. There are multiple types of functional imaging and only some of them can be discussed here. Although they are based on different technologies and different assumptions, these methods explore two key questions: (1) *how* the anatomical reading-related structures of the brain function to support reading and (2) *how* different cognitive processes that contribute to reading are enacted by the brain.

Functional imaging has been highly appealing to reading researchers because of its potential to contribute valuable data to debates about theories of reading disability. Here, factors relating to phonological, visual, and cerebellar theories are considered.

As noted in Chapter 2, the major thrust of phonological theories of reading disability is that the central deficit is related to the quality of and/or access to phonemic information (Ramus, 2004) as it is processed by, and stored, in the left superior temporal and inferior frontal cortex (Dufor et al., 2007), or perhaps even in the whole temporoparietal region including the posterior superior temporal region (Hoeft, pers. comm., 2011). Specifically, numerous studies have pointed to an impairment of left posterior brain systems that are known to be involved in the cross-modal integration of auditory and visual information and, thus, affect the realization of connections between occipitotemporal and temporoparietal circuits (Shaywitz & Shaywitz, 2008). When poor readers perform phonological tasks, these posterior systems often exhibit reduced or absent activation. These deficient patterns of activation could either be genuine, that is, first-order deficits, or derivative, that is, second-order deficits resulting from impairments in auditory processing, which could thwart the acquisition of the phoneme-grapheme maps essential for the development of accurate and efficient reading skills.

As is discussed at length in Chapter 2, the central assumption of the most popular visual theories of reading disability rests on the presupposition of the existence of low-level visual disorders related to deficiencies in the thalamic magnocellular system. These are manifested as increased thresholds for the detection of low contrast, low spatial, or higher temporal frequencies, poor sensitivity to visual motion, and jeopardized capacity for directing attention, performing eye movements, and conducting visual search (Livingstone et al., 1991; Lovegrove et al., 1980; Stein & Walsh, 1997). Studies of different aspects of visual processing in reading disability have pointed to the involvement, for primary lower-level deficits, of the thalamus (lateral geniculate nuclei), the primary visual cortex, dorsal visual areas that receive magnocellular inputs (Demb et al., 1998; Demb, Boynton, & Heeger, 1998); and, for secondary higher-level deficits, of the inferior-temporal cortex, angular/supramarginal gyri and inferior frontal gyrus (Hoeft et al., 2007; Paulesu et al., 2001; Pugh et al., 2000).

The main idea underlying the cerebellar hypothesis is that dyslexia is a type of general learning disorder that is characterized by impaired automatization of sensorimotor procedures critical to reading, but also to writing (Nicolson, Fawcett, & Dean, 2001a, 2001b). The neuronal substrate of these impairments is related to abnormal functioning in the lateral cerebellum (Doyon et al., 2002).

Functional brain studies of the "reading brain" are intimately related to structural approaches, by extending the *what* (i.e., what anatomical structures) question to that of *how* (i.e., how these structures realize reading) as well as to cognitive theories of reading disability. This is achieved by probing the cognitive processes theorized to be important for reading disability through specific experimental tasks, and by targeting specific brain regions thought to be substrates for these processes.

Positron emission tomography   Results using positron emission tomography (PET) methodology also support the impression that the patterns of activation of the brains of poor readers are different compared to controls. For example, studies of those with reading disability have reported hypoactivation in the left temporoparietal region (Rumsey et al., 1992), the left insula (Paulesu et al., 1996), the left occipitotemporal area (McCrory et al., 2005), and the frontal and parietal left hemisphere regions (Dufor et al., 2007). Of note also is that when the right frontal cortex was activated, the activated regions were larger than for controls (Dufor et al., 2007).

Functional magnetic resonance imaging   Functional magnetic resonance imaging (fMRI) is a specialized subtype of MRI used to assess changes in blood flow associated with brain neural activity. Since the early 1990s, fMRI has come to dominate the brain-mapping field in general and the field of reading in particular because of its relatively low invasiveness, relatively high availability, absence of radiation exposure, and the lack of any need to inject special tracking chemicals.

fMRI has been employed in a variety of studies of reading. First, is has been utilized to evaluate hypotheses concerning the cortical machinery substantiating typical reading (Schlaggar & McCandliss, 2007). Second, it has been used to compare this machinery in typical and poor readers to elucidate the specificity of processing reading stimuli in reading disability (Corina et al., 2001; Eden et al., 1996; Georgiewa et al., 1999; Hoeft et al., 2006; Temple et al., 2001). Third, it has been used as a source of information about brain plasticity. This has been evaluated with regard to (1) normative developmental changes (i.e., throughout the process of reading acquisition) and (2) changes that result from the introduction of specialized intervention programs (McCandliss & Noble, 2003; Simos et al., 2002).

In relation to normative development, fMRI has been utilized in studies of literate adults to register and specify the involvement of the superior temporal cortex (superior temporal gyrus/superior temporal sulcus) and auditory cortex (Heschl sulcus/planum temporale) in the integration of letters and speech sounds (Raij, Uutela, & Hari, 2000; van Atteveldt, Formisano, Goebel, & Blomert, 2004). These findings were subsequently extended by including adults with reading disability who were hypothesized to differ from controls in letter-sound integration (Blau, van Atteveldt, Ekkebus, Goebel, & Blomert, 2009). Consistent with this, the results demonstrated that poor readers underactivate the superior temporal gyrus for the integration of passively presented letter-speech sound stimuli. Behaviorally, this reduced integration was directly associated with reduced auditory processing of speech sounds, which in turn was associated with poorer performance on phonological tasks (Blau et al., 2009). Compared to the number of studies conducted with adult participants, there are still relatively few fMRI studies involving children (Richlan et al., 2011). Yet, findings from these studies consistently show that for children with a reading disability, there is evidence of hypoactivation in the perisylvian cortex and occipitotemporal gyri (Cao et al., 2006; Shaywitz et al., 2002; Temple et al., 2001) and, more specifically, the planum temporale/Heschl sulcus and the superior temporal sulcus (Blau et al., 2010). This is coupled with, in many but not all instances, deviant patterns of activation in the frontal cortex (Gabrieli, 2009; Maisog et al., 2008). Moreover, a whole-brain analysis (Blau et al., 2010) of unisensory visual and auditory group differences revealed diminished unisensory responses to letters in the fusiform gyrus in children with reading disability, as well as reduced activity for processing speech sounds in the anterior superior temporal gyrus, planum temporale/Heschl sulcus, and superior temporal sulcus. These effects are statistically significant and substantial; indicators of the neural integration of letters and speech sounds in the planum temporale/Heschl sulcus and indicators of the neural response to letters in the fusiform gyrus collectively explained almost 40% of the variance in the reading performance of participating children. These findings would appear to support the view that letter-speech sound integration is an emergent property of learning to read that develops inadequately in poor readers.

There are currently dozens of fMRI studies of reading, the majority of which, unless published by the same group, do not overlap much in terms of their theoretical platforms, their characterization of groups of typical and poor readers, their experimental tasks, and their analytical tools. Yet, regardless of their methodological and theoretical differences, studies in children and adults provide consistent evidence that those with reading difficulties, regardless of how these are defined and quantified, experience a deficient functional profile of the left posterior brain system. The essence of this deficiency is unclear but could be reflective of disruptions in either the structure of or the connections between the dorsal and ventral routes for reading (Brunswick et al., 1999; Démonet, Taylor, & Chaix, 2004; Helenius et al., 1999; Paulesu et al., 2001; Salmelin et al., 1996; Shaywitz et al., 1998; Simos, Breier, Fletcher et al., 2000; Simos, Breier, Wheless et al., 2000). Of note is that, as a group, individuals with reading disability are characterized by a shift in the pattern of activities, which, in conjunction with specific characteristics of a given study, can be defined as overbalanced toward the more anterior left regions or right temporal and perisylvian regions of the brain (Brunswick et al., 1999; Démonet et al., 2004; Georgiewa et al., 2002; B. Shaywitz et al., 2002; S. Shaywitz et al., 1998; Simos, Breier, Fletcher et al., 2000).

It is important to note that the overwhelming majority of fMRI studies of reading disability draw on the phonological deficit hypothesis. Studies underpinned by theoretical approaches that assume the presence of visual magnocellular deficit and/or auditory rate processing and cerebellar deficiencies are limited, especially among children.

PET and fMRI combined   Several meta-analytic studies have been conducted in order to provide a state-of-the-art review of PET and fMRI studies of readers with or without reading difficulty. Richlan, Kronbichler, and Wimmer (2009) carried out a meta-analysis of 17 functional imaging studies (5 PET and 12 fMRI studies). These were sampled from all those functional imaging studies conducted in the field of reading up to 2008 that met specific inclusion and exclusion criteria. Studies were included when reading or reading-related tasks involved visually presented stimuli and when results reported brain coordinates for group differences for patterns of both hypo- and hyperactivation. The majority (9) of these studies were carried out with readers of English (Booth et al., 2007; Cao et al., 2006; Hoeft et al., 2006; Hoeft et al., 2007; McCrory et al., 2005; Meyler et al., 2007; Paulesu et al., 1996; Rumsey, Nace et al., 1997; Temple et al., 2001). Four published studies (Georgiewa et al., 1999; Grünling et al., 2004; Kronbichler et al., 2006; Schulz et al., 2008) and one unpublished (Richlan et al., 2009) study recruited German readers. Other studies used an Italian (Brambati et al., 2006) and a Swedish (Ingvar et al., 2002) sample; and one study (Paulesu et al., 2001) had samples of English, French, and Italian readers.

These studies embraced a range of experimental tasks: visual letter matching and line matching, letter pair rhyme judgment, phonological lexical decision making, pseudoword rhyme judgment, word rhyme judgment, word reading and picture naming, semantic association judgment, silent reading, reading aloud, silent reading of sentences with semantically congruous or incongruous endings, and sentence comprehension. The 17 studies in the meta-analysis collectively contained 128 foci marking brain regions with under- and overactivation in individuals with reading disability (see Figure 3.2).

The following observations resulted from this meta-analysis. First, in general terms, the results supported the three-system pathway (see the beginning of this chapter) that includes the dorsal (temporoparietal), ventral (occipitotemporal), and anterior (inferior frontal) reading systems. Second, the localization of these systems in specific anatomical brain structures largely corresponded to what had been deduced in "narrative" reviews of the literature (Démonet et al., 2004; Grigorenko, 2001; Habib, 2000; Heim & Keil, 2004; McCandliss & Noble, 2003; Pugh et al., 2000; Sandak et al., 2004; Shaywitz & Shaywitz, 2005; Temple, 2002). Yet, this correspondence was not precise, and the results of this analysis led to questions about some of the regions that have been thought to be critical to reading for many years (e.g., the angular gyrus) and introduced the possibility of new regions (e.g., overactivated lingual gyrus). Third, the results featured regions with the highest levels of activation. Specifically, maxima of hypoactivation were found in inferior parietal, superior temporal, middle and inferior temporal, and fusiform regions of the left hemisphere. Moreover, maxima of hypoactivation with respect to left frontal abnormalities were placed in the inferior frontal gyrus, which was accompanied by hyperactivation in the primary motor cortex and the anterior insula. It is interesting to note that the meta-analysis did not identify specific sources of activation in the right hemisphere or the cerebellum that differentiated groups of poor and typical readers; yet, this can be explained by specific technical difficulties pertaining to fMRI of the whole brain (Hoeft, pers. comm., 2011). The analyses did reveal a number of right hemisphere hyperactivated foci, but these foci were scattered and the analyses did not result in an interpretable and reliable clustering.

Electrophysiological studies   Studies utilizing electroencephalograms (EEG) permit the gathering of important details by investigating the temporal dimension of cognitive processes as it unfolds while dealing with printed symbols. In this context, the spectrum of electroencephalograms has been studied and compared topographically with regard to the mean amplitude in each of five EEG bands (delta, theta, alpha, slow beta, and fast beta) between groups of individuals with reading disability and controls. It has been reported that multiple patterns of activity at multiple regions distinguish individuals with and without reading disability. Thus, children with reading problems show increased slow activity (delta and theta) in the frontal and right temporal regions (Arns et al., 2007). Normal readers demonstrated greater theta and beta activation at the left frontal site while individuals with reading disability showed more right-lateralized activation (Spironelli, Penolazzi, & Angrilli, 2008).

One type of EEG studies, event-related potentials (ERP), separately and in combination with fMRI studies, have offered insight into the timing and utilization of various brain structures during the process of reading (Duncan et al., 1994). Most ERP studies are devoted to electrophysiological events (i.e., specific EEG components) such as P300, N400, or mismatch negativity (MMN) that are considered to be informative for understanding the brain texture of reading disability. These studies are voluminous and often diverse in their findings. However, they appear to be rather convergent with regard to the following two observations. Patterns of brain activation in individuals with reading disability were characterized by a different time course of network activation compared to normal readers (Grünling et al., 2004; Ligges et al., 2010). Moreover, it has been observed that the network activation in the reading disability group is more diffused whereas that of the controls is more focused in the dorsal and ventral brain areas.

Magnetoencephalography Similar to those using EEG and ERP, magnetoencephalography (MEG) studies are able to provide insight into the temporal resolution of brain activity substantiating reading and reading-related processes. MEG studies (e.g., Paul et al., 2006; Salmelin, Service, Kiesilä, Uutela, & Salonen, 1996; Simos et al., 2011; Vourkas et al., 2011) have also demonstrated that poor readers utilize a different pathway while processing printed stimuli, which, compared to controls, is altered, in terms of (1) the activated brain structures (in comparison with controls, poor readers activate structures in the right hemisphere more often and in the left hemisphere less often); (2) the intensity of activation (poor readers demonstrate hypoactivation in the structures of the left hemisphere and hyperactivation in the structures of the right hemisphere); and (3) the time course of the activation.

Magnetic resonance spectroscopy Magnetic resonance spectroscopy (MRS) is a noninvasive diagnostic technique that allows the measurement of biochemical changes in the brain in response to an event (e.g., the development of a tumor) or biochemical differences between groups. This technique utilizes the same machinery as conventional MRI (see earlier in the chapter) and involves a series of tests that are added to the MRI scan to characterize the chemical metabolism in a particular area of the brain by analyzing the distribution of hydrogen ions (protons). Currently, MRS allows the reliable measurement of such metabolites as amino acids, lipids, lactate, alanine, N-acetyl aspartate, choline, creatine, and myoinositol. To illustrate, for individuals with reading disability, biochemical differences (lower ratios of choline-containing compounds to N-acetylaspartate) have been found in the left temporoparietal lobe and in the right cerebellum of controls using MRS (Rae et al., 1998). Moreover, it has been suggested that choline concentration in the angular region appears to be associated with indicators of phonological skills (Bruno, Lu, & Manis, 2013). Yet, a different study reported a group of individuals with reading disability who had a lower N-acetylaspartate/choline ratio in the right cerebellar hemisphere along with a higher choline/creatine ration in the left cerebellar hemisphere (Laycock et al., 2008). There has also been a report of a greater area of elevated brain lactate in the left anterior region (Richards et al., 1999). Similarly, phosphorus-MRS also showed that the phosphomonoester peak area was significantly elevated in a group of individuals with dyslexia, as evidenced by higher phosphomonoester/total phosphorus ratios (Richardson et al., 1997). Altogether, these findings are consistent with the hypothesis of an abnormal membrane phospholipid metabolism in individuals with dyslexia (Rae et al., 1998). In other words, reading disability appears to be associated

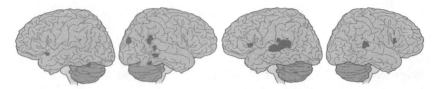

Figure 3.3 An illustration of a profound change (i.e., redistribution of activity from the right to the left hemisphere) in the pattern of brain activation evoked by a reading remediation program in a single participant. The maps were obtained using a pseudo-word rhyme-matching task before (left-hand columns) and after (right-hand columns) intensive remedial instruction. Adapted from Simos et al. (2002). (See color plate.)

with particularities of brain metabolism, but its specific signature has yet to be reliably established.

Training studies

Various imaging methods have been employed to examine the impact of various approaches to remediating reading disability upon brain functioning. Thus, fMRI, MEG, and EEG methodologies have all been used to track changes in the patterns of brain activation and to correlate these changes with those occurring at the behavioral level (Aylward et al., 2003; Kujala et al., 2001; Penolazzi et al., 2010; Richards & Berninger, 2008; Richards et al., 2000; Simos et al., 2002; Spironelli et al., 2010; Temple et al., 2003). Specifically, these studies have tracked the cerebral correlates of linguistic performance longitudinally by assessing them prior to, after, and in some cases during training protocols. All these studies have shown consistent behavioral improvement in reading and reading-related skills, with significant plastic reorganization reported in the left temporoparietal-occipital regions (Aylward et al., 2003; Shaywitz et al., 2004b; Simos et al., 2002; Temple et al., 2003) and in the left anterior brain regions, such as the left inferior frontal gyri (Richards & Berninger, 2008; Richards et al., 2000). To illustrate, during 6 months of phonological training of 14 Italian children with dyslexia, the indicators of cortical reorganization were tracked through one of the EEG components, N150 (Spironelli et al., 2010). In typical readers, N150 is generated in the left occipitotemporal cortex (Brodmann areas 39, 37, and 19), but it has been seen in right homologous areas in children with reading disability in other studies and in this sample before training. After treatment, the main N150 generator shifted to the left occipito-inferotemporal cortex (namely Brodmann areas 37 and 19) with small differences between tasks. Similarly, a pronounced shift from the right to the left hemisphere in a group of poor readers was achieved as a result of 80 hours of intensive remedial instruction (see Figure 3.3). Specifically, the improvement in reading skills was coupled with multifold activity, registered by MEG, in the left posterior aspect of the superior temporal gyrus (i.e., posterior STG) in every participant. Thus, the literature has shown that progress resulting from interventions geared to improving the accuracy and fluency of reading can be coupled with cortical plastic reorganization (Penolazzi et al., 2010; Shaywitz & Shaywitz, 2008; Temple et al., 2003; Tressoldi, Lonciari, & Vio, 2000). However, at this point, it is unclear whether the observed behavior changes are attributable to cortical reorganization, or whether indicators of such organization are merely correlates of these behavioral changes that are driven by something else.

Cross-linguistic imaging

The overwhelming majority of the studies that contain data on the brain bases of reading disability have been carried out using alphabetic languages and even then only a small number of European languages, although there is a growing number of studies involving nonalphabetic languages (e.g., Liu et al., 2013; Song et al., 2013). In other words, our current views of which parts of the brain do what when a person reads are based on individuals who are native speakers and readers of a European alphabetic language. In the last portion of the brain section of this chapter, we briefly comment on the question: Is reading disability/dyslexia "the same or different" across different languages? Here this question is reformulated so that it applies to the brain foundation of reading disability in different languages.

As data from different languages accumulate, different theories of the etiology, emergence, manifestation, and prognosis of reading disability around the world have developed (Share, 2008; Ziegler et al., 2010). These theories capture different levels of the complex theoretical representations of reading disability/dyslexia. Thus, with regard to the brain foundation of this problem, there are theories that presume that individuals with reading disability have the same type of brain abnormality irrespective of the properties of the orthographic systems of particular languages (Paulesu et al., 2001; Silani et al., 2005). This presumption, however, has been challenged as inaccurate and misleading (Hadzibeganovic et al., 2011) for two chief reasons. First, there are now multiple layers of data illustrating the presence of differences in how a given writing system connects print to spoken language (Goswami, 2002; Perfetti, Liu, & Tan, 2005; Price & Mechelli, 2005; Schlaggar & McCandliss, 2007; Siok et al., 2004). Second, even within a single orthographic system, there are many different types of reading difficulty, which, however defined, appear to differ behaviorally, cognitively, and perhaps anatomically (Kochunov et al., 2003), and are assumed to reflect differential "neural impairments" (Hadzibeganovic et al., 2011, p. 1314).

Currently, it is not possible to answer this question definitively. Seminal work by Paulesu et al (2001) used fMRI to study differences between Italian, French, and English typical readers and those with a reading disability. Reduced activation was found in the same brain areas in those with a reading problem, in comparison with typical readers. Based on these results, a universal biological foundation of reading disability was hypothesized and it was suggested that the same remediation programs should have similar effects across all three languages.

Clearly this is a bold hypothesis that needs to be verified, preferably in as many languages as possible. As mentioned earlier, brain-imaging studies in a variety of non-Western European languages, both alphabetic and nonalphabetic, have begun to emerge. For example, there are a number of studies conducted with readers of Chinese, a logographic language. In the first imaging study with readers of Chinese (Siok et al., 2004) it was found that Chinese readers (without a reading disability) appear to recruit a network of brain areas known to be utilized in response to increased visual attention; this is what is needed when logographic words are being processed. Interestingly, those with a reading disability demonstrated reduced activation in visual attention areas but not in those areas implicated in reading disability for alphabetic languages. These findings, then, directly contradict both parts of the hypothesis put forward by Paulesu and colleagues; it appears that the brain machinery supporting skilled and poor reading may differ in different languages and, moreover, remediation of reading disability might require different intervention programs in logographic versus alphabetic languages. However, a more recent study (Hu et al., 2010) generated results more consistent with the logic and findings of Paulesu and his colleagues. In this study, brain activation for semantic decisions on written words was compared in English individuals with reading disability, Chinese individuals with reading disability, English typical readers, and Chinese typical readers; all readers were monolingual. The following pattern of activation was reported: in the case of both languages, individuals with reading disability demonstrated hypoactivation in the left angular gyrus and in left middle frontal, posterior temporal, and occipitotemporal regions. Typical readers in Chinese or English, however, differed in their activation patterns. Specifically, Chinese readers demonstrated increased (compared to that normally seen in English typical readers) activation in the left inferior frontal sulcus. In comparison with Chinese readers, English readers showed increased activation in the left posterior superior temporal sulcus. The researchers referred to these differences as "cultural" and stated that they were not observed in poor readers for whom there was greater activation in both the left inferior frontal sulcus and left posterior superior temporal sulcus. The researchers claimed that this was consistent with the use of generic (i.e., culture-free) strategies when reading is less efficient. Interpreting their findings, the authors concluded that their results supported the hypothesis of a common neural basis for reading disability regardless of the language spoken and its orthography.

Brain studies: a summary

Current brain-based understandings of reading and reading disability have been derived from multiple sources of information, both structural (as evident from postmortem and in vivo studies) and functional brain research.

Early postmortem and subsequent structural imaging studies of reading disability have converged to suggest the presence of various small alterations in the structure of the brains of poor readers. The causes of these alterations are not clear, but it has been hypothesized that these are related to early stages of brain maturation and development (Galaburda et al., 2006).

Functional neuroimaging studies of those with reading disability have indicated the presence of processing deficiencies in the temporoparietal areas (Beaton, 2004), specifically of the posterior regions (Rumsey et al., 1994), and possibly of the mid-posterior cortex bilaterally (Rumsey, Nace et al., 1997). The utilization of relatively new technologies, such as VBM and DTI, has produced observations of reduced gray matter in the parietotemporal region (Brown et al., 2001; Silani et al., 2005; Vinckenbosch et al., 2005) and white matter alterations in the left parietotemporal region in poor readers (Klingberg et al., 2000). Reading disability has been most consistently associated with reduced or absent activity in the left temporoparietal regions (Hoeft et al., 2006, 2007; Shaywitz et al., 2002, 2004b; Temple et al., 2001). The engagement of imaging technologies with high temporal resolution (EEG and MEG) has demonstrated the disruption of neural processing of rapid auditory stimuli in poor readers, indicated the particular importance of the parietotemporal region in reading disability, and showed that dysfunction in posterior cortical regions leads to compensation in frontal lobe systems. Differences in brain electrical activation considered to be characteristic of typical readers and those with reading disability can be traced, at least in part, to as early as six months of age (Leppanen & Lyytinen, 1997) and perhaps even earlier (Leppänen et al., 2010).

Language involves a highly complex system of cognitive processes that engages most of the cortex. Reading is another cognitive system that is closely related to language but has links to other systems in the brain (e.g., visual) and its own brain representation and pathways. Both language (Angrilli et al., 2003; Angrilli & Spironelli, 2005; Spironelli, Angrilli, & Pertile, 2008) and reading (Aylward et al., 2003; Shaywitz et al., 2004b; Temple et al., 2003) arc highly plastic and thus can be reorganized in both adults and children throughout normal development, but also in response to systematic interventions (e.g., schooling) and asystematic events such as acquired lesions. As is discussed in Chapter 4, the acquisition of reading, however, is distinctly different from that of language; the development of reading skills requires the presence of multiple prerequisite skills and at least a decade of practice to ensure automatization of the visual associative areas that are closely connected to the linguistic regions developed early for spoken language (i.e., left temporal and frontal cortices). From an evolutionary viewpoint, the left occipitotemporal junction is the main candidate joining anterior linguistic speech areas and posterior visual cortices. It is, perhaps, particularly interesting that current evidence in the literature consistently shows functional aberrations in this particular region for those with reading disability regardless of their age (Brunswick et al., 1999; Helenius et al., 1999; Maurer et al., 2007; Paulesu et al., 2001; Penolazzi, Spironelli, & Angrilli, 2008; Penolazzi et al., 2006; Shaywitz & Shaywitz, 2005, 2008; Spironelli & Angrilli, 2006; Spironelli, Penolazzi et al., 2008). It is also of note that this system seems to be the first to come online during the acquisition of reading (Brem et al., 2010). Yet it is also of no surprise, given the complexity of reading, that some have proposed the need for a model involving multifocal brain abnormalities in reading disability. Such a model could both reconcile the diversity of findings in the field and account for the diverse deficits predicted by the different theories with a major involvement of the left superior temporal gyrus, occipital-temporal cortices, and lateral/medial cerebellum (Pernet et al., 2009).

What does neuroscience research bring to the dyslexia debate? First and foremost, this work provides a validation of the existence of a complex biological phenomenon that underlies, at the level of the brain, the cognitive and behavioral manifestations of reading disability. However, to what extent can extant knowledge in this field assist in the differential diagnosis and intervention of a dyslexic subgroup?

Brain studies of reading and reading disability can be roughly subdivided into four categories. Studies in the first (and most voluminous) category focus on typical reading in adults and attempt to understand how the "reading brain" does its job. The unequivocal conclusion from these studies is that the brain's involvement is systematic, consistently engaging specific pathways of information processing and automatizing processes as much as possible. Through these studies the field has identified "where reading happens" in the brain.

Studies in the second category examine the process of reading acquisition, the emergence of the "reading brain." These operate either cross-sectionally, looking at readers of different ages and stages of skill mastery, or longitudinally, following the same cohort of children as they acquire the skill of reading. The indisputable conclusion from this work is that the brain enters the stage of reading acquisition functionally different from its exit at the stage of fluent reading. So, things change in the brain while reading is being mastered, and then the brain maintains these changes, so that a skilled reader does not have to relearn this skill every time he or she encounters a book.

The third category of studies, featured most in this chapter, includes those in which the structural and functional properties of the "reading brain" of typical readers are compared to those of individuals with reading disability.

Such work would appear to be most valuable for resolving the dyslexia debate, yet, paradoxically, it offers comparatively little at the current time. The reason for this is because, for these studies to take place, the "target group" to be compared to typical readers has to be defined, and that very definition assumes the existence of a category of reading disability (or dyslexia) that can be reliably and validly identified. Unfortunately, the neuroscience literature of reading contains as many definitions of these terms as do the cognitive and education literatures, and the particular definition employed by each study largely depends on researcher preference. This is a hugely important issue for resolving the dyslexia debate, but one, perhaps, that is less important to neuroscience researchers.

To illustrate, one longitudinal study traced reading development in two groups of children: a group with dyslexia and a group of typical readers (Hoeft et al., 2011). The intent was to evaluate whether initial behavioral or brain measure (fMRI and DTI) can predict developmental improvements in dyslexia. Their results attracted much attention because it was brain, rather than behavioral, indicators that predicted the reading gains. Greater right pre-frontal activation during a reading task that required phonological awareness and right superior longitudinal fasciculus (including arcuate fasciculus) white-matter organization significantly predicted future reading gains in those with dyslexia. The prediction was child specific and was at 72% for these two brain areas and at >90% for the whole-brain activation pattern. This is one of the first (if not the first) example of the use of brain activation data as a type of a biomarker for the purposes of predicting individual behavioral developmental outcomes. Such biomarkers can be used either as prodermal indicators of risk for dyslexia (Black et al., 2012; Saygin et al., 2013) or as predictors of long-term outcomes of dyslexia (Hoeft et al., 2011). Yet, although the sophistication (and the success) of researchers in this field is growing, conceptual issues about what constitutes dyslexia or, indeed, reading disability, persist. It is noteworthy, for example, that to qualify for membership of the "dyslexic" group in Hoeft et al.'s (2011) study, participants needed only to score below the 25th centile on a composite score derived from a number of reading measures, and also be placed within one standard deviation of the norm on a nonverbal IQ subtest.

Unlike studies where a reading-disabled group needs to be identified before comparison with typical readers, the fourth category of brain studies has greater potential to contribute to the resolution of the dyslexia debate. This category includes brain-imaging studies that are conducted along with behavior intervention studies. Although currently boasting very few studies, this type of study has the potential to contribute to the debate by accessing whether and how the mechanics of the brain respond to a given intervention and whether behavioral outcomes are the same or differentiated for individuals with, for example, decoding difficulties as compared to individuals with reading problems of different types.

As this section has sought to demonstrate, research into the "reading brain" has contributed substantially to our understanding of reading and reading difficulty. However, it is important that we should not stray beyond the limits of our present knowledge and assume that findings from this work can currently inform diagnosis or intervention for those with reading disability. At present we cannot use understandings gleaned from neuroscience to help resolve the dyslexia debate. Certainly such work cannot enable us to identify members of a dyslexic subsample from a larger pool of poor decoders. Furthermore, there are no brain-based measures that can identify a subset of poor readers for whom a particular form of intervention would be demonstrably preferential. While neuroscience offers a potentially powerful contribution to future work with struggling readers, it has not yet enabled a resolution to the conceptual, definitional, and diagnostic dilemmas that are outlined in Chapter 1, or the problems of how best to structure targeted intervention that are discussed in Chapter 4.

Genetic bases of reading (dis)ability

Since the early clinical investigations of the late nineteenth century, reading disability has long been considered to be a condition whose pathogenesis involves hereditary factors (Hinshelwood, 1907; Morgan, 1896; Stephenson, 1907; Thomas, 1905). However, our understanding of the impact of these factors, and the biological and genetic machinery behind them, has changed significantly over the past century.

As noted throughout this book, it is widely accepted that reading involves a complex system of cognitive processes supported by multiple areas of the brain forming a particular functional system, known as the "reading brain" (Pugh & McCardle, 2009). The current view asserts that this system is established under the influence of complex genetic machinery. This brain system can be "broken" or challenged in more than one way; thus, there is no "single" way leading to reading disability (Pernet, Anderson, Paulesu, & Demonet, 2009). Similarly, it is likely that multiple deficiencies in the genetic machinery can lead to the emergence of such a malfunctioning brain system (Grigorenko, 2009).

It is important to recognize that researchers currently have only a rudimentary understanding of the components of this machinery and how these operate. Firstly, it should be noted that, when studying the genetics of reading, it is assumed that reading skills of sampled groups cannot be explained by the extent and quality of reading experience or instruction that members of these groups received. Secondly, reading skills (e.g., reading accuracy and reading speed) and reading-related processes (e.g., phonemic awareness or lexical retrieval) are continuously distributed in the general population regardless of the language in which reading is being studied (e.g., Zoccolotti et al., 2009). When examining the nature of individual differences in reading and other reading-related performance, it has been found that a substantial portion of these differences can be attributed to variation in their genetic endowments (i.e., the genomes of individuals characterized by these differences).

Estimates of the magnitude of this portion of variance vary (1) across the life span (Byrne et al., 2009), (2) for different languages (Samuelsson et al., 2008), (3) for different societal groups (Friend, DeFries, & Olson, 2008), and (4) for different classroom environments (Taylor et al., 2010). Such details are typically derived from studies of relatives and are known as heritability estimates (Sternberg & Grigorenko, 1999a). Heritability estimates can be obtained from studies of genetic relatives, where family members with differing degrees of genetic similarity – for example, identical (monozygotic) and fraternal (dizygotic) twins or other relations (e.g., parents and offspring, siblings, or members of extended families) – are assessed behaviorally (e.g., given reading tests) and correlations between their behavioral traits (i.e., phenotypic similarity) can be compared to correlations between their genetic profiles (i.e., genotypic similarity). There are numerous statistical techniques that have been developed to estimate heritability coefficients using both the behavioral data and the known degree of genetic relatedness (Elston & Johnson, 2008). Each of these techniques has its own strengths and weaknesses; correspondingly they are often used in combination so that estimation precision can be maximized.

Differences in performance have been attributed to differences in the genome at an average of 41–74% (Grigorenko, 2004) although systematic fluctuations in these estimates have been found. Although genetic influences appear to be present in virtually any process related to reading, there is some variation with regard to estimates for specific componential processes. Thus, estimates are found in the 50–80% range for various indicators of phonological processing (Byrne et al., 2009; Byrne et al., 2002), 60–87% for various indicators of orthographic processing (Gayán & Olson, 2001, 2003), and 60–67% for semantic processing or reading comprehension (Betjemann et al., 2008; Harlaar, Dale, & Plomin, 2007; Keenan et al., 2006; Petrill et al., 2007). Moreover, these estimates tend to be lower when they are obtained earlier in the child's development, for example, among preschoolers or in early school grades (e.g., Byrne et al., 2009). They also tend to vary depending on the language in which they are obtained and the specific characteristics of reading for which they are obtained, suggesting that there is tremendous variation in how genetic factors manifest themselves in the different languages in which reading is acquired (e.g., Naples et al., 2009). In addition, these estimates tend to diverge depending on the characteristics of the sample from which they were obtained, for example, SES, ethnicity, and quality of schooling (e.g., Taylor et al., 2010).

Genetic influences appear to be of even greater magnitude when one considers reading disability. When selecting samples of poor readers (e.g., Deffenbacher et al., 2004), variation is often limited, as relatives of poor readers often demonstrate similarly depressed levels of performance. Such studies typically result in higher heritability estimates.

Some researchers employ a statistical approach known as relative risk estimates. These indicate the probability that a relative of someone with a reading disability may also suffer from this problem. These estimates are then compared to estimates of the general population risk. As noted in Chapter 1, however, estimating the population risk is not an easy task as there is much variation in the literature as to cut-off points. Despite this caveat, relative risk statistics suggest that the prevalence of reading disability among relatives of those with this difficulty is substantially higher than the general population estimates. Relative risk statistics are obtained from samples that include families of individuals with dyslexia (i.e., families of so-called dyslexia probands). Multiple family constellations can be used in these studies: sibling and/or cousin units (i.e., pairs or larger groupings), nuclear families, and extended families. As is the case with heritability estimates, no particular method is preferred, and samples that include different groupings of relatives are characterized by specific advantages and disadvantages; correspondingly, multiple approaches are typically employed to maximize the accuracy and precision of findings.

Despite substantial evidence in the literature that genetic factors are important for understanding individual differences in reading acquisition and reading performance, their specific role continues to be unclear. To understand the specifics of the mechanics and magnitude of genetic factors, many researchers are engaged in so-called molecular studies of reading and reading-related processes. Unlike heritability and relative risk studies, in which only behavioral characterization of the probands and their family members takes place, molecular (or molecular-genetic) studies require the collection of biological specimens (typically either blood or saliva) from which DNA can be extracted. Molecular-genetic studies are typically one of two major types (both types can be further subdivided into subtypes), depending on the type of participants they engage, namely genetically unrelated cases/probands and matched controls, or family units such as siblings or nuclear and extended families), and the type of genetic entity they target (i.e., specific genes, specific genetic regions, or the whole genome).

The very first molecular-genetic study of dyslexia was a whole-genome linkage scan completed with a number of extended families of individuals with reading disability (Smith et al., 1983). A typical protocol for these studies is that families in which an individual has a reading disability are approached and members are requested to be evaluated behaviorally (i.e., complete a number of reading and reading-related, tasks) and to donate a biological specimen (i.e., blood or saliva). The task, once again, is to correlate the similarities in performance on various assessments to similarities in the structural variation in the genome, only now the genetic similarities are not estimated but measured using special molecular-genetic (i.e., genotyping and sequencing) and statistical (i.e., linkage and association analyses) techniques. For such studies, family units can include a variety of types of relative (e.g., siblings, parent-offspring, cousins, aunts, and uncles) and family sizes (e.g., a pair, a nuclear family, and extended family). The literature contains illustrations of different types of samples used in molecular-genetic studies of reading disability (Grigorenko, 2005).

As mentioned earlier, the very first molecular-genetic study of reading disability by Smith et al. (1983) was a whole-genome scan, although very few markers were available then, and those that were used were protein markers (the technology at that time was insufficient for work with DNA markers). Since then, much has changed, including an abundance of polymorphic DNA markers, the cost of genotyping, and computer capacity. These changes have shaped the lay of the land so much that at least 13 genome-wide investigations for reading disability/dyslexia performed using different methodologies have been reported (Brkanac et al., 2008; de Kovel et al., 2004; Eicher et al., 2013; Fagerheim et al., 1999; Field et al., 2013; Fisher et al., 2002; Igo et al., 2006; Kaminen et al., 2003; Luciano et al., 2013; Meaburn et al., 2008; Nopola-Hemmi et al., 2002; Raskind et al., 2005; Roeske et al., 2011). These studies are drastically different from the 1983 study, both technologically (hundreds of thousands or even millions of markers are now used) and in relation to sample size (hundreds of individuals are now recruited to make sure that such studies are adequately powered).

Some studies have focused on particular, selected regions of the genome. The decision concerning which regions to select will typically result from a previous whole-genome scan or a theoretical hypothesis capitalizing on a particular aspect of reading disability (Skiba et al., 2011). There are also other bases on which decisions can be made. For example, some researchers have selected their candidate regions through means such as a known chromosomal aberration. For example, in Denmark all newborns are screened for macro-chromosomal changes (e.g., large rearrangements). Databases can then be used to inform decisions about who should be screened for reading disability/dyslexia (Buon-incontri et al., 2011). The hypothesis then is that a gene affected by such an aberration, in a proband suffering from reading disability, is somehow related to the disability.

Although different accounts exist, the literature (Figure 3.4) has made reference to about 20 (Schumacher et al., 2007) potential genetic susceptibility loci that mark locations in the genome that have been "statistically linked" to reading disability/dyslexia. It is important to note that these regions are typically large, by genomic standards, and may contain many genes (i.e., more than one, and sometimes hundreds). The literature also makes reference to at least six, but often more (Grigorenko & Naples, 2009; Peterson & Pennington, 2012)

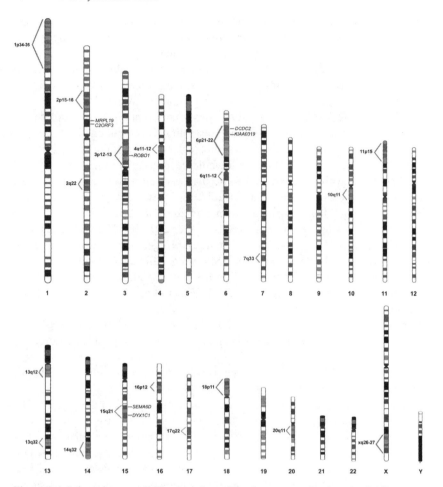

Figure 3.4 Selected susceptibility loci those (that have more citations in the literature are shown in red, and those less – shown in blue) and candidate genes identified through studies of probands with reading disability and their families. Note: often a particular susceptibility locus (e.g., 2p, 6p, and 15q) has more than one candidate gene, emphasizing both the underlying complexity of the phenotype under investigation and the imprecision of the field. (See color plate.)

so-called candidate genes for reading disability, that is, genes that, being located in the same susceptibility loci, might actually be the specific genes whose altered function is associated with the emergence of dyslexia. Yet none of these has been either fully accepted or fully rejected by the research community.

There is an ongoing debate regarding the specificity of the impact of genes related to reading disability; the issue here is whether the hypothesized candidate genes for this condition are sources of the specific genetic variation that accounts for individual differences in reading and reading-related processes only, or whether these genes have a broader impact on other types of learning (i.e., learning math) and other cognitive processes. In an attempt to address this issue, a so-called generalist gene hypothesis (Plomin & Kovas, 2005) contends that genes that affect one area of learning, such as reading performance, are largely the same genes that affect other abilities (and disabilities). Such a position is still open to debate, however.

As previously noted, approximately 20 different genomic regions are currently considered to be harboring candidate genes for reading disability, although this figure is likely to grow (Rubenstein et al., 2011). There are six candidate genes being evaluated as causal genes for reading disability/dyslexia (*DYX1C1, KIAA0319, DCDC2, ROBO1, MRPL2,* and *C2orf3*), but more genes have been reported as putative additions to this list (Buonincontri et al., 2011; Ercan-Sencicek et al., 2012; Newbury et al., 2011; Scerri et al., 2010). At the current time, there is mixed evidence for the involvement of each of these genes, and findings have proven difficult to interpret in a systematic way.

While we have some secure knowledge, there continue to be many areas of uncertainty. We can be sure that individual differences in reading performance are, at least partially, genetic, and it appears that the relationship is stronger for those with a reading disability, increasing with the severity of the deficit. Moreover, the relationship between reading and the genome appears to be stronger as the individual develops from early childhood to early adulthood. At the present time, however, there is a dearth of genetically informed studies of reading for elderly populations. Most of what is known about the genetics of reading (dis)ability is known from individuals younger than 18 years of age.

There are many reasons why our knowledge concerning the genetics of reading is still relatively rudimentary. First and foremost, reading and reading-related processes are complex in structure and are, most likely, complex in terms of their genetic sources (Smith, 2007). Second, developmental models of reading acquisition assume the involvement of both the formation and engagement of multiple psychological representations (Grigorenko & Naples, 2008), such as phonological, orthographical, morphological, and others (see Chapter 2). These representations permit the holistic process of reading to emerge. Yet, although corresponding multivariate models of reading are commonly found in the behavioral literature (Wagner & Torgesen, 1987), they are not so prevalent in the genetic literature on reading. Third, not only do environmental risk factors play an important role in the development of reading disability; they also appear to have an interactional relationship with genes (what is known as a bioecological gene by environment interaction). For example, while an association between the heritability of dyslexia and level of parental education has been found – the higher the level of education, the greater the heritability

(Friend et al., 2008; Rosenberg et al., 2012) – it is not yet known which environmental factors play a mediating role in this (Grigorenko, 2012). Fourth, it appears that many genes of small-to-moderate effects underlie the individual differences in reading and its components (Meaburn, Harlaar, Craig, Schalkwyk, & Plomin, 2008); reading is best described as a system of the related variables that quantify these components (Grigorenko, 2007). Thus, to identify the relevant genes, studies require large numbers of individuals who are homogeneous genetically (e.g., individuals with similar ancestry) and who are well characterized behaviorally with multivariate phenotypes. Unfortunately, these are not often easy to recruit.

Progressing from statistical estimates of the role of genetic factors to the identification of these factors has proven to be difficult, but these difficulties are not specific to studies of reading. Indeed, the term "missing heritability" (Eichler et al., 2010; Hemminki et al., 2011; van der Sluis, Verhage, Posthuma, & Dolan, 2010; Vineis & Pearce, 2010) has been used to refer to the many unfruitful attempts to translate the high-heritability estimates obtained for a variety of complex human conditions (i.e., disorders such as diabetes, ADHD, and autism) into their underlying genetic foundations (Avramopoulos, 2010). Research into the genetic bases of reading has the imprint of the field of the genetics and genomics of complex disorders more generally. Specifically, initial positive findings are often followed by nonreplications, suggesting either a high level of heterogeneity of the genetic mechanisms involved (Moonesinghe et al., 2008) or a high level of false positive results (Shen et al., 2005). Either of these interpretations presents a challenge to researchers. The former leads logically to the possibility that researchers have been unable to generalize effectively from specific deficiencies that might be characteristic of specific families, or from specific samples, to the general population. The latter suggests that the initial samples were too small and were lacking in sufficient statistical power to differentiate true and false findings. If this is true, much larger samples will be needed to weed out the initial field of what appeared to be promising results by marking a number of them as "false positives."

Yet, although these two possibilities appear to be the most obvious, they are not the only alternatives. So far, the field of genetic studies of reading has focused primarily on the model postulating that reading is controlled by a genetic mechanism that follows Mendelian laws (or Fisher's extension to quantitative genetics). These are the laws that determine the intergenerational transmission of a hereditary trait when that trait is controlled by a single genetic factor (i.e., a specific gene at a specific locus). This approach has focused on the idea of finding the "risk variants" that can, individually or collectively, explain a substantial portion of the high level of heritability for a condition such as dyslexia. Yet the idea that familial patterns of the transmission of reading (dis)ability will follow or be similar to patterns of traits controlled by single genes (i.e., traits to which Mendelian laws apply) is diminishing as we learn more about the structure and function of the human genome.

The last decade of genetic and genomic research has led to an explosion of studies implicating a great variety of different types of structural variation in the genome that are related to the origin and manifestation of various developmental disabilities (Miller et al., 2010). These types of structural variation range from large to small genomic events of different natures – deletions, insertions, spatial alterations (e.g., translocations and inversions), and the presence/absence of transposable elements (1000 Genomes Project Consortium, 2010; Gonzaga-Jauregui, Lupski, & Gibbs, 2012; Stankiewicz & Lupski, 2010).[1]

Different types of structural variation have been implicated in the manifestation of reading difficulties (including reading comprehension), and through analysis of these, several candidate genes for reading difficulties have been identified: *ROBO1* (Hannula-Jouppi et al., 2005), *DYX1C1* (Taipale et al., 2003), and *SEMA6D* (Ercan-Sencicek et al., 2012). All of these genes have been detected through studies of isolated families (Taipale et al., 2003) or even individual cases (Ercan-Sencicek et al., 2012). Systematic explorations of the importance of different types of structural variation in the field of reading have been few and, so far, only on large events, namely insertions and deletions larger than 1Megabases (Girirajan et al., 2011). Yet, it is important to stress that large structural variants of this kind are relatively rare (e.g., <1% of the general population), and the underlying assumption here is that the identification of these will provide a clue for subsequent studies of the gene(s) affected by this structural alteration, or the pathways involved. It is especially relevant to investigations of the genetic bases of complex traits such as reading abilities or disabilities. The idea is that once a rare variant is identified and associated with a particular trait (e.g., reading), it is necessary to investigate common variants in the gene/region impacted by this rare variant. In the field of reading, an example of such a transition from a rare variant to a set of common variants associated with a continuous trait is the research on *ROBO1* (Bates et al., 2011).

---

[1] A transposable element is a DNA sequence that can change its relative position (self-transpose). The importance of considering these (and perhaps other) types of variation has been demonstrated for autism spectrum disorder (O'Roak et al., 2011; Sanders et al., 2011, 2012), various developmental delays (Cooper et al., 2011), intellectual disabilities (Lu et al., 2007), ADHD (Lionel et al., 2011), and a number of specific genomic syndromes (Jalal et al., 2003; Roberts et al., 2004), many of which are associated with different learning disabilities. In other words, although DNA structural variations are present in individuals without reading difficulties, individuals with various neuropsychiatric disorders appear to present structural variation in their genomes to a higher degree (e.g., more variants are observed), or have variations of a particular type (e.g., deletions and insertions of larger size are observed), or at particular crucial locations (e.g., the deletion at 22q11.2 results in a well-known genomic condition, DiGeorge syndrome, one facet of which is the presentation of learning problems).

Along with the enhanced understanding of the role of structural variation in the genome, recent discoveries have identified a few other mechanisms that might be relevant to our understanding of the genetics of typical and atypical reading. Some of these are now briefly discussed.

First, it is important to note that reading skills are acquired within a developmental context. Behavior-genetic studies of typical and atypical reading and related phenotypes have indicated the presence of developmental heterogeneity in corresponding genetic bases (Byrne et al., 2009; Petrill et al., 2010). Specifically, when multiple time points of the same reading-related phenotype have been considered, results have indicated the presence of time-general and time-specific genetic factors that have contributed to the additive genetic component of the phenotypic variance (Harlaar et al., 2007). Outcomes of this type have been reported for such reading-related phenotypes as phonetic-phonological processes (Coventry et al., 2011), orthographic processes (Byrne et al., 2008), and vocabulary (Hart et al., 2009). Thus, it is important to investigate the impact of specific genetic risk factors longitudinally. It is even more important to track, at the genetic/genomic level, the impact of effective behavioral interventions.

Second, there are molecular entities, both within the DNA and separate from it, that have been found to affect DNA functioning and its products. The current estimate of genes (protein-coding sequences) is ~21,000, or 1.5% of the genome in humans (Clamp et al., 2007). However, as the accuracy of the sequence of the human genome has increased, it has become clear that genes constitute a minority in the genome compared with other types of DNA structures, for example functional conserved noncoding elements (CNEs). These are sequences within the DNA that do not code for proteins but serve other important functions. Substantial data from studies have led to the suggestion that the differentiation of species may be driven more by variation in CNEs than changes in proteins (Lander, 2011). Correspondingly, it might be important to broaden the search for the genetic bases of reading beyond protein-coding genes. The role of CNEs in reading might be directly related to the role of transposable elements, as many of the CNEs appear to be structurally derived from these (Bejerano et al., 2006).

Another recent discovery points to the importance of functional human non-protein-coding ribonucleic acids (RNAs) in humans (nb. RNA and DNA are both nucleic acids). There are many different types of RNA, and some, it has been found, regulate or modify protein synthesis through various means. In this way, the RNAs can indirectly affect such processes as cell cycle regulation, immune responses, brain processes, and gametogenesis. Moreover, and perhaps more importantly for understanding the genetic bases of reading, certain RNAs may serve as "flexible scaffolds" (Zappulla & Cech, 2006) for protein complexes (i.e., combinations of protein), which may elicit specific functions that are not carried out by any of the participating proteins in isolation.

Finally, another mechanism worthy of exploration in developmentally and intervention-oriented research is the epigenetic (or epigenomic) regulation of the genome. This concerns heritable events in genome transcription that are traceable through changes in gene expression yet are *not* caused by structural changes in DNA. In other words, what is synthesized by a particular DNA fragment may not be directly caused by changes in the DNA sequence. It has been observed that functionally active domains/components of the genome are characterized by specific epigenetic marks – that is, the presence of particular molecules (Lander, 2011) that may influence the transcription process. These marks can be recorded, cataloged, and assembled in developmental (skill acquisition) and intervention (skill reconstruction) epigenomic maps. Although the question of the tissue and cell specificity of these marks remains open, it has been shown (Thompson et al., in press) that cells from saliva and blood provide a great deal of information that indicate epigenomic maps that differentiate behavioral groups (Naumova et al., 2012) or that correlate with behavioral traits (Essex et al., 2013). There is no reason to believe that epigenomic studies will not prove to be equally if not more useful for typical and atypical reading as they have been for other complex behavioral traits.

The majority (if not all) of the samples currently used for genetic studies of reading impairment consist of individuals who have been exposed to the impact of schooling; that is, with few exceptions (Byrne et al., 2002; Petrill et al., 2010), they have been recruited while in school and after their reading disability has been identified. There is reason to believe that the severity of the phenotype (or, conversely, the degree to which a learner responds to remediation interventions) is linked to the strength of the genetic findings (Deffenbacher et al., 2004; Francks et al., 2004). Thus it seems that the success of genetic studies will depend on their capacity to "unscramble" the reading-related phenotypes from the type and amount of intervention received. It will be especially crucial to take such previous experiences into account if epigenetic analyses are to be conducted.

The promise of genetic accounts for resolving the dyslexia debate

Although work in genetics is currently unable to inform current educational practice, it is to be hoped that greater understanding of the genetic bases of learning difficulties such as reading disability/dyslexia will ultimately enable us to predict risk of academic failure more accurately and intervene at an early stage more powerfully. However, translating genetic and genomic discoveries into practical applications involves progression through a series of developmental stages. Although there are different accounts in relation to the "-omics" sciences, Khoury and colleagues (Agurs-Collins et al., 2008; Khoury, Bowen et al., 2008; Khoury, Gwinn et al., 2007; Khoury, Valdez, & Albright, 2008) indicate that for the validation of scientific knowledge to practical prevention and intervention in public health (and, most likely, to education), four stages are necessary.

The first stage, the discovery (or analytical validity) stage, involves the attempt to connect a genetic or genomic mechanism with a particular condition such as reading disability. At the second stage, the clinical validity phase, researchers seek to appraise the value of this connection for clinical purposes, validating the first-stage observations in different settings and with different samples to assess its replicability and robustness. At this stage, evidence-based guidelines connecting a genetic or genomic discovery and the particular issue concerned are developed. At the third stage, the clinical utility phase, these guidelines are introduced into clinical practice by mechanisms of knowledge transfer and delivery, as well as dissemination and diffusion practices. Only after having planted these practices into everyday application on a large scale can research, at stage four, evaluate the practical outcomes of a genomic discovery. This stage engages multiple ethical and social considerations.

Unfortunately for those seeking to apply genetic knowledge to the resolution of clinical problems, most current genome-based research is unfolding within stage one (Khoury, Valdez et al., 2008), with only approximately 3% of published studies being conducted within stage two, and very few at stage three or four (Khoury, Gwinn et al., 2007). In relation to dyslexia, most research activity is still operating at stage one. This stage defines the analytical validity (Haddow & Palomaki, 2003) of whatever genetic or genomic test needs to be conducted so that the genotype of interest for the disorder (in this case, dyslexia) may be measured accurately, reliably, and at minimum expense. Although a number of specific candidate genes for dyslexia have been identified, the mechanism that unifies these genes in their dyslexia-specific action is still far from clear. Moreover, researchers have yet to resolve the numerous hypotheses regarding the specific genomic regions and other candidate genes that are currently under consideration. In other words, stage one of the related work in the field of dyslexia is a long way from being completed. It is rapidly unfolding, but it is too early, at this stage, to ascertain any specific genetic tests that would have diagnostic validity for dyslexia.

Research on some of the candidate genes (e.g., *KIAA0319, DCDC2, ROBO1*, and *DYX1C1*) has transitioned to stage two, where the degree of association between these genes and reading disability is being validated in a variety of samples and contexts. However, the various stage-two findings have yet to be transformed into comprehensive guidelines connecting the specific genetic variants in these genes, or the specific mechanisms these genes support, to genetic vulnerability for dyslexia or its specific components. These guidelines need to be as clear and as robust as possible, presenting a list of vulnerability genetic mechanisms and identifying risks associated with these mechanisms. On the basis of current knowledge in the field of reading disability (Bates et al., 2011; Meaburn et al., 2008; Newbury et al., 2011; Paracchini et al., 2008) and of other common disorders (Khoury, Little, Gwinn, & Ioannidis, 2007), it would appear that the relative risks associated with each of these vulnerability genetic mechanisms are of small magnitude (e.g., as determined by genetic association studies, the estimated relative risk for common diseases is around 1.5 [Khoury, Little, et al., 2007]). Thus we may be confronted either by a long list of genetic risk variants for dyslexia or discover a type of clustering for these variants that results in a substantial magnification of risk when more than one variant is present in an individual.

It is likely that moving through Khoury's stages is not going to be easy. Even if the first-stage findings are convincingly validated at the second stage, and the variability of current findings can be rendered meaningful in some way, the challenges of stages three and four will need to be overcome before it will be possible to determine the ultimate value of genetic and genomic studies for the prevention and treatment of reading disability.

An unfortunate mark of the rapid development of genome-based sciences and technologies has been a popularization – to the point of hyperbole – of the scale and immediacy of the application of these developments to health-related practices (Davey Smith et al., 2005; Kamerow, 2008). The field of genetic studies of reading dis(ability) is not free of such phenomena either (for discussion, see Dorothy Bishop's blog at http://deevybee.blogspot.co.uk/2013/06/overhyped-genetic-findings-case-of.html?m=1). Such harmful popularization, coupled with commercial potential, has often resulted in ill-justified use of genetic and genomic testing for susceptibility to complex disorders, mostly with no clear application or guidance for proper utilization of this knowledge.

Summary: genetic bases

Over the past century, there has been substantial growth in our understanding of the role of genes and the genome in reading and reading disability. While it has been clearly established that reading is, in part, controlled by genes, there continues to be limited knowledge and understanding of the role genetic factors play in reading development. A proliferation of inconsistent and contrasting findings, together with recognition of the role of bioecological gene by environment interactions, has added to the complexity of this field. Recognition of such complexity, however, represents an important counter to overly simplistic and unrealistic expectations that a simple genetic account could materialize. As McCardle and Miller (2012, p. 336) note:

Genes are important, but they are not the whole story; they are not a final determination. The environment in which a child is raised, the parenting, nutrition, healthcare, peer relations, and education . . . can influence the expression of those genes. These factors can also influence in ways that are not fully understood the plasticity of the nervous system set in motion by those genes.

Although there is promise for the future arising from new developments such as the Human Genome Project, it is important to note that existing knowledge in the field of genetics cannot help resolve the dyslexia debate to any significant degree. Currently we are unable to progress beyond a recognition that reading disability has a genetic component, or even an understanding of some possible specifics of these components, to a knowledge base capable of informing differential diagnosis and individualized forms of intervention.

The promise of neurobiology for resolving the dyslexia debate

Advances in neuroscience and genetics of reading and reading disability over the past decade have been substantial. As this chapter has shown, we now have far greater insight into the biological bases of reading and reading failure. However, this has highlighted the immense complexities involved and the inappropriateness of simple explanations or recommendations. As is often the case, the more we learn, the more we appreciate the limits of our understanding. For this reason, scientists in these fields have needed to be circumspect about the steps that must be progressed before insights from their work can be used to inform educational and clinical applications. Work in the fields of neuroscience and genetics offers great potential for assisting the resolution of the dyslexia debate. However, we are still a long way from reaching that position.

4 Assessment and intervention

Introduction

A 22-year-old woman was condemned to 'temporary menial tasks', the High Court heard. P.P. claims that she is of average intelligence but because her learning difficulty was not discovered until two months before she left school, she never learned to read and write properly.... Tests were carried out at infant, junior and comprehensive schools. At the age of 10 she was found to be four years behind in reading and writing skills but the reason was never identified. (*The Guardian* newspaper, July 27, 1997, p. 5)

The much publicized Pamela Phelps (P.P.) case in the United Kingdom seems to provide a perfect illustration of the key difficulties arising from debates on the existence and utility of the concept of dyslexia and the relevance of such a diagnosis for intervention. The case centered on the assertion that if a diagnosis of dyslexia had been forthcoming at an earlier stage of Phelps's school career, her difficulties would more likely have been overcome. However, there was no suggestion that her literacy difficulties had not been recognized. An educational (school) psychologist had assessed her at primary school and on transfer to secondary school at age eleven; further assessment indicated that she had a reading accuracy age equivalent of 7 years and 3 months. She left school with a reading age equivalent of 8 years.

Although there have been cases of children with severe reading disabilities failing to receive specialist assistance, this was evidently not the case here; Phelps had received remedial help in English and mathematics. The grounds for the claim did not center on the presence or absence of psychological assessment and in-school support, but rather the failure to diagnose Phelps's dyslexia. Such a diagnosis, it was claimed, would have pointed to the most appropriate form of intervention – a highly structured, multisensory approach to the teaching of reading. The key issue arising from this case in relation to the dyslexia debate is whether there are forms of intervention particularly designed for dyslexic children that are not also appropriate for all children who experience word reading difficulties.

In examining how intervention relates to the dyslexia debate, it is necessary to pose the following questions: (1) How can we best identify young children at risk of word reading difficulties and use this information to prevent later problems? (2) What can be done to help those who are resistant to initial interventions? (3) Is there anything special about specialist dyslexia teaching that is particularly effective for a subgroup of poor readers? Prior to considering each of these issues, it is first necessary to consider the claims of two very different philosophies concerning how reading should be best taught.

The reading wars

In many ways the fierce controversy over the teaching of reading, sometimes described as the "great debate" (Chall, 1996) or the "reading wars," reflects broader value-laden disputes between traditionalist and progressive approaches to education. In the traditionalist reading camp were those who emphasized bottom-up approaches dominated by phonics, defined as "an approach to, or type of, reading instruction that is intended to promote the discovery of the alphabetic principle, the correspondences between phonemes and graphemes, and phonological decoding" (Scarborough and Brady, 2002, p. 326). In contrast, the progressives, with a heritage stretching back to Deweyian-inspired child-centered approaches (Pearson, 2004) advocated top-down whole-language approaches in which an emphasis on textual meaning had primacy. For this latter group,

phonics is regarded as the polar opposite of whole language; it is rigid, authoritarian and fanatically concerned with the acquisition of skills such as spelling. Phonics is seen as deeply anti-democratic, and its critics, defenders of whole language, find it inconsistent with the abstract values of progressive education. (Anderson, 2000, p. 5)

Underpinning the debate were clear differences between the camps as to the extent to which reading was seen as a natural process. Advocates of the whole-language approach tended to argue that children learn to read naturally even in the absence of explicit or systematic instruction. Thus, Goodman (1986, p. 24) stated:

Why do people create and learn written language? They need it! How do they learn it? The same way they learn oral language, by using it in authentic literacy events that meet their needs. Often children have trouble learning written language in school. It's not because it's harder than learning oral language, or learned differently. It's because we've made it hard by trying to make it easy.

Goodman contended that the use of structured skills-based approaches, largely divorced from any meaningful context, were inadvisable. However, this position, widely espoused by advocates of the whole-language approach, does not reflect contemporary scientific understandings in which reading, unlike speech, is not naturally acquired (Liberman, 1999; Perfetti, 1991; Share, 1995, 1999; Stanovich, 2000; Tunmer & Nicholson, 2011). Language – an evolved behavior that developed from the origins of humanity – is very different from literacy, a cultural invention that has only featured in the past few millennia (Pennington & Olson, 2005). Steven Pinker, the celebrated neuroscientist, notes:

Language is a human instinct, but written language is not. Language is found in all societies, present and past. . . . All healthy children master their own language without lessons or corrections. When children are thrown together without a usable language, they invent one of their own. Compare all this with writing. Writing systems have been invented a small number of times in history. . . . Until recently, most children never learned to read or write; even with today's universal education, many children struggle and fail. A group of children is no more likely to invent an alphabet than it is to invent the internal combustion engine.

Children are wired for sound, but print is an optional accessory that must be painstakingly bolted on. This basic fact about human nature should be the starting point for any discussion of how to teach our children to read and write. (Pinker, 1998, p. ix)

The debate as to whether children learn better with an initial method that emphasizes meaning or one that stresses learning the code has a long history stretching back to the nineteenth century (Chall, 1996; Snow & Juel, 2005) and is closely associated with the rising and waning influence of a diverse range of interest groups (Song & Miskel, 2002). In the United States, whole word, sight reading was the dominant methodology from the 1920s until the 1960s. However, in a highly influential text, *Why Johnny Can't Read*, Flesch (1955) attacked the "look and say" whole-word approach because, he argued, a lack of skill in phonics limited children's ability to read books that did not contain the carefully controlled vocabularies that were being used.

Supported by a broad spectrum of U.S. conservative interest groups (Burnett, 1998), phonics gained influence throughout the 1960s and 1970s. However, by the 1980s, whole-language approaches, fueled by the seminal writing of Smith (1971) and Goodman (1965, 1969, 1970), and backed by the vigorous support of university education departments and professional associations for teachers of English, had regained their former influence. The dominant picture was one whereby reading was primarily a linguistic, rather than a perceptual, process (Pearson, 2004). Goodman's (1967) description of the reading process as a "psycholinguistic guessing game" reflected a view of the skilled reader as one who drew on contextual clues and background knowledge to enable the identification of words. Teachers were trained to undertake "miscue analysis" in which the child's oral reading errors were classified on the basis of semantic, syntactic, or graphophonic factors. This information could then be used to help children become more skilled in the guessing process. However, numerous research studies have now established that prediction on the basis of contextual information has tended to be overemphasized as a means of facilitating word identification (Adams, 1990; Gough, 1983; Snow & Juel, 2005). Indeed, it appears that contextual cues are more likely to be relied on by poorer readers who need to find ways to compensate for their poor decoding skills (Stanovich, 1980; Tunmer & Chapman, 2003). As Pressley (2006, p. 164) observed:

[P]erhaps the most disturbing conclusion that comes from this research is that teaching children to decode by giving primacy to semantic-contextual and syntactic-contextual cues over graphemic-phonemic cues is equivalent to teaching them to read the way weak readers read!

By emphasizing the communicative function of written language (Stahl & Miller, 1989) the whole language approach proved popular with classroom teachers. Its use of bright and appealing children's literature – so-called real books – compared favorably with the often visually and linguistically sterile texts that were typically used as basal readers. In contrast, phonics approaches were seen to be taking meaning and context out of reading and replacing these with lists and drills that reduced children's interest and motivation. However, with all the polemic, the need to achieve balance was overlooked, and in some cases, whole-language proponents seemed to concentrate on increasing children's interest in reading rather than on how to make them better readers. Zane (2005), for example, cites a teacher survey in which respondents tended to see research into motivation to read as more important than conducting scientific investigations into how to best improve reading comprehension.

Whole-language approaches also played out differently in terms of teacher identity. Unlike the heavy prescription and structure of phonics instruction, teacher professionalism and autonomy were emphasized by the whole-language approach (Snow & Juel, 2005), leading Goodman (1992) to claim that teachers were regaining confidence in their professional evaluations of themselves and their pupils. Unfortunately, appeal to teacher professionalism often took place in a climate that was antagonistic to scientific research approaches and dismissive of notions of objectivity.

During the 1990s, the debate became particularly polarized and often heated on both sides of the Atlantic (Chall, 2000). As Calfee and Norman (1998) remarked, "A battle is raging" (p. 244). In the United Kingdom, the government's Department of Education and Science refused to publish its sponsored teacher training package, *Language in the National Curriculum*, to an outrage from many teacher education departments, partly because "it didn't bang on sufficiently about phonics" (Goddard, 1991, p. 32).

By the turn of the century, the pendulum was swinging away from the whole-language camp. A range of factors was involved in the demise of this previously

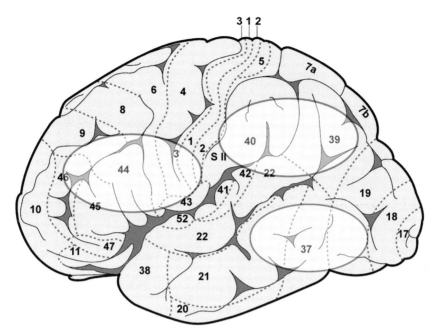

Figure 3.1 The consensual view of the neuronal network of reading: left inferior frontal (anterior component region, recruiting, partially, Brodmann areas, BA, 44, 45, and 6), posterior dorsal (temporoparietal region, recruiting, partially, BA 39 and 40), and posterior ventral (ventral occipitotemporal, recruiting, partially, BA 19, 21, and 37) brain areas. Adapted from Démonet, Taylor, and Chaix (2004).

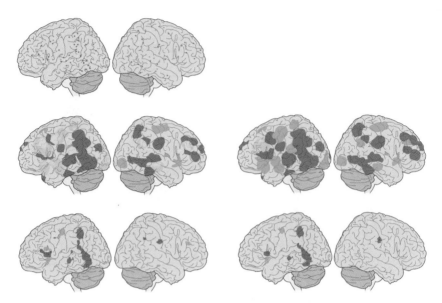

Figure 3.2 **(Top left)** Surface rendering of all input foci with underactivation (69) in red and overactivation (59) in green meta-analyzed by Richlan, Kronbichler, and wimmer (2009). **(Middle left)** Overlays of the separate maps for under- and overactivation, respectively; regions displayed in both maps are shown in yellow. **(Middle right)** Surface rendering of the difference map (after subtracting underactivation indicators from overactivation indicators). The blurred coloring results from discrepant activations at surface and deeper regions. **(Bottom left)** Surface rendering of the unthresholded difference map. **(Bottom right)** Surface rendering of the thresholded difference map. Adapted from Richlan, Kronbichler, and Wimmer (2009).

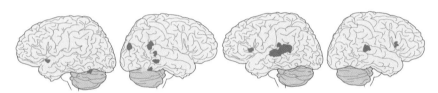

Figure 3.3 An illustration of a profound change (i.e., redistribution of activity from the right to the left hemisphere) in the pattern of brain activation evoked by a reading remediation program in a single participant. The maps were obtained using a pseudo-word rhyme-matching task before (left-hand columns) and after (right-hand columns) intensive remedial instruction. Adapted from Simos et al. (2002).

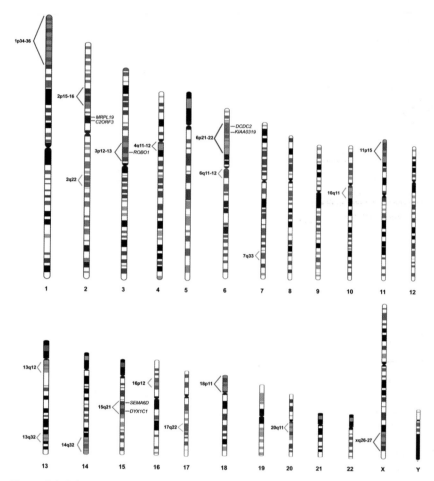

Figure 3.4 Selected susceptibility loci those (that have more citations in the literature are shown in red, and those less – shown in blue) and candidate genes identified through studies of probands with reading disability and their families. Note: often a particular susceptibility locus (e.g., 2p, 6p, and 15q) has more than one candidate gene, emphasizing both the underlying complexity of the phenotype under investigation and the imprecision of the field.

dominant approach, several of which were primarily ideological. Particularly relevant was the widespread political and, in some quarters, professional, mistrust of the qualitative, interpretivist research tradition with its embrace of individual classroom ethnographies and teacher action research. In its place

a "new" brand of experimental work began to appear . . . with great emphasis placed on "reliable, replicable research," large samples, random assignment of treatment to teachers/and or schools, and tried and true outcome measures. It finds its aegis in the experimental rhetoric of science and medicine and in the laboratory research that has examined reading as a perceptual process. (Pearson, 2004, p. 225)

This trend was clearly evident in the convening of a National Reading Panel in the United States in 1997 that was charged with providing a scientific review of reading research. Its heavily quantitative focus (utilizing meta-analytic techniques wherever possible) and exclusion of nonexperimental studies (e.g., ethnographic studies of students learning to read) clearly reflected the decline in influence of the interpretivist tradition.

The subsequent National Reading Panel Report (2000) considered research undertaken in five key areas between 1966 and 1997: alphabetics, fluency, comprehension, teacher education, and technology. In the alphabetics section the Panel gave close attention to instruction in phonemic/phonological awareness, as this, together with letter knowledge, appeared to be the best predictor of children's early reading progress. The results of a meta-analysis of 52 studies that satisfied the panel's demanding scientific criteria were described as "impressive." Findings showed that incorporating phonemic awareness training in instruction improved children's reading significantly more than programs that did not use such an approach. The Report also indicated that systematic phonics instruction enhanced children's ability to learn to read and noted that this was more effective than instruction that taught little or no phonics. While the impact of phonics was strongest in the early years, it also proved beneficial for older students who struggled to learn to read. However, echoing a conclusion from another major review produced two years earlier by the National Research Council (Snow, Burns, & Griffin, 1998), it was emphasized that a balanced approach to the teaching of reading was necessary in which phonemic awareness training and phonics instruction were important components.

The outcome of the reading wars was widely perceived to represent a victory for those who emphasized skills instruction but, as noted earlier, this outcome was generally tempered by agreement that a balance of approaches was necessary (although see Stanovich [2000], for a discussion about the fierce resistance to notions of scientific evidence by whole-language advocates). Of course, balance is a rather slippery concept, and as Calfee and Norman (1998) observe, no one in this debate has argued for an unbalanced position, and those in both camps have tended to see their opponents as holding extreme views.

Further evidence that teachers need to look to a balanced approach in which phonics instruction is but one element was provided in a research synthesis of reading programs for children in the elementary grades (Slavin et al., 2009). Beginning reading programs that were found to be effective or promising had a strong focus on teaching phonics and phonemic awareness, although caution was expressed against any assumption that a heavy emphasis on phonics can prove sufficient to achieve positive effects (see also van der Leij (2013) for the limitation at a narrow emphasis upon phoneme awareness). Increasing the amount of time devoted to phonics will not necessarily result in further significant gains (Gamse, Tepper-Jacob, Horst, Boulay, & Unlu, 2008; Moss et al., 2008). Of significant importance are the way that reading is taught and the skills of teachers in delivering programs (Connor, 2010; Slavin et al., 2009). The content of programs is also influential and it generally understood that teachers should address the key components of linguistic awareness – phonological, orthographic, and morphological – that are important for learning to read (Berninger, Abbott, Nagy, & Carlisle, 2010).

For children at risk of reading disability, the rejection of systematic skills instruction by the more extreme advocates of the whole-language movement was particularly unhelpful. The tedious and decontextualized drills of the 1970s may have been far from ideal for motivating young readers, yet, in the shift toward "authenticity," balance was sacrificed and the advantages of structured instruction in basic skills were often overlooked (Pearson, 2004). In the heat of the reading wars it was not always acknowledged that approaches to the teaching of reading may not be uniformly appropriate for all levels of ability. Those with reading difficulties, irrespective of whether these are predominantly of biological or environmental origin, are more likely to be undermined by whole-language approaches that neglect explicit instruction of letter-sound relationships (Juel & Minden-Cupp, 2000; Stanovich, 2000; Tunmer & Nicholson, 2011; Tunmer & Prochnow, 2009). They are less able than their normally achieving peers to discover letter-sound patterns as a consequence of reading, and for this reason, more explicit teaching is required (Calfee & Drum, 1986). Such instruction should not leave essential skills and knowledge to be discovered by the child on their own (Torgesen, 2004).

Whereas "attention to small units in early reading instruction is helpful for all children, harmful for none, and crucial for some" (Snow & Juel, 2005, p. 518), a very high level of structured intervention may not be necessary or, indeed, ideal for all (Arrow & Tunmer, 2012). Thus, in a comparative study of stronger and weaker readers, Juel and Minden-Cupp (2000) found that first grade children with limited reading skills made more progress in classrooms where there was greater emphasis on word recognition instruction. In contrast, those with stronger skills benefited more from a literature-rich environment with reduced emphasis on basic decoding. Similarly, in a study of first graders, Connor,

Morrison, and Katch (2004) found that an emphasis on explicit teaching of decoding skills was beneficial for those children with low initial decoding skills but had no effect for those with high initial scores. Interestingly, and underlying the importance of this debate for reading-disabled children, the influence of classroom instruction, positive or negative, was greater for those with poor decoding skills and weaker vocabulary than for those with strengths in these areas. Thus, the suggestion that a common balanced approach is suitable for all children is overly simplistic and potentially misleading. Instead, the available evidence suggests that the particular emphasis of differing instructional strategies in any given context should be adjusted to reflect students' differing skill levels (Connor, 2010; Connor et al., 2007 and particular domains of reading difficulty (Connor et al., 2009).

Irrespective of the child's reading skills, however, it is now widely accepted that a systematic phonics approach usually leads to superior reading skills when compared with a non-phonics or nonsystematic phonics approach. This appears to be true for both opaque (Ehri, Nunes, Stahl, & Willows, 2001) and transparent (de Graaff, Bosman, Hasselman, & Verhoeven, 2009) languages. However, rather than providing phonics teaching in a narrow, decontextualized fashion, teachers need to root such instruction within a broad-based literacy curriculum that includes reading for meaning and writing (Torgerson, Brooks, & Hall, 2006), and the development of oral and written language comprehension skills (Bianco et al., 2010).

Identifying young children at risk of word reading difficulties and using this information to prevent later problems

Identifying those at risk of reading disability

While research has consistently demonstrated that the development of reading competence can be maximized by the provision of effective instructional experiences in the early years (Francis et al., 1996; Snow et al., 1998), high-quality whole class inputs are not sufficient for all (Brooks, 2007). For those children most at risk of difficulty, some form of preventive supplementary intervention appears to be superior to waiting to conduct remedial interventions with those subsequently identified as reading disabled (Ehri, Nunes, Willows et al., 2001).

A focus on intervening early where a child has special educational needs has long been recognized by practitioners, researchers, and policy makers. In the United States, support for such children was boosted by the passage in 2002 of the No Child Left Behind Act (NCLB) and, in 2004, by the Individuals with Disabilities Education Act (IDEA; U.S. Department of Education, 2004). NCLB placed a great emphasis on early intervention, high-quality evidence-based instruction, and accountability for educational outcomes.

IDEA provided encouragement for early intervention and permitted a model of service delivery that involved screening children for academic and behavioral problems, close monitoring of progress, and, where deemed necessary in light of the child's progress, the provision of increasingly intense interventions. Such legislation has helped fuel the development of highly structured and sophisticated programs of reading intervention for very young children who are at risk of developing reading difficulties. It has also highlighted the importance of conducting high-quality research to evaluate program effectiveness.

While traditional "wait to fail" models have meant that children with reading disability have typically not been identified until they reached second grade or higher (Schatschneider, Wagner, & Crawford, 2008), with all the deleterious motivational consequences that can ensue (Snowling & Hulme, 2011), the accountability provisions of the U.S. No Child Left Behind legislation and the widespread take-up of responsive approaches to instruction have resulted in attempts to provide screening in kindergarten (Santi et al., 2009). As discussed in Chapter 1, a tiered system, Response to Intervention (RTI), typically but not exclusively of three levels, has been increasingly adopted in many countries as a means to provide a swift response as early in the child's educational career as possible. At the level of primary intervention (Tier 1), forms of instruction that have been shown to be most effective are provided by classroom teachers. It is anticipated that such provision will be appropriate for the majority of children. Those who fail to make adequate progress receive secondary intervention (Tier 2), which usually takes the form of supplemental small-group instruction with systematic monitoring of children's progress to ascertain its effectiveness. For those who continue to experience difficulty, tertiary intervention (Tier 3) involves more intensive small-group or individual instruction with a significant emphasis on ongoing assessment, feedback, and monitoring. In practice, the distinction between Tier 2 and Tier 3 is often more of degree than of kind, and the major differences between the tiers usually concern the intensity of the intervention and the precision of the measurements (Reschly, 2005). While there are many debates and controversies about this approach, particularly its ability to predict outcomes for particular subgroups (Stuebing, Fletcher, & Hughes, 2012; Tran et al., 2011), it does appear that it can generally help to improve the performance of those with reading disabilities.

While RTI approaches were principally designed to identify children who were failing to respond to instruction, the approach has also been used to assist in the identification of those who may be at risk of future learning difficulty (Santi et al., 2009; VanDerHeyden, 2011). However, accurately ascertaining risk status for very young children is a problematic enterprise (Catts et al., 2009; Fuchs et al., 2008; Puolakanaho et al., 2007) with estimates of false positives ranging from 20% to 60% (Jenkins & O'Connor, 2002; Torgesen, 2002) and false negatives between 10% and 50% (Catts, 1991; Scarborough, 1998; Torgesen, 2002). False positives refer to decisions that children are at risk when they are not; false negatives are decisions that children are not at risk when, in actuality, they are. The proportion of true and false positives and negatives will be a function of the cut-off point used for screening, but such points have yet to be established and validated (Tannock, 2013). Most likely, these will be arbitrary as a response to intervention would seem to be best located on a continuum (Fletcher & Vaughn, 2009). However, the more lenient the cut-off, the more likely that a larger number of positive cases, both true and false, will be identified. False negatives can result in children at risk failing to receive the additional intervention that they require (Jenkins, Hudson, & Johnson, 2007). In contrast, the identification of false positives can lead to the inappropriate use of scarce resources (Jenkins & O'Connor, 2002), although some (Scanlon et al., 2005) are less concerned about this on the grounds that wrongly identified kindergarten children will still benefit from specialized interventions. Moreover, interventions focusing on emergent literacy skills are often less intensive than may be necessary in the later years and thus relatively inexpensive.

In seeking to identify children at risk at as young an age as possible there is risk that initial assessments will be undertaken before children have had sufficient experience of literacy-based activities, thus likely increasing the number of false positives. At this age, literacy experience and instruction have a significant influence on performance on measures of letter knowledge and phonological awareness that are typically found in screening assessments (Catts, Petscher, Schatschneider, Bridges, & Mendoza, 2009). The difficulty of screening for skills that are often in rapid development has been likened to hitting a moving target (Speece, 2005). It is important to note in this respect that a significant proportion of children in kindergarten and Grade1 who are progressing appropriately in the development of early literacy skills, such as phonemic segmentation and knowledge of letter sounds and names [variables that predict response to reading intervention in kindergarten (Hagan-Burke et al., 2013)], later demonstrate word reading problems, particularly when multisyllabic words are introduced (O'Connor et al., in press).

For such reasons, it has been argued that it is better to delay screening until the first grade (Fletcher et al., 2002; Hurford, Potter, & Hart, 2002) when, it is easier to draw on measures that are more closely aligned to real reading. Experiences in kindergarten will often have reduced the differential impact of language and literacy experience in the home, and later measurement will be more accurate, given that precision typically increases in line with maturation (Compton et al., 2006).

An alternative option that is increasingly being advocated by RTI researchers is to avoid making screening decisions on the basis of a one-off measure and, instead, utilise multistage assessment.[1] Assessment on the basis of progress is also not without its methodological problems particularly when used with very young children. Some infants may not have sufficient cognitive, linguistic, or attentional maturity to respond to the tasks in ways that will reveal their true potential. For others, significant gains may be made in kindergarten, which cannot be sustained in later years, particularly where the home environment is suboptimal (Kieffer, 2012). Thus Al Otaiba et al. (2011) found that a good response on a variety of language and literacy measures in kindergarten, across a diverse range of schools, was not a good predictor of first grade performance. They suggested that this was probably because low-scoring children tended to have more room for growth when entering kindergarten than did their more advantaged peers. Such gains may mask the true extent of some children's difficulties, and as a result, their need for specialized support in first grade may not be recognized.

Measures of growth can also be problematic in first grade. Using an oral reading fluency measure, Schatschneider, Wagner, and Crawford (2008) examined first grade performance gains over four time points. Growth failed to add unique information to the prediction of future reading skills beyond that which could be obtained from a one-off, end-of-year assessment. However, a more encouraging finding is reported by Zumeta, Compton, and Fuchs (2012) who employed a measure of word identification fluency (WIF), involving the reading of isolated words, rather than words in connected text as typically found in oral reading fluency measures. This approach, utilizing regular weekly measurements, appeared to be useful for both screening and monitoring progress. The value of WIF for monitoring the progress of poor readers in first grade has also been demonstrated by Clemens et al. (in press).

Allocations to good or poor responder groups can vary according to the particular measures and criteria that are applied (Beach & O'Connor, in press), and prediction can be aided by the use of multiple measures, the particular nature of which will vary as a function of grade level (Fletcher et al., 2002), yet the time involved to administer these can be prohibitive for the purposes of universal screening. One option is to introduce a two-stage approach to assessment in which an initial measure given to all children is used to identify those who may be at risk of developing reading disability; this smaller group would then receive a multivariate screening battery. Such an approach was utilized by Compton et al. (2010), who found their "two-step gated procedure"

---

[1]   RTI assessment should also involve examination of children's progress in performance over time, although this issue has received far less researcher attention than has screening, perhaps because the latter tends to be easier and less expensive to conduct (Fuchs & Vaughn, 2012).

to be an effective means of increasing screening efficiency for first grade children.

There are many measures available for screening young children at risk of reading disability. These can be divided into those that directly address underlying reading skills and others, often explicitly seeking to identify underlying dyslexia, that introduce other, supposedly related, skills. Those of the former approach tend to include measures of phonemic awareness, letter-naming fluency, concepts about print, word reading, and oral language fluency (Compton et al., 2010). Examples of such approaches in the United States include the Texas Primary Reading Inventory (TPRI; Foorman, Fletcher, & Francis, 2004) and the Dynamic Indicators of Basic Early Literacy Skills (DIBELS; Good & Kaminski, 2003).

The TPRI, designed for kindergarten through to third grade, comprises both a screening and an inventory component. The screening section is designed to identify children at risk of reading disability and employs measures of knowledge of letter sounds and names and phonemic awareness. The measure was reported as scoring highly on all indices of reliability, with few false negatives – estimated at less than 10% in the measure's Technical Report (Foorman et al., 1998, p. 8). However, it was acknowledged that relatively high false positive rates (below 45%) were found for kindergarten and first grade children (Foorman et al., 1998).

The DIBELS was originally designed to measure progress over time for children from kindergarten to sixth grade but is now widely used within RTI models of practice as a screening tool to identify children who may be at risk of reading disabilities (Office of Inspector General of the U.S. Department of Education, 2007). This tool initially consisted of seven measures, five of which directly address underlying decoding skills: two involving phonological awareness (fluency in identifying initial sounds of given words and segmenting the phonemes in a word), two involving knowledge of the alphabetic principle (fluency in letter naming and nonsense word reading), and oral reading fluency of connected text. Reported reliabilities are sound (Good et al., 2004), although concern has been expressed about the equivalencies of some of the reading passages. If these differ in demand, it is possible that the particular passage selected at a given measurement point might affect perceptions as to whether a child's performance has changed substantially, for the better or the worse (Scanlon, 2011). Zumeta et al. (2012), for example, found that for low-achieving first grade children, a measure with a broad range of high-frequency words appeared to be a better predictor than one using a more narrowly sampled list. Since its inception, DIBELS has been regularly revised and updated, and is currently operating a seventh edition, DIBELS Next.

Catts et al. (2009) surveyed findings from DIBELS screening in relation to progress for more than 18,000 children enrolled in the Florida Reading

First program. They found significant floor effects that obscured individual differences between those at the lower end of the distribution, and poor predictability. These difficulties were not tied to a particular grade level but were a feature of initial administrations of the measures. Predictability improved as further administrations took place, although problems remained with the initial sound and phoneme segmentation tasks. Noting that other measures of phonological awareness (e.g., the Comprehensive Test of Phonological Processing [Wagner, Torgesen, & Rashotte, 1999] and the Phonological Awareness Test [Robertson & Salter, 1997]) also show floor effects at the beginning of kindergarten, the authors emphasized the importance of not only selecting the correct screening instrument but also ensuring that this is administered at the right time. Although delaying the assessment may help, this leaves open the possibility that identification of children at risk of reading disability will also be delayed.

Exactly when screening takes place within the kindergarten year may not be greatly important, however. In a large-scale study of more than 3,000 children (Santi, York, Foorman, & Francis, 2009), it was found that the timing of screening during the kindergarten year appeared to have little impact on the results. This finding supports the observation of Catts et al. (2009) that it is familiarity with the test content and procedures, rather than the particular age of the child, that is most important. Difficulties concerning the accuracy of DIBELS when used as a screening tool with very young children, in particular the problem of identifying an excessive proportion of false positives, are discussed in detail by E. S. Johnson et al. (2009).

Dyslexia screening tests often include a broader range of items than are typically found in academic screening programs. Thus, in its 12 subtests, the Dyslexia Early Screening Test – 2nd edition (DEST; Nicolson & Fawcett, 2004), designed for children 4.5 to 6.5 years, includes measures of rapid naming, memory, shape copying, postural stability, and bead threading. Interestingly, a variant of this measure with very similar items (for children aged 3.6 to 6.5 years), primarily geared for the U.S. market, "Ready to Learn" (Fawcett, Nicolson, & Lee, 2004), makes no reference to dyslexia in its publisher's description. Instead, it is stated that this tool is designed to identify children at risk of reading difficulty. This terminological distinction reflects the conceptual and definitional tensions raised in Chapter 1. This research group has also produced the Pre-School Screening Test in the United Kingdom (Lee, Nicolson, & Fawcett, 2001) with items similar to those in DEST. However, its description also makes no reference to dyslexia but instead refers to its purpose of identifying children aged 3.6–4.5 years who might require additional support in their education.

Fine and gross motor skills of various kinds feature in many dyslexia checklists, although their role in screening and diagnosis has long been contentious (see Chapter 2). According to Crombie and Reid (2009), early identification of future literacy difficulties can be made from observations of very young children, with early pointers including a "lack of coordination and sequencing skills as the baby struggles to learn to crawl (or simply does not bother to crawl)" (p. 72). Such indicators might form part of a wider range of signs, including poor early rhyming and alliteration skills and a known family history of dyslexia (Molfese et al., 2008; Viholainen et al., 2002). However, despite the appeal of motor assessment to many, the evidence base for its predictive validity in relation to reading disability is weak (Barth et al., 2010). Although the DEST authors claim that postural stability is "one of the best predictors of resistance to remediation" (Nicolson & Fawcett, 2004, p. 15), Barth and colleagues found little evidence to link performance on either of the two motor subtests to reading proficiency or to response to intervention. The most powerful predictors proved to be phonological awareness and rapid naming of letters. Similarly, Simpson and Everatt (2005) found that some DEST subtests – sound order (a measure of auditory perception), rapid naming (of familiar outline pictures), and knowledge of lowercase letter names – proved to be better predictors of reading and spelling performance than did the total score.

Identification of "at risk" status can help prevent early difficulties from impairing subsequent academic progress. Screening may be used not only to identify children who are at risk but also to highlight those poor readers who are likely to struggle even when additional help is given. Such children may need to be given more intensive support at an earlier stage than would typically be the case (Al Otaiba & Fuchs, 2006).

Several studies have been undertaken to identify the variables that can best identify those young children who will struggle to progress despite being provided with additional help. Most have pointed to difficulties with phonological awareness, rapid naming, vocabulary, and oral language skills as the most common cognitive attributes of poor responders (Fletcher et al., 2011). Al Otaiba and Fuchs (2002) reviewed 23 studies and identified phonological awareness as the strongest predictor of poor responsiveness. Another review, involving a meta-analysis of 30 studies (Nelson, Benner, & Gonzalez, 2003) – many of these having also been selected by Al Otaiba and Fuchs (2002) for their own review – highlighted rapid naming, phonological awareness, and letter knowledge as the strongest predictors (see Torppa et al., 2013, for a similar finding in the case of Finnish children). It also has been suggested that dynamic assessment approaches, which assess students' response to assistance provided during the testing procedure (Elliott, 2003; Grigorenko & Sternberg, 1998), can add predictive power in relation to individuals' responsiveness to small group (Tier 2) intervention (Cho et al., in press).

In seeking to identify methods and measures that can be used to predict subsequent reading disability, it is easy to forget that a significant variable will be the classroom environment, involving such elements as the influence of classmates, the nature of the curriculum, and the level of teacher skills. Accordingly, Compton et al. (2010) have suggested that future prediction models might be enhanced by examination of both child- and classroom-level effects. However, research on the influence of particular teacher variables on student learning suggests only weak or inconsistent relationships (Goe, 2007), and teachers' domain-specific knowledge about reading-related skills does not appear to influence reading outcomes in kindergarten (Cirino et al., 2007; Hagan-Burke et al., 2013).

Interventions for those at risk of reading disability

The goal of secondary interventions is that struggling readers will be enabled to catch up with their peers. While the precise balance of activities needs to be tailored to the particular strengths and weaknesses of the student, key elements of literacy instruction are as follows (Vaughn & Roberts, 2007):

- phonemic awareness
- phonics
- spelling/writing
- fluency
- vocabulary
- comprehension

Over the past two decades, a vast raft of studies utilizing structured approaches to intervention have generally produced positive outcomes showing that young children at risk of reading disability can be helped to make significant gains in basic reading skills (Denton et al., 2010; Duff, Hayiou-Thomas, & Hulme, 2012; Foorman et al., 2010; Fuchs et al., 2008; Hatcher et al., 2006; Kamps et al., 2008; Mathes et al., 2005; Ryder, Tunmer, & Greaney, 2008; Scanlon et al., 2005; Torgesen, 2007; Torgesen et al., 1999; Vadasy, Sanders, & Abbott, 2008; Vellutino et al., 2006, 2008; Wanzek & Vaughn, 2007). Most studies have stressed the particular value of phonics-based approaches, a finding emphasized in a recent analysis of one-on-one tutoring programs for struggling readers (Slavin et al., 2011), where it was reported that those schemes with less emphasis on phonics (e.g. *Reading Recovery* [Clay, 1985]) tended to have smaller effect sizes. However, this finding is rather more relevant to young children as the use of phonics tends to be less powerful for older struggling readers (Flynn, Zheng, & Swanson, 2012). In addition, it should be noted that there is some evidence that training in phonics for struggling readers is rendered more powerful by additional instruction in sight word reading (McArthur et al., 2013).

Beyond basic decoding, improving poor performance in other areas of reading has proven to be more of a challenge. While some progress in helping students with weaknesses in reading fluency and/or comprehension has been reported (Begeny et al., 2011; Fuchs et al., 1997; Hasbrouck, Ihnot, & Rogers, 1999; Pressley & Wharton-McDonald, 1997), developing automaticity and fluency in respect of the component skills of reading has often proven to be particularly problematic for children who struggle with decoding (Blachman et al., 2004; Denton et al., 2010; Rashotte, MacPhee, & Torgesen, 2001; Ryder et al., 2008; Torgesen, 2000, 2007).

In a series of intervention studies, Vellutino and colleagues (Scanlon et al., 2005; Vellutino, Scanlon, & Jaccard, 2003; Vellutino, Scanlon, & Lyon, 2000; Vellutino et al., 1996; Vellutino, Scanlon, & Tanzman, 1998) have repeatedly demonstrated the powerful effect of early intervention. In their 1996 study (Vellutino et al., 1996), daily one-on-one tutoring was provided to first grade children scoring below the 15th percentile on measures of word and pseudoword reading. Those who failed to make adequate progress received further help in second grade. The total amount of assistance ranged from 35 to 65 hours. It was found that 67.1% of the tutored children could be brought to within the average range of reading ability in just one semester of remediation and most could maintain this level of functioning when reassessed at the end of the fourth grade.

Vellutino, Scanlon and their colleagues (Scanlon et al., 2005, 2008) have also examined interventions in kindergarten for children at risk of reading difficulty. It was found that small-group instruction, with a heavy emphasis on the development of phonological processing skills, provided for two 30 minute sessions each week throughout the school year (and continued in first grade), reduced the number of children who qualified as poor readers in first grade (Scanlon et al., 2005). Moreover, this intervention reduced the number of children who were still struggling with reading at the end of first grade (treatment resisters). Indeed, at the end of first grade, none of the children who had received the kindergarten intervention, plus a first grade program emphasizing the development of phonological skills, obtained a standard score below 85 on the Basic Skills subtest of the Woodcock Reading Mastery Test (WRMT-R; Woodcock, 1987). In light of their findings, the authors suggest that a powerful means of reducing treatment resistance is to provide modest amounts of small-group intervention in kindergarten before early differences in literacy skills are exacerbated by subsequent failure to profit from classroom instruction. These should be followed up in first grade by an intensive intervention with a particular focus on the development of phonological skills.

However, it is important to note that the gains that arise from such work will not necessarily persist into the upper elementary grades unless structured classroom interventions continue to operate (Slavin et al., 2011). This appears to apply equally to socially disadvantaged children (Connor et al., 2013). Few longitudinal intervention studies of early readers have followed students into Grades 2 and 3 to ascertain how those with difficulties progress as they are confronted by more complex reading demands. One such study involving a lay-ered approach to reading intervention from kindergarten to third grade found that gains achieved at the end of Grade 2 had diminished somewhat the fol-lowing year, arguably as a result of more complex reading demands in third grade (O'Connor, Fulmer, Harty, & Bell, 2005). An important finding was that the needs of individual children for specialist help fluctuated over time and constant vigilance of their changing circumstances proved necessary. Indeed, only a minority of the children scored consistently below the cut-off at every point in the testing cycle. Prediction was not clear-cut as the reading measures employed were unable to identify which of the kindergarten children would respond well or poorly to the intervention. However, by the end of first grade, all those who would eventually be labeled "learning disabled" were receiving additional intervention. Other researchers (Catts et al., 2012; Leach, Scarborough, & Rescorla, 2003; Lipka, Lesaux, & Siegel, 2006) have similarly shown that reading difficulties are not demonstrated by some children until third or fourth grade. In some cases, this may be explained by the late emergence of problems that are not readily identified by early literacy screening assessments (Compton et al., 2008), although some such children demonstrated mild weaknesses in certain other language and nonverbal cognitive domains (Catts et al., 2012). To some extent, later recognition of reading difficulties can reflect the changing nature of task demands in school, with phonological skills proving adequate for the challenge of the infant years but insufficient to cope with the increased demands of third and fourth grades (Lipka et al., 2006).

Wanzek and Vaughn (2007) conducted a synthesis of reading interventions for students enrolled in kindergarten through to third grade, which had been conducted between 1995 and 2005. Their focus was on extensive interventions, aspects that had not been specifically examined in previous syntheses (Foorman, 2003; McCardle & Chhabra, 2004; Pressley, 2006). For the purposes of this investigation, extensive interventions were defined as those occurring for 100 sessions or more. A further noteworthy aspect of their study was the desire to focus on the relative contributions of standardized and individualized approaches. Standardized approaches are those where instruction is provided in a relatively uniform fashion to all the students, but with some adjustments to ensure appropriateness of challenge to those of differing ability levels. Individualized approaches involve more of a problem-solving approach in which children's skills are assessed, the nature of the form of intervention for each child is determined individually, close monitoring of progress is conducted, and, in light of regular feedback, the nature of the intervention is amended as necessary. In practice, the authors were unable to locate any extensive intervention studies utilizing an individualized approach, and as a result, their synthesis compared approaches categorized as high versus low standardization. Low standardization lessons were those with less clear prescription where teachers had more freedom to modify their approach in the light of emerging student needs. Eighteen studies met the criteria for inclusion in the synthesis.

Results indicated that higher effect sizes were associated with early intervention (beginning in first grade) and smaller group sizes. No difference was found between high and low standardization groups. While this finding is based on a relatively small number of studies, it is consonant with outcomes reported by Mathes et al. (2005) and by Vaughn et al. (2011) in the case of struggling middle school students. Mathes and colleagues found only one difference between more and less standardized approaches; here, the former group scored rather more highly on a measure of word attack. However, as these researchers note, while there may be scope for teacher choice about which approach to use, this does not mean that the content of supplementary instruction is unimportant. In comparing two very different approaches (behavioral versus cognitive-apprenticeship) that proved to be equally effective, they point out that both

provided for instruction in key reading skills, balanced with opportunities to apply reading and writing skills in connected text, and they both provided students with explicit instruction and practice in skills related to phonemic awareness, decoding, fluent word recognition and text processing, and spelling. Likewise, both approaches provided instruction in comprehension strategies applied to connected text. (Mathes et al., 2005, p. 179)

What can be done to help those who are resistant to initial interventions?

Intervention programs for older children have proven to be considerably less successful than those operating for young children (Denton & Vaughn, 2008; Flynn, Zheng, & Swanson, 2012; Shaywitz, Morris, & Shaywitz, 2008; Vaughn, Denton et al., 2010; Wanzek and Vaughn, 2007; Wanzek et al., 2013), and, unfortunately, a significant proportion of students continue to struggle despite having received early, high-quality, intensive research-based interventions (Torgesen et al., 1999).

Although the proportion of poor readers found in the later years is likely to decline as a result of the increase in early intervention programs, growth rates for this diminishing and, correspondingly, more intransigent group of treatment resisters are likely to prove poorer as a result (Torgesen, 2005). Furthermore, the importance of other reading skills, such as reading fluency and comprehension, becomes more salient, and problems are more difficult to overcome, as the child passes through school (Blachman et al., 2004; Rashotte, MacPhee, & Torgesen, 2001; Ryder et al., 2008).

There is also a thorny issue concerning maintenance of performance. As has been noted, a small proportion of children initially make sound progress but then drop back in third grade and in subsequent years (Vellutino et al., 2008), a period of time when reading demands increase significantly. Torgesen (2005) reflected on the difficulties encountered by some children when they were engaged in an intensive intervention for fourth grade students with severe reading disabilities (Torgesen, Alexander et al., 2001). While the results were seen to be "very impressive" (Hulme & Snowling, 2009, p. 87), a significant proportion (between one-third and one-half) were unable to score within the normal range (a standard score of 90 or above) on a test of reading accuracy. Furthermore, the gains made could not be sustained by all; over the following two years, approximately one-quarter of the sample lost most of the standard score gains they had achieved. Only slightly more than half of the sample succeeded in sustaining or improving their gains once the intervention had been completed. Improving reading fluency was also a challenge for most of the students, and although many made progress, their standard scores failed to increase. Student factors that seemed most important for prediction of progress after the intervention were teachers' ratings of attentional behaviors, receptive language, and socioeconomic status.

Estimates of the proportion of those who continue to struggle despite receiving high-quality intervention vary, although a figure of 4–6% of the school population is quite common (Kamps et al., 2008; Mathes & Denton, 2002; Mathes et al., 2005). Vaughn and Roberts (2007) offer a more optimistic estimate in which less than 10% of the 20% to 30% of children who require supplemental, research-based instruction are deemed likely to make little or no substantial progress. Scanlon et al. (2005) suggest a slightly higher figure of 15–20% of remediated readers. In a randomized controlled trial intervention undertaken in the United Kingdom involving individual and small-group input, approximately one-quarter of the participants failed to respond to the intervention (Hatcher et al., 2006). Singleton's (2009a) review concludes that between 1.5% and 3% of children are likely to require further help after the provision of secondary intervention. Torgesen (2004) has suggested that if all children were given the most effective interventions when needed, the incidence of early reading difficulties might range from 1.6% to 6% of the total population.

The appropriate intensity and length of Tier 2 intervention for the primary grades continues to be subject to debate, and the *What Works Clearinghouse* (Gersten et al., 2008) was unable to identify the period that Tier 2 should operate prior to providing a more intensive Tier 3 intervention, stating merely that it should be "a reasonable amount of time" (p. 26). The notion that initial interventions should, in the first instance, be of modest intensity has been questioned by Denton et al. (2011) and Vaughn, Denton, and Fletcher (2010). Denton and colleagues compared outcomes of a Tier 2 intervention of varying intensity with three groups of first grade students at risk for reading difficulties. No group differences in reading outcomes were found in respect of intervention duration or of scheduling. This finding led the authors to conclude that many of the students in the study required more intensive Tier 3 intervention.

The rapid growth of Response to Intervention initiatives has resulted in young children moving rapidly through to Tier 3 provision within the first years of schooling rather than having to wait many years to receive such assistance. In general, Tier 3 involves individual or very-small-group instruction and provision of more frequent, longer sessions over a greater period of time. Given the lack of success at the earlier Tier 2 phase, it is also likely that a more individualized program, albeit still focusing primarily on the development of decoding skills, will be valuable. Employing a randomized controlled trial, Denton et al. (2013) examined the operation of a Tier 3 intervention with second graders. The intervention was provided to groups of 2 or 3 students a day in 45-minute sessions over a 6-month period. Instruction was based on a structured program, *Responsive Reading Instruction* (Denton & Hocker, 2006) and, where appropriate, an additional fluency program, *Read Naturally* (Ihnot et al., 2001). Those providing the intervention were encouraged to use these programs' evidence-based instructional activities provided within a framework of lesson components in a flexible fashion tailored to individual student needs. Compared with controls who received typical school instruction, children in the intervention group made significantly greater progress on measures of word identification, phonemic decoding, word reading fluency, and a measure of sentence and paragraph reading comprehension. However, statistically significant differences between the groups were not found for pseudoword reading, text reading fluency, and comprehension of extended passages of text. While these findings are generally promising, it should be noted that for many of the children in the study, severe problems, particularly in respect of reading fluency and reading comprehension, remained. Furthermore, a statistically significant difference was not found between the control and intervention groups in respect of the proportion who demonstrated the benchmark performance considered to represent an adequate response to intervention. In general, those who were inadequate responders to the Tier 3 intervention demonstrated greater impairments on a range of language measures that had been evident prior to an earlier Tier 2 intervention.

As children move into middle childhood, the importance of reading fluency and comprehension becomes greater (Speece et al., 2010). However, the requirements of this particular age group may differ from those of older students as well as those in elementary school. In this respect, Wanzek et al. (2010) note that struggling readers in the later elementary/junior school years (aged 9–11 years) are often treated as having similar needs to adolescents, and question whether this is actually the case. Their synthesis of the rather sparse number of experimental studies evaluating reading interventions for children in the middle years found only small to moderate effect sizes for studies that focused on word-reading skills. Equally disappointing findings following a small group intervention with fourth grade struggling readers are reported by Wanzek and Roberts (2012). They note that even high-quality research studies have proven largely incapable of indicating how to help those who have not benefited sufficiently from earlier high-quality interventions.

In many ways, identifying and addressing the precise nature of reading-related difficulties in adolescents is more complex than for young children. Where an RTI model operates, there may be a need for some students to progress directly to a more intensive third-tier intervention (Compton, Gilbert et al., 2012; Fuchs, Fuchs, & Compton, 2010; Vaughn & Fletcher, 2012), although, as noted earlier, this strategy is also increasingly advocated for young children. Rather than using poor responsiveness to intervention to determine the level and intensity of support needed, as tends to be the case for younger children, it may be more appropriate to base decisions on current performance on measures of reading accuracy, fluency, and comprehension.

Interventions need to be tailored to changes and fluctuations in student performance. Such variation renders standardized small-group intervention problematic (Leach, Scarborough, & Rescorla, 2003; Vaughn et al., 2008; but see Vaughn et al., 2011). Some students continue to experience significant word-reading difficulties that require help at the letter-sound level; others have few problems with single-syllable words but struggle with those that are multisyllabic (Archer, Gleason, & Vachon, 2003). For this latter group, more advanced word study involving a variety of word analysis skills will be more appropriate (Curtis, 2004; Roberts et al., 2008). Others, who have made gains in basic word reading skills, may lack reading fluency and can struggle with the consequences of earlier problems, for example, limited vocabulary and concept knowledge, or difficulties with regard to reading comprehension and poor motivation (Biancarosa & Snow, 2006). For these reasons,

Older students with reading difficulties may need instruction in any of a range of reading components from beginning phonics skills to decoding multi-syllabic words and practicing reading for fluency, depending on their degree of development and corresponding areas of need. In addition, many students benefit from multiple opportunities to read text aloud and to engage in activities that involve reading fluency. . . . Even older students who require instruction in the basic elements of decoding and word-level reading should not be precluded from receiving instruction in vocabulary, concept development, and reading comprehension. (Vaughn et al., 2008, p. 339)

Others have emphasized the difficulties that some poor readers encounter with executive functions and argue that helping children develop metacognitive and self-regulatory strategies is also likely to prove beneficial (Berninger et al., 2008).

Motivation to read is a particular problem for many adolescent poor readers. A history of struggle and embarrassment is often compounded by classroom environments in which reading material becomes increasingly more complex, and the importance for teachers to foster motivation to read is de-emphasized (Guthrie & Davis, 2003; Roberts, Torgesen, Boardman, & Scammacca, 2008). At this age, students with difficulties may seek to protect themselves from public humiliation by appearing unmotivated and dismissive of the value of learning (Covington, 1992). The ability of interventions to engage and motivate older students is, of course, crucial. As was noted by proponents of the whole-language approach, the highly structured nature of work in the development of basic reading skills is not easily rendered intrinsically appealing. One factor that may help increase engagement is peer endorsement and mediation, although our understanding of the means to operate such an approach effectively with poor readers is still rudimentary (Fuchs et al., 2010).

Scammacca et al. (2007) conducted a meta-analytic review of instruction for struggling adolescent readers. This investigation, involving 31 studies, considered a number of reading-related skills but, as would be expected for students of this age, reading comprehension was adjudged to be the most important indicator of the effectiveness of the interventions. Across all the various reading studies included in the analysis, an overall effect size of 0.95 was found. However, many of these studies utilized non-standardized measures that are more likely to be closely aligned to the aims of the specific interventions and which tend to provide higher effect sizes than traditional assessments (Swanson, Hoskyn, & Lee, 1999). Although concluding that adolescence is not too late to intervene, Scammacca et al. (2007) raised a number of issues that served to temper their findings. These include large confidence intervals that, in relation to the standardized assessments, do not wholly rule out the possibility of a "true" effect of 0. Large differences between the effect sizes obtained by standardized and other measures employed, and differences in effect sizes between research and teacher-implemented interventions, were also notable. In particular, an overall effect size of 0.21 for teacher-implemented interventions using standardized measures raises many questions about generalization and transfer. As is commonly the case in the reading disability intervention literature, the authors attempted to build upon these findings by suggesting that more intensive interventions may prove productive. A similar conclusion is reached by Wanzek et al. (2011), who found only modest gains resulting from a year-long reading intervention in 50-minute sessions provided on a daily basis to moderately sized groups (10–15) of middle school students with learning disabilities.

Scammacca et al. (in press) undertook a follow-up meta-analysis of reading-related interventions involving the same age range. They found that, for papers published between 2005 and 2011, the overall effect size of 0.49 represented a drop from the 0.95 figure reported in their earlier 2007 publication. For standardized measures alone, the figure dropped from 0.42 to 0.21 across these two periods. In seeking to explain these reductions, Scammacca and colleagues listed several possible contributory factors: the recent use of more scientifically rigorous and complex research designs, greater use of standardized measures, changes in the characteristics of participants in the studies (perhaps involving a broader range of struggling readers), and likely improvements in the reading instruction received by the "business as usual" comparison groups. The authors conclude that while the magnitude of effects of reading interventions for struggling readers may be less than was thought previously, there is strong evidence that these can lead to improvements. However, an effect size of 0.21 should be recognised as a very modest figure that is only a little higher than the effect size found in another meta-analysis undertaken by Wanzek et al. (2013) (see later in the chapter for further discussion).

There are further complications when students with significant reading difficulties are attempting to cope in a school system in which the medium of instruction is not in their first language. Such children have a unique set of challenges, being more likely to have reduced understanding of the meaning of words and, in many cases, having reduced access to high-quality and sustained educational experiences (Denton, Wexler, Vaughn, & Bryan, 2008). However, there are very few interventions reported in the literature for such students and results from these are not encouraging (e.g., Denton et al., 2008).

Approaches recommended for reading-disabled students are similarly advocated for children with intellectual disabilities. Thus, phonemic awareness training, phonics instruction, and teaching letter-sound correspondence to students with moderate intellectual disabilities have proven beneficial when operated as part of a comprehensive reading program that should not be merely limited to sight-word memorization (Allor et al., 2010; Hoogeven, Smeets, & Lancioni, 1989).

In addition to helping children read single words accurately, many interventions also target reading fluency. The ability to read text with both speed and accuracy is important because this can enable decoding to become a largely automatic process and free up cognitive resources to focus on higher-order meaning-related text processing (Wolf et al., 2003). Unsurprisingly, therefore, fluency has a strong relationship to reading comprehension, although evidence of a causal relationship, whether unidirectional or reciprocal, is scanty (O'Connor, White, & Swanson, 2007). Somewhat neglected in studies of English, where the primary focus is typically on reading accuracy (Share, 2008), this skill is often central in transparent languages where letter-sound decoding is less problematic and reading rate is typically a primary concern for teachers.

It has generally been found easier to improve word-reading accuracy than fluency (Lyon & Moats, 1997; Torgesen, 2005), and, despite long-lasting assumptions to the contrary, gains in alphabetic decoding do not necessarily lead to improved fluency or reading comprehension (Moats & Foorman, 1997; Torgesen, Rashotte, & Alexander, 2001). Older students, who have struggled with reading for many years, read less than normal readers, and their reduced exposure to print (Cunningham & Stanovich, 1998; Pfost, Dörfler, & Artelt, 2012) is likely to reduce the number of words that can be read automatically

(Ehri, 2002; Share & Stanovich, 1995) – an example of the Matthew Effect (Stanovich, 1986) whereby the gap between good and weak readers increases over time. Thus weak readers will continue to struggle to "catch up" with their classmates, and even significant gains in word-reading skills may still be insufficient to enable them to read as fluently as their peers (Torgesen, 2005; Torgesen, Rashotte et al., 2001).

Findings from Scammacca et al.'s (2007) meta-analysis highlighted a number of difficulties with fluency interventions. Studies that explicitly sought to increase fluency (primarily by means of repeated reading) were found to be largely ineffective, with effects not reliably different from zero. Wexler, Vaughn, Edmonds, and Reutebuch (2008) similarly undertook a synthesis of fluency interventions for struggling adolescent readers conducted between 1980 and 2005. They noted that there had been few high-quality empirical investigations and, where gains in fluency had been found, these did not easily transfer or generalize to other reading-related activities (see also Huemer et al., 2010).

Subsequent investigations have continued to demonstrate the complexities of this area. Thus neither a repeated-reading nor a wide-reading approach proved effective in raising performance in word reading, fluency, or comprehension of 9th and 10th grade students with severe reading problems (Wexler et al., 2010). It was concluded that for older students with significant reading disabilities more intensive approaches that include a variety of other components are likely to be necessary. Adding to this dispiriting picture, Vaughn et al. (2009) similarly found that students experienced significant difficulty in improving fluency even when intensive intervention was provided. While there is some evidence from a small-scale study that providing fluency practice at a variety of levels (sounds, single words, short phrases, and whole passages) on a one-on-one basis with a paraprofessional may lead to fluency gains (Spencer & Manis, 2010), important methodological limitations were reported. At the present time, it appears that research has yet to determine powerful ways of increasing reading fluency in ways that can have a positive and meaningful effect on the everyday skills of struggling adolescent readers.

Building on their theoretical work, Wolf and colleagues have developed an approach to the development of children's reading fluency and comprehension that draws on several linguistic systems. Their *Retrieval, Automaticity, Vocabulary, Engagement with language, and Orthography* (RAVE O) program (Wolf, Miller, & Donnelly, 2000) is based on the premise that the more the child understands about a word (i.e., in relation to phonemes, orthographic patterns, semantic meanings, syntactic uses, and morphological roots and affixes) (see also Berninger et al., 2008, 2010]), the more speedily it will be decoded, retrieved, and comprehended. In addition to focusing on identified core words each week and relating these to each of the various linguistic systems in a connected fashion, RAVE-O places an emphasis on a variety of metacognitive strategies geared to helping children segment words into common orthographic and morphological units. A multi-site intervention (1 hour daily for 70 days) in which RAVE-O was combined with a another program focusing on letter-sound knowledge and blending skills (*Phonological Analysis and Blending*; PHAB), and utilizing direct instruction approaches, resulted in significant gains in a variety of reading skills, compared with control programs. Similar gains were found for another multiple-component program (PHAST) employed in a study that also utilized a combination of phonological and strategy-based approaches. For both programs, the gains found continued to be evident at follow-up one year later and were unrelated to the children's race, SES or IQ (Morris et al., 2012). Morris and colleagues conclude that interventions that incorporate multiple components of language and that address a variety of core deficits are more likely to lead to gains in a range of reading skills, including those found to be the most difficult to remediate: fluency and comprehension. However, despite these encouraging gains, unadjusted standard score means for reading efficiency (i.e., reading rate) at the end of the 70-hour intervention were 80.97 (RAVE-O/PHAB) and 81.21 (PHAST), a picture that was relatively unchanged a year later. Further studies involving variants of these programs, but of significantly longer duration, are currently under way, with preliminary results described as "encouraging" (Lovett, Barron, & Frijters, 2013, p. 344).

Further research is needed to help understand the effects of different elements of multiple component interventions in relation to differing levels of student need and local capacity (Scammacca et al., 2007). While this approach would seem to be one that holds much promise, the appropriate balance of activities is difficult to determine and, with some notable exceptions, guidance in the research literature has often focused more on the need for intensive, individualized approaches than specifics about the balance of content.

Shaywitz, Morris, and Shaywitz (2008) state that there is no evidence for the existence of any program that is appropriate for all struggling readers. Neither have any specific programs been identified that are beneficial for particular groups of dyslexic readers. For these authors, there is a need to focus on contextual or procedural factors rather than on the particular content of intervention programs. They suggest that greater understanding is required in relation to instructional intensity, program fidelity, teacher skills, program focus, and the influence of student-related variables such as prior experience and current abilities (see also Foorman et al., 2008).

There has been some debate in the literature as to whether standardized programs are more helpful than individualized interventions. However, the number of empirical investigations examining the relative benefits of the two approaches for reading disability is sparse (Vaughn et al., 2008). While the clear and defined structure of standardized approaches would seem to be helpful to teachers, instruction that can be adapted to meet individual students' changing requirements may also prove to be powerful. As noted earlier (see pp. 138–139), there is little evidence of differences in outcome between standardized and individualized approaches in the early grades (Wanzek & Vaughn, 2007), although it is likely that the latter may be more relevant for Tier 3 intervention (Denton et al., 2013) and for older children. Gelzheiser, Scanlon, Vellutino, Halgren-Flynn, & Schatschneider (2011) evaluated the effects of a responsive and comprehensive program (i.e., one tailored to address students' individual needs in relation to word- and text-level skills) for fourth grade struggling readers. Significant gains were found for reading accuracy and comprehension, but not for fluency, perhaps reflecting the nature of the program content in which comprehension may have taken primacy over fluency. Reflecting on the findings, the authors pointed to the potential of more responsive, individualized approaches but noted that these place significant demands on teacher skills and school resources. The expectation that individualized approaches are likely to prove more effective than standardized interventions with older poor readers was not supported by findings from a year-long, daily, small-group Tier 3 intervention with seventh and eighth grade poor readers (Vaughn et al., 2011). It was found that while both types of intervention group performed better on measures of reading fluency and comprehension than did a comparison group that received no researcher intervention, differences between the standardized and individualized intervention groups were not statistically significant. In addition, and counter to the researchers' expectations, the individualized treatment also failed to be more effective than the standardized input for children with low English proficiency.

It has often been assumed that fidelity of implementation of structured reading programs is a critical component of success, and there is some supportive evidence for this (e.g., Benner et al., 2011). However, fidelity is a more complex element than is always recognized. While it is important to draw on programs that have been empirically verified, it seems that a certain degree of flexibility is required to accommodate the particular needs of differing contexts and diverse student populations (Harn, Parisi, & Stoolmiller, 2013).

A significant concern relates to our continuing inability to find practical ways to help those with the greatest problems beyond advocating "more of the same." Thus, while a recent research synthesis (Wanzek et al., 2013) indicates that extensive reading interventions for post-Grade 3 students with reading difficulties can have a positive effect, the dispiriting finding is that mean effect sizes are small (0.15 for word reading and 0.16 for fluency). The picture outlined by Scammacca et al.'s (2013) meta-analysis is only a little rosier.

Although the overall picture supports arguments for the provision of extensive reading interventions in the upper grades (see also Vaughn et al., 2012), it is not clear exactly how the interventions can be rendered more powerful. Taking a lead from findings with younger children, researchers have been largely confined to speculating on the possible benefits of more intensive and more prolonged forms of intervention for older students (Vaughn, Denton et al., 2010). For example, in reflecting on the modest gains achieved following a lengthy intervention with Grade 6 students (Vaughn, Cirino et al., 2010), involving more than 100 hours of instruction per child, two of the authors (Vaughn & Fletcher, 2010) were unable to offer further guidance other than to emphasize the need to focus resources and intensity on those students (estimated to be 2–5%) who prove to be most resistant to evidence-based practices. However, "intensity" has proven to be a rather problematic construct. Wanzek et al.'s (2013) review was unable to demonstrate that either increasing the time of interventions or decreasing instructional group size (both considered to be ways of increasing intensity) were effective with older children. These authors caution against any assumption that these strategies, which are supported by research in elementary classrooms (Harn, Kame'enui, & Simmons, 2007; Harn, Linan-Thompson, & Roberts, 2008; Wanzek & Vaughn, 2008), will apply equally for students in secondary education. For adolescents, finding alternative ways to boost intensity may prove necessary.

D. Fuchs et al. (2013) question whether quantitative approaches to increasing intervention intensity (i.e., increasing time and/or duration or reducing group size) will prove effective when students have already failed to progress in response to earlier, similar interventions. Instead, they argue that an approach to increasing intensity is called for that is qualitatively rather than quantitatively different. This might involve making changes to the curriculum, instructional approaches, teaching personnel (e.g., the use of a peer rather than a teacher), forms of feedback, and motivational drivers. To inform and evaluate these modifications, their approach uses an ongoing process of data-driven hypothesis testing that Fuchs and colleagues term "data-based individualization." This involves ascertaining, in light of data systematically gathered over several time points, what works best for a given individual who appears not to be responding to particular instructional approaches. These researchers note that, for such an approach to work, educators need to acquire a range of high-level skills that may be rarely delivered by current teacher preparation programs.

It is clear that many questions remain about the best way to organize and structure intervention for those with the most intransigent problems, what constitutes the most effective ways to engage those with histories of school failure, what are the changing instructional needs of children from different age groups, and what are the critical academic targets that will maximize successful adult futures for such students (Fuchs et al., 2010).

There has been some debate in the literature as to whether specialized interventions for children with reading disabilities need to be undertaken by qualified teachers. Several studies suggest that this is not necessarily the case (Gunn et al., 2005; Hatcher et al., 2006; Vadasy & Sanders, 2010; Vadasy et al., 2008). Vadasy and colleagues, for example, found that paraeducators were able to provide effective supplemental code-oriented intervention to first grade children with reading scores initially in the bottom quartile. However, they observed that for those children who fail to respond to this level of intervention, more differentiated instruction from highly skilled teaching staff may be necessary. One of the benefits of using paraeducators in the early stages is that this may free up specialist time for those children who subsequently need more intensive, individualized assistance. On the other hand, the use of poorly trained or ineffective classroom aides can be deleterious to the progress to those with learning difficulties (Rubie-Davies et al., 2010). In the United States, tertiary-level interventions are sometimes undertaken by specially trained staff brought in from outside of the school (Torgesen, Alexander et al., 2001). However, it has been argued that this is not necessary where school staff have appropriate training and sufficient resources (Kamps et al., 2008).

Finally, the debate as to whether children with reading and other learning disabilities are better catered for in fully inclusive or in resource room settings continues to rage (McLeskey & Waldron, 2011). However, it seems likely that it is not the physical location of provision that is critical, but rather the appropriate utilization of mainstream and specialist teacher skills. In mainstream classrooms it has been found that general education is often sound but may lack sufficient individualized and structured programing to address sufficiently the learning-disabled child's specific needs (McLeskey & Waldron, 2011) while ensuring that other students in the classroom are working productively (Denton, 2012). Education in resource settings has been frequently criticized for being undemanding, insufficiently tailored to individual needs, lacking accountability, and leading to reduced student engagement (Moody et al., 2000). However, as evidence-based programs for children with reading disabilities operating within an RTI model become more widely employed, the somewhat simplistic mainstream versus resource-setting debate is likely to become increasingly irrelevant.

What is special about specialist dyslexia assessment and teaching?

The origins of several interventions for children with reading disability can be traced back to the work of Samuel Orton, in the 1930s. Although Orton's emphasis on hemispheric difficulties as the underlying cause of reading disability has been superseded by more recent scientific advances, his multisensory teaching approach (influenced by the work of Fernald) is still widely employed today. Orton worked with an educator, Anna Gillingham, to develop the highly structured Orton-Gillingham multisensory teaching method (Gillingham & Stillman, 1997), which underpins many present-day programs (Moats & Farrell, 1999, 2005). While the sequence of activities can vary from one variant of the approach to another, the key elements are as follows; individual letters are paired with their sounds using a Visual-Auditory-Kinesthetic-Tactile (VAKT) procedure that involves tracing the letter while saying its name and sound.[2] Repetition is stressed as a means of gaining mastery between letters and sounds. The technique of overlearning involves constant repetition in order that newly acquired skills become automatized and readily recalled when needed. Letters are blended together to enable the child to read words and sentences. Spelling is advanced by means of dictation. Finally, short stories that contain the taught sounds are read. With more complex texts tackled subsequently.

In a review of specialist approaches to dyslexia teaching, Singleton (2009b) highlights common features as outlined by Townend (2000) and Thomson (1990). Townend emphasizes the following elements, which, with the exception of the multisensory component, are strongly supported by research evidence:
1. a structured approach involving small steps
2. a multisensory approach
3. reinforcement of learned skills with an emphasis on automatization
4. an emphasis upon the learning of skills rather than facts
5. developing metacognitive approaches in which students reflect on appropriate strategies for use in particular circumstances

Despite the enthusiasm for multisensory approaches held by many specialist dyslexia teachers (Kelly & Phillips, 2011), the theoretical grounds and scientific rationale for their use are questionable (Moats & Farrell, 2005). Most research evaluations have taken the form of case studies (Riccio, Sullivan, & Cohen, 2010), and while these have often proven to be positive (Fernald & Keller, 1921; Strauss & Lehtinen, 1947), high-quality research evidence for the multisensory component of a broader structured phonological approach is sparse (Everatt & Reid, 2009; Snowling & Hulme, 2011) and not overly convincing. The National Reading Panel (2000) review found only four studies using the Orton-Gillingham approach that had sufficient methodological rigour for inclusion. Only two of these demonstrated positive effect sizes. For Vaughn and Linan-Thompson (2003), research has "offered no compelling evidence" (p. 142) that a multisensory approach can benefit children with reading difficulties.

One of the difficulties of evaluating the utility of the multisensory approach is that it contains a number of elements commonly found in everyday classroom contexts, but only some of which may be important. One (auditory) component, reading aloud, is found in almost all initial reading approaches, and another

---

[2] Teaching both letter names and sounds to early readers has proven controversial (Adams, 1990), although more recently, this approach has received some empirical support. However, explicit instruction in letter sounds remains the more important element for children with poor phonological abilities (Piasta & Wagner, 2010).

element, silent reading, described as an ideovisual component (Watkins, 1922), has not thrived (Brooks, 1984).

Fletcher et al. (2007) observe that traditional multisensory components appear not to be crucial (Clark & Uhry, 1955; Moats & Farrell, 1999; Wise, Ring, & Olson, 1999) and contend that the strengths of such programs may lie in the use of an intense systematic approach focused on the particular needs of individual students. Recently published reviews of "what works" (e.g., Brooks, 2007; Singleton, 2009a) point to the generally favorable value of structured programs that have an emphasis on phonological skills training, but there is little evidence pointing to any significant contribution of multisensory aspects. Interestingly, although Singleton notes in the opening section of his review that multisensory teaching is "a core feature" (p. 19) of specialist dyslexia teaching, because his remit was to consider only published evidence, this approach is not subsequently discussed or evaluated.

The use of computers and assistive technology

Computers and other electronic devices have the potential both to help remediate reading difficulties and to assist those for whom reading and writing will continue to prove to be a significant struggle despite being in receipt of intensive, high-quality educational interventions.

However, it is a notable feature that the introduction of information and communications technology (ICT) has largely failed to deliver the anticipated gains in reading development that have long been foretold (Cheung & Slavin, 2012). Such unfulfilled potential appears to apply to instruction for those with reading disability (MacArthur, 2013). Slavin et al.'s (2011) review of interventions for struggling readers reported that computer-assisted instruction had minimal effects on reading achievement. Similarly, a large randomized controlled trial using a number of commercial packages (Campuzano et al., 2009; Dynarski et al., 2007) found almost no evidence of effectiveness in comparison with regular classroom experiences. However, it is possible that the potential of computers has been undermined by poor pedagogic practice, with computer-based instruction being insufficiently integrated into everyday classroom practice (Torgesen et al., 2010).

Some evidence for the value of computerized interventions for children with reading disabilities is provided in longitudinal studies in Finland (Saine et al., 2011) and Sweden (Fälth et al., 2013). In Saine and colleagues' study, computer-assisted reading intervention, in combination with small-group teacher instruction, led to significant gains for young children deemed to be at risk of reading failure. However, the sample comprised mainly middle-class children scoring in the lowest 30% of all participants in the study. The respective contribution of the computerized instruction, and that provided in small-group sessions, cannot be discerned. Another confounding factor was that these children were taught by their regular class teachers and thus may have received additional attention in ordinary lessons. Fälth et al. (2013) found that children who received computerized phonological and comprehension training showed greater improvement in a number of reading-related activities than typical readers and poor readers receiving ordinary forms of special instruction. However, it should be noted that the participants were identified by their teachers as those who would benefit from the intervention. In addition, the cut-off point for allocation to the reading disability group was a mere 0.75 SD below the mean sight word reading score of the typically developing reader group. Furthermore, each child's computer sessions involved one-on-one training sessions with a special education teacher. Despite this advantageous scenario, gains were insufficient to bring the poor readers up to the baseline level of their peers.

Interestingly, researchers emphasizing the problems of visual attention for reading difficulties have reported findings suggesting that 12 hours of play with commercially available action video games can improve the attention and reading performance of Italian dyslexic children (Franceschini et al., 2013). Irrespective of the impact of such an intervention on deeper orthographies such as English, it seems unlikely that this approach will prove to have a widespread, significant, and long-standing impact on the performance of struggling readers.

Complementary and Alternative Approaches to Treatment

The field of dyslexia, similar to other developmental difficulties (Jacobson, Foxx, & Mulick, 2005), has been subject to claims of effectiveness for a variety of alternative non-curriculum-based interventions. Usually these are promoted as tackling some hypothetical underlying physical or cognitive problems rather than academic or behavioral difficulties. These alternative therapies, sometimes touted as miracle cures, can receive much media attention and, understandably, are often attractive to parents and professionals who are eager to discover any program that may help with seemingly intractable difficulties (Bull, 2009; Favell, 2005; Stephenson, 2009). However, rigorous scientific studies of such interventions have been consistently unable to demonstrate significant efficacy in relation to the primary problems of concern.

Perceptual-motor training

One set of approaches to tackling reading disability involves participation in differing types of kinesthetic exercise as part of a long tradition of perceptual-motor training that has sought to improve cognitive functioning in children with developmental disorders. In relation to children with poor neurological functioning, the work of Doman and Delacato (Delacato, 1959; Doman & Delacato, 1968) and Ayres (1963, 1979) has been highly influential. However, much of this early work, and later variants of it (e.g., Blythe, 1992), has been criticized for relying on testimonials, case studies, and emotional appeal rather than on rigorous peer-reviewed scientific examination (American Academy of Pediatrics, 1982; Balow, 1996; Fawcett & Reid, 2009; Holm, 1983; Silver, 1987). Rarely have studies in this area employed control groups in order to rule out confounds such as test-retest effects (McArthur, 2007). Irrespective of their low scientific credibility, published studies have failed to yield promising findings. Kavale and Mattson's (1983) meta-analysis of 180 studies of perceptual-motor programs, for example, found no important effect sizes for academic skills and, indeed, only a small effect (0.17) for perceptual-motor skills themselves.

Despite reduced influence in the 1980s (Hallahan & Mercer, 2001), perceptual-motor skills training subsequently regained a degree of popularity at the beginning of the new millennium, in part because of its supposed association with developing insights and understandings about brain functioning. Of the various kinesthetic initiatives for children with learning difficulties, perhaps the most prominent in recent years has been the DORE program (also known as the Dyslexia, Dyspraxia, Attention Treatment Program (DDAT) (Dore & Brookes, 2006). This is based on the notion of cerebellar developmental delay as the primary cause of dyslexia (Nicolson, Fawcett, & Dean, 2001a, 2001b). Intervention involves the child undertaking a series of physical exercises for approximately 10 minutes, twice daily. Although claims of the success of the program have largely relied on personal testimony, two highly controversial publications in a specialist dyslexia journal (Reynolds & Nicolson, 2007; Reynolds, Nicolson, & Hambly, 2003), in which results from a UK primary school intervention were reported, have drawn much ire from the scientific community. These two papers testified to the success of the intervention with one of the authors (Reynolds), a well-known British professor of education, stating on BBC Radio that "it's the closest thing to a cure that I have ever seen" (cited in Rack et al., 2007, p. 98).

Despite such enthusiasm, a series of research papers identified serious design flaws in this study (Bishop, 2007; McArthur, 2007; Rack, 2003; Rack et al., 2007; Snowling & Hulme, 2003), criticisms that were not abated by the response of the original authors (Nicolson & Reynolds, 2007). Among a lengthy list of problems, perhaps the two most influential were a failure to compare sufficiently the subsequent performance of the control group and questions about the true weaknesses of the children in the study; the pretest performance of the treated group indicated that many did not have a significant reading problem at the outset. In reviewing the relevant literature, Bishop (2007) has concluded that one should be skeptical of claims that the intervention improves any skills other than those that are trained in the exercises.

An alternative movement approach to the enhancement of children's academic skills has been pioneered by McPhillips and colleagues in Northern Ireland. This work is derived from interventions that seek to remediate abnormal primary reflexes (Blythe, 1992; Goddard Blythe, 2005), but, cognizant of the poor quality of previous evaluations in this field, McPhillips and his team have endeavored to undertake more rigorous, scientific evaluations and published their findings in some highly respected scientific journals (although criticism of the approach used for assessing children's reflexes is offered by Hyatt, Stephenson, and Carter, 2009).

Of particular interest to McPhillips and his team is the asymmetrical tonic neck reflex, with persistence of this into the school years having been found to be associated with literacy difficulties (McPhillips & Jordan-Black, 2007). However, these authors readily acknowledge that not all children with reading and spelling problems demonstrate persistent reflexes, and some children with clinically high levels of persistent reflex are good readers.

In an attempt to reduce the proportion of children with academic difficulties, McPhillips devised the *Primary Movement Programme* that involves children undertaking a series of movements designed to mimic the early reflex movements of the fetus. The exercises are hypothesized to stimulate the major motor centers in the brain, including the cerebellum. Research findings from two intervention studies undertaken by this team (McPhillips, Hepper, & Mulhern, 2000) have indicated gains for the intervention groups in reading and mathematics, although there is no suggestion that such interventions can help children overcome severe reading disabilities. In reviewing this work, Hyatt et al. (2009) note that reported gains are modest and conclude that this approach is unlikely to be any more successful than earlier perceptual-motor programs in remediating reading disabilities.

Despite the paucity of evidence, advocates of kinesthetic approaches continue to make claims that are not justified by the evidence, and some programs maintain a strong following among practitioners. In concluding their wide-ranging review of perceptual-motor training programs, Kavale and Mattson (1983) comment on the "remarkable" resistance to the weight of evidence against the approach, in part a consequence of its "deep historical roots and strong clinical tradition" (p. 172):

Process training has always made the phoenix look like a bedraggled sparrow. You cannot kill it. It simply bides its time in exile after being dislodged by one of history's periodic attacks upon it, and then returns, wearing disguises or carrying new *noms de plume,* as it were, but consisting of the same old ideas, doing business much in the same old way. (Mann, 1979, p. 539)

The perceived viability of perceptual-motor programs has persisted in the new millennium, buoyed by the allure and promise of neuroscience. Despite Kavale and Mattson's (1983) expectation that findings from their review might finally undermine its popularity, the approach is still being actively promoted. However, it appears that there is growing awareness that the supposed bases for some well-known approaches often bear little relationship to current understandings of brain functioning (Howard-Jones, 2007; Hyatt, 2007).

Visual interventions

As noted in Chapter 2, there are a variety of theories that suggest that dyslexia is, in part, a result of visual processing difficulties. While researchers interested in the role of visual processing are beginning to examine possible intervention approaches, there is currently very little evidence to justify the introduction of any large-scale initiatives.

Perhaps the most widely known current form of visual intervention is that relating to scotopic sensitivity syndrome (Meares-Irlen syndrome) (see pp. 73–74). Treatment typically involves the use of individually prescribed colored lenses designed to reduce visual stress and increase reading speed. While such lenses have been widely promoted as a "cure" for dyslexia, advocates of this technology such as Wilkins (2003) and Singleton (2009a, 2009b, 2012) have emphasized that resolving the primary problems of reading disability is not an appropriate aim for such treatments. For Singleton, visual stress is likely to be a disorder that is often found to be comorbid with dyslexia, these having a multiplicative detrimental effect on reading performance. As noted earlier, those who struggle with reading may be more susceptible to visual stress, perhaps because they typically need to focus on the visual components of the text more than do skilled readers (Shovman & Ahissar, 2006). For this reason, Wilkins (2012) and Singleton (2012) both contend that those who are susceptible to visual stress (whether reading-disabled or not) can be helped make the reading process less uncomfortable, and this should lead to gains in reading speed.

Research has failed to show a clear causal relationship between the use of colored lenses or overlays and reading gains, although attempts to evaluate such tools (e.g., Cardona et al., 2010) have not been helped by poor design and methodological flaws (Hyatt et al., 2009; Parker, 1990; Zane, 2005). Particular concerns in this respect include the use of anecdotal reports, poor controls, failure to determine equivalence of groups at the pretest phase, potential researcher bias, inappropriate measurement metrics and statistical analyses, and likely placebo effects.

A systematic review of the literature on the use of colored lenses for reading difficulty (Albon, Adi, & Hyde, 2008) found that more than half of the 23 studies identified were hampered by severe methodological weaknesses. The review concluded that there was "no convincing evidence" (p. 93) to support the argument that colored filters could improve the reading ability of dyslexic children. A subsequent, more rigorously designed intervention study, examining the effects of Irlen filters with children of below-average reading ability

(Ritchie et al., 2011, 2012), also found little evidence to support their value for reading progress. This was the case at both the end of an initial trial period and, then again, at one year follow-up. Similarly, a study of university students with dyslexia (Henderson, Tsogda, & Snowling, 2013) also found no differences in improvement in reading rate or comprehension of connected text in comparison with controls, when both groups were provided with colored overlays. Reviews by McIntosh and Ritchie (2012) and Hyatt, et al. (2009) have both concluded that the efficacy of this approach has yet to be demonstrated.

In 2009, a joint statement was provided on dyslexia and vision by the American Academy of Pediatrics, Section on Ophthalmology, the Council on Children with Disabilities, the American Academy of Ophthalmology, the American Association for Pediatric Ophthalmology and Strabismus, and the American Association of Certified Orthoptists (see also p. 74 for discussion). This stated that various forms of vision therapy for dyslexia were not supported by the available evidence. The statement resulted in a rebuttal by an optometrist, Lack (2010), who fiercely criticized the statement's "false, confusing and contradictory statements" (p. 540). The debate served to highlight ongoing professional disagreements between medical (ophthalmologists) and other vision professionals (optometrists) about the appropriateness of vision-based interventions for learning disabilities.

The American Academy of Pediatrics' 2009 statement was subsequently updated in a joint technical report produced by these same medical academies (Handler et al., 2011). Taking a similar stance to that before, the report endorsed the view that various forms of vision therapy for dyslexics had not been scientifically validated:

Scientific evidence does not support the claims that visual training, muscle exercises, ocular pursuit-and tracking exercises, behavioral/perceptual vision therapy, training glasses, prisms, and colored lenses and filters are effective direct or indirect treatments for learning disabilities. There is no evidence that children who participate in vision therapy are more responsive to educational instruction than those who do not participate. The reported benefits of vision therapy, including nonspecific gains in reading ability, can often be explained by the placebo effect, increased time and attention given to students who are poor readers, maturation changes, or the traditional remedial techniques with which they are usually combined. (p. e847)

Fatty acid interventions

Scientific findings concerning the efficacy of various dietary approaches to reading disability are similarly unconvincing. Findings from research claiming that unsaturated fatty acid dietary supplementation may help dyslexics (Cyhlarova et al., 2007; Richardson, 2006; Richardson & Montgomery, 2005) have been criticized for their poor research design, the use of correlational data, and a lack of clear focus on the development of reading skills. In an attempt to remedy these weaknesses, an experimental study (Kairaluoma et al., 2008) sought to ascertain the effects of fatty acid supplements on the reading skills of dyslexic children. After a period of treatment, gains on a variety of measures of reading and spelling were made by both intervention and control (placebo) groups, and parents reported that their children's reading skills had improved. Tellingly, however, no differences were found between the two groups on any of the measures, indicating that it was not the nature of the supplement itself that could explain any improvements. While some have argued for the benefits of supplements for all children, a study using omega-3 supplementation with a mainstream school population (A. Kirby et al., 2010) found no gains in reading ability. Despite findings from a more recent study (Richardson et al., 2012), which has indicated a small positive effect on poor readers, evidence supporting the use of fatty acids as a means of remediating complex reading difficulties continues to be unpersuasive (Everatt & Reid, 2009).

Auditory interventions

As noted in Chapter 2, there has been significant interest in the possibility that auditory processing deficits have a negative influence on the development of phonological awareness. While new auditory theories and models are currently being proposed, existing intervention programs have largely been developed from Tallal's seminal work. Initial studies examining the effectiveness of a computer training program used with children with language impairments (Merzenich et al., 1996; Tallal et al., 1996) led to claims that such an approach could be beneficial, although these met with strong opposition from Tallal's former colleagues at the influential Haskins lab (Mody, Studdert-Kennedy, & Brady, 1997). In light of this early work, a commercial product, *Fast ForWord*, consisting of a suite of computer programs, was launched in 1997. The programs involve the auditory presentation of acoustically modified speech that is initially slowed down and gradually modified as the child becomes more skilled on various tasks. This product, geared to improve both language and reading skills, has proven popular, having been used over the subsequent decade with more than 570,000 children in the United States alone (What Works Clearinghouse, 2007). The program involves a significant commitment on the part of participants who are required to spend 30 to 100 minutes a day, 5 days a week, for 4 to 16 weeks. Interestingly, the claims on websites that promote this approach, often drawing on findings from the *Fast ForWord's* publisher's "privately conducted and non-peer reviewed studies [Scientific Learning Corporation, 1999; 2003]" (Strong, Torgerson, Torgerson, & Hulme, 2011, p. 225), are not generally supported by independent, peer-reviewed studies published in the scientific literature. In one case, publishers have referred to a research study on its website as supporting the theory underlying the program when, according to its author, it provides an opposing position (http://deevybee .blogspot.co.uk/2011/12/pioneering-treatment-or-quackery-how-to.html).

Strong et al. (2011) undertook a systematic meta-analysis of 6 studies, taken from a larger pool of 13, all of which met appropriate scientific criteria. They found that when compared with untreated or alternative treatment controls, there was no evidence for the effectiveness of *"Fast ForWord"* for the treatment of either reading or language. In addition, the only study in the meta-analysis that included a measure of auditory temporal processing (Gillam et al., 2008) failed to result in significant gains on the auditory processing task for the *Fast ForWord* intervention group. On the basis of their review, Strong and colleagues concluded that their findings cast considerable doubt on the claims that *Fast ForWord* training can remediate auditory processing problems, or that this intervention offers significant benefits for reading and language development.

One of the criticisms of meta-analytic approaches is that their inclusion of solely those studies with high-quality scientific designs can result in the discarding of other investigations that may provide contrasting findings. Strong et al. (2011), for example, included only 6 studies for their meta-analysis from 13 that were identified as potentially appropriate. To address the possibility that this might underestimate meaningful effects, Stevenson (2011) considered the seven papers that had been excluded. He noted that of these, only one study (Troia & Whitney, 2003), excluded because of the absence of baseline group equivalence, showed any evidence of significant gains for the program, and this was in just one of the four measures employed. Stevenson also remarked on the potential for publication bias whereby studies with negative findings tend to be less likely to be published in peer-reviewed journals. However, as is pointed out, the conundrum here is that the inclusion of studies without positive outcomes would only have served to reduce the overall effect size reported in the meta-analysis.

McArthur (2009) reviewed the evidence from six studies of auditory training programs that included a focus on either nonspeech sounds or simple speech sounds. She concluded that such programs appeared to help increase performance on auditory tasks of those with marked deficits but had little effect on the literacy performance of poor readers. At the present time, there is insufficient evidence that any current auditory training program is able to serve as a means of tackling severe reading difficulties.

Biofeedback

The use of various forms of biofeedback/neurofeedback with those with a variety of developmental difficulties, including reading disability, has persisted for a long time (Tansey, 1991), but the effect of this approach on reading accuracy has not proven persuasive. In a single blind study with dyslexic adults, Liddle, Jackson, and Jackson (2005) provided feedback from each participant's cardiac cycle. Comparison with controls indicated no subsequent gains for reading accuracy, although there was a small but significant effect for reading speed.

Two studies have claimed that neurofeedback can assist poor readers (Thornton & Carmody, 2005; Walker & Norman, 2006), although sample sizes were very small and neither study employed a control group. Breteler et al. (2010) conducted what they claimed to be the only randomized controlled treatment neurofeedback study with dyslexics but failed to find an improvement in reading. Gains were found in spelling for the experimental group, most likely, according to the authors, because of improved attention. However, it should be noted that group sizes were small (n=10 experimental and n=9 control), and there was no attempt to measure whether the gains observed were maintained for any period once the experiment was completed. Although it has been suggested that advances in quantitative EEG techniques may lead to improved neurofeedback interpretations and interventions (Walker, 2010), practitioners will currently need to look elsewhere. Certainly, Breteler and colleagues' conclusion that "Neurofeedback can make an important contribution to the treatment of dyslexia" (p. 10) would best be understood as an aspiration rather than as an established finding.

The allure of complementary treatment approaches

In writing about those with the most intractable forms of reading disability, Snowling (2010) notes that families may often turn to alternative or complementary therapies despite the fact that there is no evidence that any of these are effective. In popularizing many of these alternative approaches, there has been an overreliance on personal testimonials, anecdotes, and in-house studies – sources that are often associated with pseudoscientific thinking (Hyatt et al., 2009; Park, 2003). Greenspan (2005) highlights several factors that can lead to gullibility and credulity in respect of treatment fads, and stresses the need for professional service providers to maintain a strongly scientific approach to the validation of new approaches.

Obviously science advances in sometimes unexpected ways, and a blind and knee-jerk skepticism can sometimes cause legitimate advances to be resisted and delayed. But the dangers of an unwarranted belief are much greater than the dangers of unwarranted skepticism, and a central tenet of the scientific method is to be skeptical of new claims until they are demonstrated, replicated, and hopefully, explained. (p. 137)

Despite the continuing difficulties in finding effective means to help those with severe reading disability and the temptation to look elsewhere, it seems that alternative approaches have yet to be proven effective, and until scientific findings suggest otherwise, our best option is to continue to focus on the search for the most efficacious intensive and systematic approaches to reading instruction. These are most likely to involve phonologically based reading interventions that are embedded within the context of a broad and balanced literacy curriculum (Duff & Clarke, 2011).

The pedagogic value of a diagnosis of dyslexia

A key question for the dyslexia debate is whether such a diagnosis offers guidance for intervention. Given the widespread recognition of the need for early intervention for all children with reading difficulties, one might question whether it is helpful to differentiate between dyslexic and nondyslexic poor decoders. To justify such a stance, we would need to demonstrate that each of these groups requires different forms of intervention and, if this were shown to be the case, that such groupings could be reliably identified in the case of very young children. Both of these preconditions are problematic. For example, while the Rose Report (2009) in the United Kingdom advocates early identification of dyslexic difficulties, it also notes that for most young children in the first years of schooling, "it would be very difficult to be certain which of them have dyslexia, and which do not" (p. 15).

Neither is it easy to determine the extent to which any individual's reading difficulty has a biological basis. In practice, it is impossible to differentiate between those whose poor reading and reading-related skills are a result of inherent neurobiological weaknesses and those whose difficulties are fundamentally a consequence of limited and impoverished learning experiences at home and at preschool (Torgesen et al., 2010, p. 54). Furthermore, differentiation on the basis of supposed etiology appears to have little relevance for early years' intervention:

We currently have no scientific evidence that effective prevention of reading difficulties in students with dyslexia depends on accurate differential diagnosis of the disorder in kindergarten or first grade. What *is* critical is that difficulties learning to read are identified as early as possible, and that intensive and well-targeted interventions be provided to students who are lagging behind, no matter what the cause. (Torgesen, Foorman, & Wagner, n.d., p.5; emphasis as in the original)

When considering the needs of older students, it is similarly unclear how a diagnosis of dyslexia can inform intervention beyond those approaches that are deemed appropriate for any child struggling with reading accuracy and fluency. In a UK Web-based discussion between special-needs teachers on the topic of dyslexia (SENCO Forum, 2005), for example, it was widely reported that a decision to refer children to specialist agencies was largely motivated by a desire for advice on how best to help the child's reading. However, the guidance subsequently received from specialists was perceived as offering little that could be added to those practices that were already in widespread use. In similar vein, Vellutino et al. (2004) criticize clinicians' reports for often having little prescriptive value for educational or remedial planning. These authors argue that clinicians should concern themselves less with the use of psychometric tests for the purposes of categorical labeling (e.g., "specific reading disability") and instead devote their energies to providing guidance to educators to help with the implementation of appropriate remedial interventions that are tailored to each child's individual needs.

The ways in which a diagnosis of dyslexia might lead to differential forms of intervention was an issue specifically explored by the UK House of Commons Science and Technology Committee (2009). In taking oral evidence from those advocating the need for such a diagnosis, repeated attempts were made by the chairperson to ascertain how provision for such a group would be "different" from that of other poor readers (see Q. s97–102, pp. Ev 28–29). The Select Committee, seemingly unconvinced by the claims of some expert witnesses, subsequently concluded that it was not useful from an educational point of view to differentiate between the dyslexic and other poor readers:

There is no convincing evidence that if a child with dyslexia is not labelled as dyslexic, but receives full support for his or her reading difficulty, that the child will do any worse than a child who is labelled dyslexic and then receives special help. That is because the techniques to teach a child diagnosed with dyslexia to read are exactly the same as the techniques used to teach any other struggling reader. There is a further danger than an overemphasis on dyslexia may disadvantage other children with profound learning difficulties. (p. 28)

Clearly, it is important to differentiate between children who have decoding difficulties and those who, while accurate and fluent readers, struggle with other reading-related problems such as spelling and comprehension. It is also helpful to identify those with adequate reading skills but whose progress is hampered by low motivation or lack of enthusiasm for reading (Morgan & Fuchs, 2007). In undertaking clinical assessment, the assessor will also wish to ascertain whether there are other co-occurring difficulties (e.g., language impairment, attentional difficulties) the provision for which may need to be incorporated into intervention programs. There is some evidence, for example, that medication may help the reading performance of children with co-occurring RD and ADHD (Sumner et al., 2009), although the picture is far from conclusive (Sexton et al., 2012). There is an important distinction to be drawn, however, between identifying and addressing commonly found comorbid features of reading disability and understanding these as underlying indicators of dyslexia.

It is sometimes argued that biologically or cognitively based origins of reading difficulties require a different approach to those where reading problems are primarily a consequence of poor experiences in the home and school (although, as noted earlier, achieving a valid differentiation is difficult). In reality, such a distinction appears not to be important for determining the main form of intervention (although outreach work with the family may prove additionally helpful where domestic circumstances are disadvantageous [Foorman et al., 2002]). Instead, the child's response to high-quality intervention would appear to "provide guidance as to his or her long-term instructional needs, *regardless of the origin of his or her reading difficulties*" (Vellutino et al., 2004, p. 31; emphasis added). Persistent difficulties may lead the child to "be justifiably classified as 'reading disabled' *for whatever official purposes such classification is needed*" (Vellutino et al., 2008, p. 471; emphasis added). As this statement suggests, a dyslexia label may operate for bureaucratic and resource-related reasons rather than guide particular forms of intervention beyond that which is considered appropriate for all poor decoders. In the United Kingdom, for example, the dyslexia label is often a means to gain additional resources and special assistance for college and university students. In the United States, a diagnostic label (e.g., learning disability) is required to access special education provision.

A common concern of parents of poor readers is that teachers may inappropriately consider their child to be lazy or unmotivated, and in so doing, their expectations of, sensitivity towards, and desire to encourage and help the youngster may be reduced (Gwernan-Jones & Burden, 2010). Many parents believe that a diagnosis of dyslexia, portraying the child as suffering from a biological condition of some kind, may dispel any tendency of teachers to blame the child for poor academic performance. However, the relationship between motivation and ability is more complex and multilayered than this picture suggests (Lackaye & Margalit, 2006; Morgan, Fuchs, Compton, Cordray, & Fuchs, 2008) and overly simplistic analyses involving unmotivated/dyslexic dichotomies are unlikely to help our understanding of the interactions between interest, agency, self-concept, self-efficacy, and engagement, factors that are likely to have a significant bearing upon such situations.

Some students conceal the true extent of their reading difficulties from their teachers and underachieve further as a consequence of this (Wadlington, Elliot, & Kirylo, 2008). A desire to create a systemic approach to resolving associated academic and emotional problems underpinned the creation of the "dyslexia-friendly" schools movement in the United Kingdom (Coffield et al., 2008). However, here the term "dyslexia" is used in a general fashion that is intended to incorporate a wide range of literacy problems. The key components of this initiative – to assess accurately the academic needs of children with literacy difficulties, to intervene with appropriate learning instruction, to recognize that word-reading difficulties and likely progress are unrelated to intellectual capacity, to be sensitive to student anxieties and insecurities, and to recognize that reduced motivation is often a consequence of a history of struggle with print, rather than a primary cause of difficulties – are all relevant to any child struggling with reading (Riddick, Wolfe, & Lumsdon, 2002).

The dyslexia debate is exemplified by the Pamela Phelps case outlined at the beginning of this chapter. As was pointed out, the fact that severe reading difficulties were hampering Ms. Phelps's learning and development were not in dispute; rather, the issue centered on the potential value of a diagnosis of dyslexia to help her overcome her difficulties. In such a dispute it would seem important to ascertain whether:

a) there was appropriate intervention to address Ms. Phelps' reading difficulties;
b) teacher expectations and general academic demands were inappropriately reduced because of misattribution of the origins of her difficulties (e.g., intellectual weakness);
c) an insufficient level of resourcing to address her difficulties was made available because of the failure to provide the diagnosis;
d) the failure to provide the label resulted in Ms. Phelps not receiving an alternative or complementary therapy that would have resolved her difficulties.

None of the above is dependent or conditional on a diagnosis of dyslexia. As noted in this chapter, educational interventions for those with reading accuracy or fluency difficulties are not further informed by the application of this label. No judgment of a child's intellectual abilities should be based on their performance on word-reading skills. Instead, teachers' academic expectations and demands should be dependent on the child's performance across multiple domains. While in some contexts, such as the United States, there are resource-related issues concerning the designation of certain labels (e.g., learning disabilities), this is not true of the United Kingdom, and Ms. Phelps received remedial intervention in the light of assessment of her special educational needs. Finally, as this chapter has indicated, non-educational interventions have yet to demonstrate academic effectiveness. Thus, if Ms. Phelps had been diagnosed as dyslexic, it is unclear how this could have led to her receiving any additional therapy that would have helped resolve her difficulties.

Perhaps the key message from this chapter in relation to the dyslexia debate is that categorical labeling *within* the population of children with decoding difficulties offers little guidance for intervention:

If we want to identify children with problems in reading, then identified problems in reading should serve as the basis for identification. There is no need to distinguish between "reading disability" and "poor reading." One need only identify problems in reading and treat them accordingly. (Sternberg & Grigorenko, 2002, p. 82)

Given this position, one is left to question what benefits are served by investing significant resources in a search to ascertain, from within the population of poor decoders, who is, and who is not, dyslexic.

Summary

The debate over the teaching of reading was, for many years, influenced by polemic and ideology rather than findings from high-quality scientific investigations. The whole-language approach, based on a misunderstanding that reading is naturally acquired, often decried or de-emphasized structured, phonics-based approaches on the grounds that these were decontextualized, artificial, and demotivating. With the advent of more rigorous research approaches it has become clear that children at risk of reading disability require highly systematic and structured educational approaches.

It has been repeatedly demonstrated that systematic instruction, incorporating a strong emphasis on phonemic awareness and phonics as part of a broad range of reading-related activities, in small groups or individually as necessary, can significantly reduce the proportion of children who are later considered to be reading disabled. However, initial gains in the first years of schooling are not always sustained, some problems only emerge in later years, and individual children's circumstances are subject to fluctuation as they mature and encounter changing reading demands.

While it is important that intervention should commence as early as possible, predicting which children will struggle with reading is complex and typically generates a significant proportion of false positives and negatives. To date, there is no clear consensus as to the most appropriate measures, methods, or timing. Screening tests for dyslexia often include a wider range of measures than the more narrow tools used for identifying reading problems. The former are more likely to assess fine and gross motor skills, although the predictive validity of these measures for reading appears to be weak.

Although structured interventions with young children have proven helpful, there continues to be a proportion of children (approximately 2–6%) who continue to experience significant difficulties in reading ("treatment resisters"). In the later school years, reading difficulties are compounded by increasingly complex reading demands and, in some cases, reduced motivation to read. To date, work in genetics, neuroscience, and cognitive science is not sufficiently advanced to be able to generate additional guidance for educational practice with such children. At the current time, other than recommending "more of the same," researchers are uncertain about how to assist those with the most complex and intractable reading difficulties.

There is little evidence to support the use of any special approaches for dyslexia, as key elements of dyslexia teaching programs are typically the same as those routinely employed in the reading disability literature. Complementary approaches such as motor training, auditory and visual interventions, the use of fatty acids, and biofeedback have yet to demonstrate significant evidence of effectiveness.

Contrary to the beliefs of many, once a reading difficulty is identified, a diagnosis of dyslexia offers little or no further benefit for guiding the nature of any intervention. In some societies such a label, irrespective of its questionable scientific rigor or validity, is necessary in order to receive additional educational resources. In respect of pedagogy, however, the crucial task is to identify the individual's particular reading strengths and weaknesses and address these directly.

5   Conclusions and recommendations

The debate about how we should understand the concept of developmental dyslexia has sometimes become oversimplified to the point that the very existence of a biologically based reading disability has been questioned. Such a position is untenable, yet it is not always understood that criticism of the scientific rigor of a given label or construct does not necessarily imply that the problems it seeks to encompass are not real or meaningful. Thus, critical concerns expressed about the value of the dyslexia construct have been incorrectly understood or reframed by some as reflecting a perception that the term serves as an "excuse" for laziness, stupidity, or poor teaching. While there remain some commentators who certainly hold such views, the great majority of critiques in the academic literature (Elliott & Gibbs, 2008; Soler, 2010; Stanovich, 1994) have sought to provide a more nuanced perspective that eschews such notions.

In 2005, the dyslexia debate gained prominence in many countries as a result of widespread coverage given to a British television program, *The Dyslexia Myth* (http://topdocumentaryfilms.com/dyslexia-myth/). The main assertion of this program was that there were many myths surrounding the nature of dyslexia and its treatment. Existing practice, where only a limited proportion of struggling readers were identified as having dyslexia, typically on the basis of extensive cognitive assessments, was resulting in delays in intervention for some and no intervention for other candidates who also needed help. The program's message, largely reflecting the perspective of the response to intervention movement, was misperceived by some as stating that biologically based reading difficulties were a myth (see, for example, Nicolson [2005] and a subsequent response to this by Elliott [2005]). Surprisingly, this perception flew in the face of clear statements to the contrary that were offered throughout the program. What was actually being questioned were the rigor, utility, and added value of a clinical diagnosis of dyslexia, not the existence of the very real underlying problems that those with complex reading difficulties typically encounter. Rather than focusing on expensive assessments, often more accessible to children from socioeconomically advantaged families (Sternberg & Grigorenko, 1999b), and usually undertaken after long-term failure had been established, it was recommended that intervention should be conducted as early as possible with all those who were potentially at risk of reading difficulty, irrespective of etiology.

In the United Kingdom, the Rose Report (2009) was conceived to provide expert guidance to practitioners, which was underpinned by current under-standings in the research literature. However, within its apparent reporting of secure knowledge, many of the underlying complexities were ignored. Thus, having confidently asserted that dyslexia "exists" (p. 9), the Report neglected the difficulty of moving from a broad conceptual definition to an operational definition that could be consistently and uniformly employed in education con-texts. Instead, its position rather blithely suggested that research could clearly show what dyslexia is and is not, and the implicit message was that rather than focusing further on conceptual clarification, the key task was now to build greater professional expertise in identifying the condition so that effec-tive intervention could take place. This implied that (1) all parties shared a common understanding as to what dyslexia is, (2) there was a broad consensus on how it could be reliably identified in clinical and educational contexts, and (3) such identification was an important precursor to appropriate intervention. All of these propositions are highly questionable, and it is the consideration of these, not the existence or otherwise of dyslexia, that truly constitutes "the dyslexia debate."

The use of the term "dyslexia," both in research and in clinical and educa-tional practice, has been compounded by multiple problems and differences of opinion in relation to:

a) conceptualization and operationalization;
b) the ability to provide meaningful subgroup classifications or individual diagnoses on the basis of genetic or neurological biomarkers;
c) the ability to specify to any significant degree of precision the nature, role, and influence of underlying cognitive and sensory processes in dyslexia;
d) the relationship between existing biological and cognitive insights into the nature of dyslexia and evidence-based understandings about the most appro-priate forms of intervention.

Conceptualization and operationalization

The demise of the IQ discrepancy model, by which the dyslexia label was used to differentiate between one group of poor readers marked out by their higher intelligence from other, "garden variety" poor readers, resulted in a conceptual lacuna. If the term was no longer a means of identifying intellectually able poor readers, what was its purpose? Add to this vacuum the understandably strong desire of many struggling readers and their families to avoid inappropriate attributions of low intelligence for their difficulties, and it is unsurprising that the belief that those with dyslexia are high-functioning poor readers, rather than those who represent the full continuum of intellectual ability, has continued to persist despite all evidence to the contrary (O'Donnell & Miller, 2011; Stanovich, 2005).

For those who have accepted the scientific evidence about IQ and reading disability, agreeing on a new explanatory role for dyslexia has proven difficult (Wadlington & Wadlington, 2005). As noted in Chapter 1, dyslexia is often used interchangeably with such terms as "reading disorder," "reading difficulties," "specific reading difficulties," "reading disabilities," or "specific reading disabilities," with decoding rather than reading comprehension clearly being the issue of concern (Vellutino & Fletcher, 2007). Some contend that "dyslexia represents the lower end of a normal distribution of word reading ability" (Peterson & Pennington, 2012, p. 1997). Others understand the term as describing a subgroup of poor readers whose difficulties have a neurobiological basis marked by various cognitive or behavioral features (e.g., a phonological impairment [Spear-Swerling, 2011]). Some suggest that dyslexia should be a term reserved to describe problems of single-word decoding (Fletcher, 2009), others contend that it should concern difficulties of both reading accuracy and fluency (Snowling & Hulme, 2012), and yet others consider poor reading to be only one particular element of a more pervasive dyslexic disorder manifested by a range of cognitive and self-regulatory difficulties. For example, Wilkins, Garside, and Enfield (1993) state that individuals with dyslexia have difficulties not only with reading and spelling but also "understanding language that they hear, or expressing themselves clearly in speaking or writing" (p. 2).

The International Dyslexia Association fiercely contested the proposed deletion of the term "dyslexia" from the DSM-5 framework, to be replaced by Specific Learning Disorder, on the grounds that dyslexia should be treated as more than a reading difficulty:

If it remains unelaborated, the term "specific reading disorder" implies a condition that is limited to reading problems. Dyslexia affects more than reading, although reading difficulty is the primary marker. The disorder encompasses language processing, language production, related symbolic learning (such as second language learning), and often adaptive skills in daily living and in social and emotional functioning. (International Dyslexia Association Advisory Board, 2012, para. 6)

For some, dyslexia reflects "an alternative way of thinking – a learning preference" that can have an impact on the acquisition of literacy and numeracy skills (http://www.dyslexiafoundation.org.nz/d_assessment.html). Indeed, for those who understand dyslexia in this broad sense, it is possible to be dyslexic even in the absence of decoding difficulties. Tunmer and Greaney (2010), for example, have criticized the working definition provided by the New Zealand Ministry of Education on the grounds that this enables a diagnosis of dyslexia for those with difficulties in numeracy or musical notation but with no problems in reading, writing, or spelling.

It has been suggested that the dyslexic child should show signs of average or high ability in other domains (a "sea of strengths"); for others, the particular underlying processes that result in reading failure are likely to be prevalent across the ability range, and thus it is quite conceivable that a dyslexic individual may demonstrate low achievement across the board. Some argue that there must be an unexpected element to the reading difficulty, adjudged on the basis of the individual's performance in other domains; others contend that the unexpected component should instead reflect the individual's poor response over time to high-quality educational intervention. Some point to the high proportion of individuals with dyslexia who are delinquent and incarcerated (Dyslexia Action, 2005) while others view dyslexic individuals as having particular creative gifts that often mark them out for success in life (Davis, 1997; Eide & Eide, 2011; Geschwind, 1982), particularly as entrepreneurs (Logan, 2009; Marazzi, 2011):

Usually when people hear the word dyslexia they think only of reading, writing, spelling and maths problems a child is having in school . . . but learning disability is only one face of dyslexia. Once as a guest on a TV show I was asked about the "positive" side of dyslexia. As part of my answer, I listed a dozen or so famous dyslexics. The hostess of the show then commented, "Isn't it amazing that all those people could be geniuses in spite of having dyslexia?" She missed the point. (Davis, 1997, p. 3)

Despite such claims, a recent research study suggests that the success of high-performing dyslexic adults is unlikely to be a function of particular cognitive factors (supposedly superior creative and visuo-spatial abilities were not found in a sample of university students and graduates). Rather, outstanding success would seem to depend more on personality and motivational factors (Łockiewicz, Bogdanowicz, & Bogdanowicz, in press).

Confusion about the manifestation of dyslexia is reflected in a huge variation in prevalence rates ranging from 5–8% (Mather & Wendling, 2012) to as much as 20% (Shaywitz, 2005). Employed as a dimensional term, there will necessarily be an arbitrary cut-off in those contexts where a label of some kind is required, but there is little agreement as to how and where such a cut-off should be made and how permanent the label should be. Given that an individual's reading performance relative to others often fluctuates over time, one might query whether is it possible to be dyslexic, then improve to the point that one is no longer dyslexic, but then subsequently perform poorly on standardized measures and thus become dyslexic once more.

It has been argued that the "true" dyslexic can be revealed by their poor response to reading assistance over time – a figure of 4–5% equating to that proportion of the population that appears to be resistant to the best forms of evidence-based reading intervention currently available. At a clinical level, the restriction of the term to treatment resisters might have some merit as this could identify those who are likely to require long-term technological and ancillary support (Elliott & Gibbs, 2008). Treatment resistance has been suggested as a key criterion for reading disability and also the broader conception of learning disability (Berninger & Abbott, 1994; Fuchs & Fuchs, 1998; Speece & Shek-itka, 2002) – propositions that sit easily with RTI approaches where access to immediate help and support is not conditional on a diagnosis ("wait to fail") but is provided as soon as difficulties emerge.

As this book has sought to demonstrate, it has proven impossible to identify a dyslexic subgroup in any consistent or coherent fashion that would be accept-able to the majority of the scientific and professional community. While many would be agreeable to its use as a synonym for poor decoding, others would reject this position on the grounds that the construct would then no longer add anything to other commonly used terms.

The ability to provide subgroup classifications or individual diagnoses of dyslexia on the basis of genetic or neurological biomarkers

Given that demonstrating the constitutional origins of "hidden" impairments is widely seen as a primary means of proving their legitimacy (Riddick, 2000), it is not surprising that the biological basis of dyslexia is frequently cited when the scientific rigor of the construct is raised. Nicolson (2005), for example, distinguishes between dyslexic and other poor readers (seemingly on the basis of their level of general intelligence) stating: "The fact that 50 per cent of the variance in dyslexia is genetic means that dyslexia does have a clear and distinct basis" (p. 658). Certainly, knowledge of genetics and brain functioning in relation to typical and atypical reading (including reading disability) has increased exponentially during the past decade. However, as has been pointed out in Chapter 3, what is often overlooked is that the reading-disabled/dyslexic samples in these studies are generally comprised of participants selected on the basis of their having obtained a score below an arbitrary cut-off point on one or more measures of reading, not subgroups of poor readers selected on the basis of a particular underlying cognitive profile indicative of dyslexia.

There is often a flawed line of reasoning offered in the literature, which runs as follows:

1. Studies from genetics and neuroscience (whose participants are typically selected on the basis of performance on a standardised reading test) suggest that biological factors play a role in both poor and good reading.
2. Dyslexic individuals are those whose reading difficulties have a biological basis.

3. Those with dyslexia can be differentiated in practice from other poor readers on these grounds.

In reality, the key conclusions that can be offered from relevant work in genetics and neuroscience are that (a) there often appears to be a genetic component to typical and atypical reading although specific mechanisms are still unclear; (b) we can identify certain areas of the brain that appear to be associated with typical and atypical reading but these findings, although offering promise for the future, cannot be used for diagnostic purposes; and (c) findings from such studies are often difficult to generalize (it is especially the case for genetic findings), suggesting a remarkable amount of heterogeneity in the etiology of both typical and atypical reading.

Although research has demonstrated that complex reading difficulties typically have a neurobiological basis, in practice, distinguishing between the dyslexic (with an inherent disability) and other poor readers (whose problems may be deemed to be environmentally determined) is a task predicated on a problematic dichotomization. While there may be instances of widespread reading failure in cultures and contexts where the teaching of reading is nonexistent or lamentable, or in particular situations where a child has missed a significant amount of schooling, in most advanced societies it would generally be highly difficult to conclude that a child's prolonged difficulty with reading is primarily environmental in origin. Similarly, the current state of affairs does not allow the separation of poor readers into clear causal groups based on biological phenomena – there are no established biomarkers, either genes or brain-based, that could be used for such purposes of differentiation.

As was shown in Chapter 4, certain educational approaches to the teaching of reading have generally proven less helpful to those with reading disabilities, but here, of course, there is often an important interaction – a biologically based problem may be greatly exacerbated by inappropriate provision. If a child with a biologically based difficulty encounters an educational environment that fails to deliver structured and explicit teaching of reading, the likelihood is that limited progress will ensue. Clearly it would be an error to conclude that the child's problem is merely the consequence of poor teaching. In other cases, a young child struggling to develop basic literacy skills may subsequently make rapid progress once high-quality teaching is introduced. In such circumstances one might conclude that here the origin of the difficulty was essentially related to inadequate early learning experiences, whether at home or at school. However, it is not clear what the extent of any gain in performance should be for such a judgment to be made, and indeed, in such cases, a label or classification would no longer be required, for the primary problem would no longer exist. Add to this complexity the fact that socially disadvantaged children are not always able to sustain reading gains made during the first years of schooling (Kieffer, 2012), and it becomes clear that making such a judgment is largely arbitrary.

Given that we cannot make a meaningful distinction between the relative influence of those factors that predispose a particular pattern of brain development (i.e., genetic patterns), those patterns that are derivative of specific characteristics of the brain and emerge only when reading is being acquired (i.e., specific neural signatures differentiating the "reading" from the "non-reading" or "poor reading" brain), and those systematically socially derived factors (i.e., reading-related learning at home and at school) that are key for reading development, perhaps the way forward is to focus on the individual's unique biological characteristics. Unfortunately, it is not yet possible to utilize advances in genetics or neuroscience to provide individual assessments of poor readers. Often misunderstood is the fact that the colorful images produced to show areas of the brain that are engaged when various cognitive tasks are being tackled are typically composites reflecting the activity of multiple participants, not an accurate picture of an individual's functioning that can be used to inform individualized intervention. Moving from group average differences to individualized assessment represents one of the major challenges for such approaches (Giedd & Rapoport, 2010). Although prediction and individual profiling on the basis of genetics and neuroimaging may yet become a possibility at some time in the future, particularly if this is combined with behavioral indicators and environmental measures of an individual's learning (Black & Hoeft, 2012), it should also be borne in mind that the cost of such assessments is likely to prove prohibitive for many years to come.

Conceptions of complex developmental disorders such as reading disability have become increasingly sophisticated, with greater recognition that these are heterogeneous conditions underpinned by multiple genetic and environmental risk factors (Willcutt et al., 2010), which all play a role in the rate of growth in reading (Petrill et al., 2010). Findings indicating, for example, that SES appears to have an influence on brain structure (Jednoróg et al., 2012), and that heritability declines linearly in relation to decreased levels of parental education (Friend, DeFries, & Olson, 2008; Rosenberg et al., 2012), have rendered increasingly untenable the suggestion that we can, in practice, differentiate a biologically based dyslexic subgroup from others who also struggle with decoding.

The ability to specify to any significant degree of precision the nature, role, and influence of underlying cognitive and sensory processes in dyslexia

Despite having accumulated a vast wealth of research findings on the many sensory, cognitive, and motor processes that have been associated with reading disability/dyslexia, we have achieved only rudimentary understandings and even less consensus about how causal mechanisms operate. While it is generally agreed that the core causes of reading difficulty are primarily linguistic, the role of visual factors, seen largely as irrelevant a decade ago, and still deemed peripheral by many researchers and leading medical associations (American Academy of Pediatrics, 2009; Handler et al., 2011), has emerged once more to become a topic of interest in scientific laboratories (Dehaene, 2009). However, despite evidence that some poor readers appear to suffer from low-level sensory deficits, there is still a dearth of evidence of a causal relationship between these and difficulties in learning to read (Vellutino et al., 2004).

Although the phonological deficit theory continues to dominate, the notion of a single homogeneous deficit is now recognized as inadequate (Snowling & Hulme, 2012). Phonological weakness, seemingly the most influential cognitive component, cannot account for the difficulties of all those with reading disability; not all those with word-reading difficulties demonstrate a phonological weakness, and not all those with such a weakness demonstrate a reading difficulty. This syllogistic complexity applies equally to the many other cognitive and sensory processes that have been put forward as causal factors in dyslexia.

Given that individuals with dyslexia cannot be identified purely on the basis of their having an identifiable phonological or some other cognitive deficit, an alternative approach is to specify a particular combination of processes that would enable individuals to be matched to a particular dyslexic profile. Systematic studies have failed to support such an approach (Kavale & Forness, 1984; Kramer et al., 1987; Stuebing et al., 2012), although these findings have not deterred efforts to find an alternative solution. Le Jan et al. (2011), for example, argue that not all poor readers are dyslexic: "[S]ome garden-variety children may have poor reading/spelling as dyslexic children [*sic*] but cannot be 'labelled' as dyslexics" (p. 2). They suggest that their complex multivariate predictive model, incorporating a range of underlying processes (including measures of phonological awareness, attention, memory, morphology, and auditory discrimination), can help practitioners "clarify the type of dyslexia and identify the appropriate remediation to consider" (p. 16). However, not only are they unclear about what they consider to be the characteristics of "garden variety" readers; they also offer no explanation as to how information from their approach can be utilized in practice – an unfortunate omission given that there is little evidence that profiles of this kind can inform the nature of intervention programs. As is so often the case in the dyslexia literature, there is a chain of argument that includes assumptions and suppositions that are not adequately followed through.

Arguing that dyslexia is a "clinical diagnosis," Shaywitz and Shaywitz (2013, p. 645) assert that the condition cannot be determined on the basis of a single score on a test. In their opinion, the clinician needs to take into account multiple features of a given individual's strengths and weaknesses. Seemingly, this position can be contrasted with that commonly held by reading researchers whereby dyslexia is defined by one's position at the tail end of a distribution curve of scores on a reading test. One immediate difficulty with Shaywitz and Shaywitz's perspective is that, as has been shown throughout this book, there are no clear understandings as to what particular constellations of features would either result in such a diagnosis or, instead, in a determination that the individual was a nondyslexic poor reader. Neither is it clear what would be the educational implications of making such a distinction for any such individual.

The relationship between existing biological and cognitive insights into the nature of dyslexia and evidence-based understandings about the most appropriate forms of intervention

It is often assumed that a diagnosis of dyslexia can point to a particular form of intervention that is best suited for those with the condition. Ideally, data sourced from genetic, neuropsychological, and cognitive assessments could be used for the purposes of preparing bespoke interventions directly addressing a given dyslexic individual's strengths and weaknesses (see Figures 1.1 and 1.2). The reality, however, is that there is a clear disjuncture between the information that can be derived from such sources and the use that can be made of this for educational planning. Given that diagnosis is primarily designed to inform action, clinicians continue to be best advised

to shift the focus of their clinical activities away from emphasis on psychometric assessment to detect cognitive and biological causes of a child's reading difficulties for purposes of categorical labeling in favor of assessment that would eventuate in educational and remedial activities tailored to the child's individual needs. (Vellutino et al., 2004, p. 31)

In such a scenario, the child's response to an appropriately tailored remedial intervention "would provide guidance as to his or her long-term instructional needs, *regardless of the origin of his or her reading difficulties*" (p. 35) (emphasis added).

Of course, it is possible that future advances in neuroscience will ultimately lead to the development of new, effective, and innovative pedagogic practices for those with reading difficulties. However, despite indications that it may ultimately be possible to offer helpful information about likely response to intervention in struggling readers (Hoeft et al., 2011; Rezaie et al., 2011), the value of neuroimaging for tailoring clinical or educational interventions is currently negligible (Grant, 2012), and for the foreseeable future it is likely that the main focus of educational neuroscience will be on seeking greater understanding of the underlying mechanisms involved in human development, and subsequently gaining insights into why certain existing educational practices often prove valuable (Goswami, 2012; Goswami & Szucs, 2011). Certainly, we need to be cautious about our expectations of neuroscience in the short term, if not the long term, recognize the hype and overblown claims that are currently so prevalent in the scientific literature (Bishop, 2013; Turner, 2012), and accept that we are many years from achieving a neuroscience that can inform pedagogic responses that are individually tailored to address the particular needs of given children.

The science and politics of dyslexia

In determining the scientific value of the dyslexia construct, it is important to recognize the differing perspectives and agendas of diverse stakeholders. Geneticists, neuroscientists, medical practitioners, cognitive psychologists, clinical psychologists, school/educational psychologists, speech and language therapists, education researchers, mainstream teachers, special education teachers, education consultants and trainers, lobby and advocacy groups, and, of course, struggling readers and their families, may each appropriate the dyslexia label, ascribing to it different meanings and utilizing it for differing purposes. When the construct is questioned, the reaction can often be puzzlement or bemusement, as members of such groups typically each have their own understandings that act as received wisdom. Thus, Siegel and Mazabel (2013) express the view that dyslexia and reading disability are synonymous terms with identical meanings, adding that they are puzzled as to why "dyslexia . . . is often viewed as if it were a four-letter word, not to be uttered in polite company" (p. 187). What they fail to fully grasp, however, is that their use of this construct is not shared by many others who, as Table 1.1 illustrates, may hold alternative conceptions and understandings, and therein lies a fundamental problem.

The conception of learning disability (and, by extension, dyslexia) has been criticized for having been heavily shaped by historical and cultural influences that range far beyond the medical account of a biologically grounded condition (McDermott, Goldman, & Varenne, 2006; Reid & Valle, 2004; Soler, 2009). Others (Lopes, 2012) have criticized the dominance in the literature of biological explanations, and complain that cultural and educational factors are underrepresented in explanatory accounts. However, while there is some explanatory merit in sociocultural perspectives (Riddick, 2001; Soler, 2010), one must guard against permitting the pendulum to swing too far to an equally flawed radical social constructionist position in which biological argument is replaced by a social and cultural account. Here the notion of disability is reduced to a wholly sociological construct in which those with disabilities appear to be devoid of any biological features (Anastasiou & Kauffman, 2011) – a position that is hardly consonant with the advances of research into reading difficulty.

Being labeled dyslexic can be perceived as desirable for many reasons. Some are attracted by its potential to attract extra educational resources or support (Macdonald, 2009). It offers the promise (although not the reality) of tailored forms of intervention or treatment, and it can reduce the shame and embarrassment that are often an unfortunate consequence of literacy difficulties (Burden, 2008; Cooke, 2001). It may help exculpate the child, parents, and teachers from any perceived sense of responsibility, or even guilt, for literacy difficulties (Ho, 2004; Warnke et al., 2012), and, for similar reasons, it may result in more patient and sensitive handling from professionals. It may fulfill the common need that many of us have to secure a label for our physical and psychological problems. Teachers may find the notion of the dyslexic child as one who is intellectually able helpful in considering how best to provide appropriate learning activities and in offering greater understanding of the particular frustrations that such children are likely to encounter (Regan & Woods, 2000). However, this misunderstanding of the relationship between intellectual ability and decoding skill may act as a two-edged sword, for such teachers may be less well disposed to accept a diagnosis of dyslexia when a child is seen to be intellectually weak, and they may make inappropriate attributions of low intelligence to poor readers who do not have this label. In these cases the outcome may be lowered expectations leading to reduced teacher efforts to boost the child's performance.

The many problems associated with dyslexia, in all its various manifestations, sustain a vast industry geared to providing assessments, diagnoses, and treatments. Commercial pressures are such that professionals may feel obliged to give parents the label that is desired (Sternberg & Grigorenko, 1999b) and this can easily result in the conceptual inflation of attractive labels such as dyslexia. Schools, seeking to avoid potential conflict and litigation, are unlikely to question such diagnoses, and special education teachers can see these as providing additional resources (Senco Forum, 2005). It has even been argued (Garner, 2004) that UK universities have encouraged the over-diagnosis of dyslexia for their own gain (see also Soler, 2009, for a discussion of this issue). Business, professional, and parent groups all seek to influence public understanding and government legislation through various lobbying activities, the political and adversarial aspects of which can have a distorting effect on scientific research (Kauffman et al., 1998; Nicolson, 2005; Stanovich, 1998).

As noted earlier, decisions concerning dyslexia, like so many aspects of special education, are not neutral and value-free, but instead reflect a myriad of differing political and social agendas:

> The definition of dyslexia, and the assessment and classification of literacy difficulties are discursive spaces for ongoing resistance, challenges and contestation, because they are key aspects in the construction of social and personal identities associated with dyslexia and LD/SpLD (Learning Difficulties/Specific Learning Difficulties) . . . they are central to the professional practice/discourse surrounding dyslexia because of their inextricable links to professional identity, power relationships and the access to resources. (Soler, 2010, pp. 190–191)

Of course, there is less difficulty if the term "dyslexia" is not expected to offer additional diagnostic information beyond that of reading disability and, as Stanovich (1994) has argued, where this happens, arguments about the validity of a dyslexia label largely disappear. However, if this were to be the case, the construct would no longer offer the conceptual added value that is often sought from it, and many would surely rail against any narrowing of its explanatory field. Alternatively, perhaps we should accept that there are many types of dyslexia, social constructs that are each created by, and reflect the values and agendas of, differing groups? However, to accept such a position must surely be to dispense with any suggestion of scientific rigor.

The end of dyslexia?

Parents of students with dyslexia continually face challenges within our educational system, experiencing frustration, disappointment, and anger due to a lack of understanding about dyslexia. All too often students with dyslexia are misdiagnosed, misunderstood, or just plain ignored. As a result, their skills and abilities often are overlooked. These students begin to doubt themselves and their abilities; they feel stupid, lazy, and worthless. This lack of knowledge about dyslexia often means schools do not provide the necessary identification, instruction, intervention, and accommodations that students with dyslexia need to succeed. From the time a student's dyslexia is first identified to the implementation of an IEP or 504 plan, it is essential that educators understand the potential of our students when given appropriate instruction and accommodations. (Steinberg & Andrist, 2012)

It may seem paradoxical that while highlighting the needs of children with reading difficulties, the authors of this book are recommending that the use of the term "dyslexia" should be discontinued. However, the difficulties of operationalizing the commonly used yet often contrasting definitions of dyslexia in a way that is clear, rigorous, and consistent for educational practice are such that the uncertainties generated serve to exacerbate rather than reduce the very problems and misunderstandings that are described in the section-opening quotation.

The term "dyslexia" has surely outgrown its conceptual and diagnostic usefulness. This assertion may seem puzzling given the increasing use of the construct around the world. In the United States, where the popularity of the term has fluctuated since the 1930s (Rooney, 1995), dyslexia currently features in the legislation of several states, with dyslexia laws progressing through the legislative process in a number of others, and is predicted to become more widely used (Mather & Wendling, 2012). The extent to which the term's deletion from DSM-5 will halt this trajectory, if at all, is currently unclear, especially as clinicians can still use "dyslexia" as a specifier within the DSM framework. Furthermore, and despite the fierce resistance of lobby groups such as the U.S.-based International Dyslexia Association, to the DSM-5 proposals, the majority of professionals operating in the field of reading disability are unlikely to be greatly influenced by changes within the field of psychiatry.

Irrespective of its popularity and usage, the dyslexia construct should be recognized as inadequate for both classification and diagnosis. In science, classification acts as a tool to enable communication between researchers so that when they discuss a feature, it means the same thing to everyone (Taylor & Rutter, 2008). As this book has demonstrated, this is far from the case for dyslexia. Researchers who use the term solely to describe decoding difficulties (Fletcher, 2009; Fletcher et al., 2011; Peterson & Pennington, 2012) may not perceive the construct as unduly problematic, but not all researchers share this understanding, and important differences of conceptualization are rarely made explicit when sample characteristics are described in research publications. Discrepant and inconsistent understandings tend to be even more problematic in clinical work where there is no clear consensus as to the basis on which a diagnosis of dyslexia would be reliably and consistently offered above and beyond the actual reading behavior itself.

Differences of opinion exist in psychiatry about the value of separate systems of classification for researchers and clinicians (see Pine (2011) and Rutter (2011) for a discussion of this in relation to DSM-5). Within the field of special education tensions can exist between researchers who typically desire tight, precise definitions and clinicians for whom loose flexible definitions offer greater opportunity for maximizing the number of those who might profit from additional resource allocation (Lloyd, Hallahan, & Kauffman, 1980; Mellard, Deshler, & Barth, 2004). However, where resources are limited, dyslexia is a diagnosis that may have adverse consequences. Rather than opening up access to resources in an inclusive fashion, the label may serve to exclude those with reading difficulties who for various reasons (social, economic, political) fail to obtain the label. Furthermore, its conceptual remit is sometimes so broad that teaching resources are poorly targeted, away from those most in need and wasted on complex, wide-ranging assessments that do not meaningfully inform intervention.

In respect of word-reading difficulty, the construct *reading disability* is surely preferable for use by both researchers and clinicians. This term dispenses with much of the conceptual and political baggage associated with dyslexia. At a stroke, it highlights the fact that the core problem is reading rather than a myriad of other associated or comorbid cognitive and behavioral features.

Reading disability can best be understood as a particular type of reading difficulty – a problem of single-word decoding (Fletcher, 2009). The difficulty should not be able to be explained by severe visual or hearing impairment, although other potential exclusionary factors such as low intelligence, poverty, opportunity to learn, or emotional well-being should not feature in any individual judgments. While the origins of complex reading disability (like dyslexia) will usually have a biological basis (Spear-Swerling, 2011), there should be no requirement to make a nature/nurture distinction for the purposes of identifying this condition. The interaction of multiple factors is such that a clear-cut judgment would be impossible to make in practice.

An individual's single-word reading ability, and the extent of any reading disability, could be relatively easily assessed using appropriate measures (Fletcher et al., 1994). As noted earlier, such disability is best understood as a dimensional construct, and any arbitrary decision to use one or more cut-off points for the purposes of research or intervention should not be suggestive of a categorical classification (Branum-Martin, Fletcher, & Stuebing, in press).

For the purposes of educational assessment and differentiated intervention, measures of reading fluency, reading comprehension, and spelling should also be routinely undertaken, although difficulties for each would, like reading disability, be conceptualized as differing forms of reading difficulty (see Fletcher et al. (2011) for a rationale for understanding reading fluency as distinct from reading accuracy, Snowling and Hulme (2012) for spelling, and Kamhi (2009) for a discussion of the problems resulting from confusing word reading with comprehension). Such a procedure sits well with DSM-5 where a psychiatric diagnosis of Specific Learning Disorder subsequently leads to specification of the particular domain (e.g., reading) and subskills (e.g., word reading accuracy) involved. However, it is often necessary to go beyond these basic descriptors, and further assessment can usefully examine the individual's unique reading profile (Valencia, 2011). The key point to recognize here is that such assessment is undertaken for the purpose of guiding appropriate intervention, not for classification or diagnosis. Ultimately, it is knowledge about an individual's skills on each of these aspects of reading, together with their strengths and weaknesses on a range of other academic and cognitive skills, that will inform educational practice (Gormley & McDermott, 2011; Snowling & Hulme, 2012).

Although IQ tells us little about intervention and prognosis in relation to severe decoding difficulties, this does not mean that assessment of cognitive functioning is unimportant for educational planning. Clearly it is essential for teachers to have a sound understanding of their students' cognitive abilities in order that they might ensure that the level of intellectual challenge of classroom activities is appropriate across all subjects in the school curriculum. It would, of course, be a grave error to base academic demands solely on the child's performance in basic skill areas. Similarly, tracking or streaming based on performance in tests or examinations should not result in intellectually able poor readers being placed in classes where the educational diet is insufficiently challenging. However, one of the more confused understandings of the dyslexia debate results from a failure to grasp that there is a major difference between undertaking cognitive assessment to inform decisions regarding the intellectual content and challenge of a broad range of curricular activities, and its use in relation to the widely discredited IQ-reading discrepancy diagnosis.

The use of the term "reading disability" would be appropriate for work in genetics and neuroscience where, as has been noted throughout this book, participants are typically selected on the basis of their performance on standardized reading tests. Similarly, it would sit well with the literature on reading intervention where, again, samples are largely determined on the basis of reading performance. Distinguishing between accuracy and fluency more specifically would not only assist efforts to understand the nature and relationship of these two elements but also reduce the conceptual and empirical confusion that results from the differing use of these in the dyslexia literature.

Given that reading disability would be identified at the behavioral level, there would be no need to test for prerequisite underlying cognitive skills in order to legitimize a judgment that such a difficulty exists. A dimensional approach should be employed as the longitudinal stability of reading disability is low (Wagner et al., 2011) and, for this reason, one-off categorical labeling is not advisable (Snowling & Hulme, 2012). Rather than having a label for life, any such designation would depend on an individual's current reading performance. Thus, a child might fluctuate from having a reading disability or not, while also having other forms of reading difficulty or not, as he or she moves through school.

Some might wish to argue that the term "dyslexia" could be employed in a similar fashion, seeing this as preferable because of its appeal to the wider public. However, such a position would be predicated on an assumption that the historical, social, and political factors that have rendered the dyslexia debate so problematic for many decades can be overcome by a reframing of this kind. Such an outcome is highly unlikely as this would both include some and exclude others in ways unacceptable to many.

Of course, dispensing with the term "dyslexia" would be difficult to achieve in practice. The field of special education has seen the demise of many labels that were once in everyday use in various education systems – spastic, cretin, delicate, deaf and dumb, mentally retarded, mongol, educationally subnormal. In the majority of cases, these terms disappeared rapidly because they were widely perceived to be demeaning or offensive. Although dyslexia is a term that is also ready to be consigned to the history books, it offers a diagnostic label that is typically sought after rather than shunned, and its advocates will surely put up a strong fight to retain its use. In defending the use of the term, Stein (2012b, p. 189) states: "Knowing that his dyslexia is a respectable neurological diagnosis, and not another word for laziness or stupidity can transform a child's self-image." However, creating a Manichean division between those poor readers who might be deemed worthy, or not worthy, of holding a positive sense of self, on the basis of the supposed etiology of their difficulties, is not consonant with the goals of those who seek to help all children who struggle to learn. Many poor readers, quite understandably, find it difficult to maintain desirable levels of motivation when their learning is arduous and gains are difficult to sustain. Attributing reading failure to a lack of intelligence is never productive for any child.

Rather than sustaining the current poorly defined and operationalized construct of dyslexia in the belief that children so labeled will develop more positive views of themselves as learners (Burden, 2008), the perceived link between reading disability and intelligence or laziness should be wholly severed. Unfortunately, current diagnostic procedures only serve to fuel such divisions between poor readers. The unintended consequence of this is that struggling readers, not adjudged to be dyslexic, are likely to be perceived in a more negative light and may have greater difficulty in accessing specialist service and resources. It is surely the responsibility of researchers, clinicians, and education practitioners to directly address and overcome common misunderstandings, rather than to use labels such as dyslexia to help some, but not all, individuals who suffer as a result of widespread ignorance about the nature and origins of reading difficulties.

Some four decades ago, a UK government's Committee Report on the teaching of reading in schools provided very similar criticisms to those outlined in the present text. The Committee commented upon a:

group of children who experience a difficulty in learning to read that cannot be accounted for by limited ability or by emotional or extraneous factors. The term "dyslexic" is commonly applied to these children. We believe that this term serves little useful purpose other than to draw attention to the fact that the problem of these children can be chronic and severe. *It is not susceptible to precise operational definition; nor does it indicate any clearly defined course of treatment.* (Department of Education and Science, 1975, p. 268; emphasis added)

The Committee's views were heavily influenced by findings from a large-scale epidemiological study on the Isle of Wight. Reflecting on the growing understandings of the time, one of the study's lead researchers (Yule, 1976, p. 176) commented:

The era of applying the label "dyslexic" is rapidly drawing to a close. The label has served its function in drawing attention to children who have great difficulty in mastering the arts of reading, writing and spelling but its continued use invokes emotions which often prevent rational discussion and scientific investigation.

Yule's prediction failed not because a clear and consensual understanding of dyslexia as a discrete condition subsequently emerged (which, as has been shown, it clearly did not), but because the term continues to meet the psychological, social, political, and emotional needs of so many stakeholders. One must recognize that the truth value of an idea can often be secondary to other factors. Kamhi (2004) has pondered why it is so often more desirable to have dyslexia than a reading disability. He suggests that dyslexia is a classic example of a *meme*, a unit of cultural transmission, complementary to genetic transmission, in which ideas and behaviors are passed on from one person to another (Blackmore, 1999; Dawkins, 1976). The meme's ability to survive by means of replication does not depend on whether it is true, useful, or even potentially harmful. What is crucial is that it is "easy to understand, remember, and communicate to others" (Kamhi, 2004, p. 106) – characteristics that apply readily to everyday conceptions of dyslexia. The fact that these understandings are often impoverished, misleading, or incorrect has had little bearing on the dyslexia meme's capacity for survival as "an unfortunate consequence of. . . selection forces is that successful memes typically provide superficially plausible answers for complex questions" (Kamhi, 2004, p. 105).

The term "dyslexia" is so rooted in everyday discourse that, for some, the articulation of theoretical and ethical concerns about its use can do little to reduce its hold (Reason & Stothard, 2013). However, researchers, educationalists, and clinicians should surely not fail to accept their responsibility to challenge the use of constructs that lack scientific precision and rigor, however popular and embedded these are within society. Stanovich (2000), one of the leading researchers in the area of reading and reading difficulties over the past three decades, expresses faith in the ultimate ability of science and logic to counter misleading memes. It is in line with such optimism that the present authors seek to present the scientific evidence surrounding the dyslexia debate. In taking issue with the recommendations outlined in this chapter, some might argue that rather than discontinuing its use, a truly scientific approach should result in the establishment of a more rigorous understanding and deployment of the term "dyslexia." However, in this particular case, the power of the meme may prove too powerful for such scientific endeavor.

In his earlier writings, Stanovich (1996) called for a tightening up of the use of the dyslexia construct. However, in light of subsequent experience, he has come to the conclusion that this is impossible, and instead the field should, "retire the term dyslexia permanently [because] . . . whatever small purpose it serves is swamped by the confusion it causes" (Stanovich, personal communication, March 21, 2012).

Whether science will ultimately resolve the many contradictions in the field of reading difficulty is uncertain. However, it is hoped that the present book will, in some small way, help contribute to this end, for clear, rational, and rigorous understandings will surely prove essential in our ongoing attempts to serve those who struggle to master the reading process.

References

1000 Genomes Project Consortium. (2010). A map of human genome variation from population-scale sequencing. *Nature, 467*, 1061–1073.

Ackerman, P. T., Holloway, C. A., Youngdahl, P. L., & Dykman, R. A. (2001). The double-deficit theory of reading disability does not fit all. *Learning Disabilities Research & Practice, 16*, 152–160.

Adams, M. J. (1990). *Beginning to read: Thinking and learning about print.* Cambridge, MA: MIT Press.

Adlof, S. M., Catts, H. W., & Lee, J. (2010). Kindergarten predictors of second vs. eighth grade reading comprehension impairments. *Journal of Learning Disabilities, 43*, 332–345.

Agurs-Collins, T., Khoury, M. J., Simon-Morton, D., Olster, D. H., Harris, J. R., & Milner, J. A. (2008). Public health genomics: translating obesity genomics research into population health benefits. *Obesity, 16*, S85–S94.

Ahissar, M. (2007). Dyslexia and the anchoring-deficit hypothesis. *Trends in Cognitive Sciences, 11*, 458–465.

Ahissar, M., & Oganian, Y. (2008). Response to Ziegler: The anchor is in the details. *Trends in Cognitive Sciences, 12*, 245–246.

Ahissar, M., Protopapas, A., Reid, M., & Merzenich, M. M. (2000). Auditory processing parallels reading abilities in adults. *Proceedings of the National Academy of Sciences, 97*, 6832–6837.

Al Otaiba, S., Folsom, S. J., Schatschneider, C., Wanzek., J., Greulich, L., Meadows, J., et al. (2011). Predicting first-grade reading performance from kindergarten response to Tier 1 instruction. *Exceptional Children, 77*, 453–470.

Al Otaiba, S., & Fuchs, D. (2002). Characteristics of children who are unresponsive to early literacy intervention: A review of the literature. *Remedial and Special Education, 23*, 300–316.

Al Otaiba, S., & Fuchs, D. (2006). Who are the young children for whom best practices in reading are ineffective? *Journal of Learning Disabilities, 39*, 414–431.

Albon, E., Adi, Y., & Hyde, C. (2008). *The effectiveness and cost-effectiveness of colored filters for reading disability: A systematic review.* Birmingham, AL: University of Birmingham Department of Public Health and Epidemiology.

Aleci, C., Piana, G., Piccoli, M., & Bertolini, M. (2012). Developmental dyslexia and spatial relationship perception. *Cortex, 48*(4), 466–476.

Allor, J. H., Mathes, P. G., Roberts, J. K., Jones, F. G., & Champlin, T. M. (2010). Teaching students with moderate intellectual disabilities to read: An experimental examination of a comprehensive reading intervention. *Education and Training in Autism and Developmental Disabilities, 45,* 3–22.

Alloway, T. P., Bibile, V., & Lau, G. (2013). Computerized working memory training: Can it lead to gains in cognitive skills in students? *Computers in Human Behavior, 29*(3), 632–638.

Alloway, T. P., Gathercole, S. E., Kirkwood, H. J., & Elliott, J. G. (2009). The cognitive and behavioral characteristics of children with low working memory. *Child Development, 80,* 606–621.

Al-Yagon, M., Cavendish, W., Cornoldi, C., Fawcett, A. J., Grünke, M., Hung, L., Jiménez, J. E., Karande, S., van Kraayenoord, C. E., Lucangeli, D., Margalit, M., Montague, M., Sholapurwala, R., Sideridis, G., Tressoldi, P. E., & Vio, C. (2013). The proposed changes for *DSM-5* for SLD and ADHD: International perspectives – Australia, Germany, Greece, India, Israel, Italy, Spain, Taiwan, United Kingdom, and United States. *Journal of Learning Disabilities, 46*(1), 58–72.

American Academy of Pediatrics (Section on Ophthalmology & Council on Children with Disabilities, Ophthalmology, American Academy of Ophthalmology, American Association for Pediatric Ophthalmology and Strabismus, & American Association of Certified Orthoptists). (2009). Learning disabilities, dyslexia, and vision. *Pediatrics, 124,* 837–844.

American Academy of Pediatrics. (1982). The doman-delacato treatment of neurologically handicapped children: A policy statement by the American Academy of Pediatrics. *Pediatrics, 70,* 810–812.

Amitay, S., Ben-Yehudah, G., Banai, K., & Ahissar, M. (2002). Disabled readers suffer from visual and auditory impairments but not from a specific magnocellular deficit. *Brain, 125,* 2272–2285.

Amitay, S., Ben-Yehudah, G., Banai, K., & Ahissar, M. (2003). Visual magnocellular deficits in dyslexia: Reply to the Editor. *Brain, 126,* e3.

Amtmann, D., Abbott, R. D., & Berninger, V. W. (2007). Mixture growth models of RAN and RAS row by row: Insight into the reading system at work over time. *Reading and Writing, 20,* 785–813.

Anastasiou, G., & Kauffman, J. M. (2011). A social constructionist approach to disability: Implications for special education. *Exceptional Children, 77,* 367–384.

Anderson, K. (2000, June 18). The Reading Wars – A look at the report of the National Reading Panel, "Teaching Children to Read," and the debate over what reading strategy works best in the classroom, *Los Angeles Times,* p. 5.

Andrews, J. S., Ben-Shachar, M., Yeatman, J. D., Flom, L. L., Luna, B., & Feldman, H. M. (2010). Reading performance correlates with white-matter properties in preterm and term children. *Developmental Medicine & Child Neurology, 52,* 505–506.

Angrilli, A., Elbert, T., Cusumano, S., Stegagno, L., & Rockstroh, B. (2003). Temporal dynamics of linguistic processes are reorganized in aphasics' cortex: An EEG mapping study. *Neuroimage, 20,* 657–666.

Angrilli, A., & Spironelli, C. (2005). Cortical plasticity of language measured by EEG in a case of anomic aphasia. *Brain and Language, 95,* 32–33.

Archer, A. L., Gleason, M. M., & Vachon, V. L. (2003). Decoding and fluency: Foundation skills for struggling older readers. *Learning Disability Quarterly, 26,* 89–101.

Arnoutse, C., van Leeuwe, J., & Verhoeven, L. (2005). Early literacy from a longitudinal perspective. *Educational Review and Research, 11,* 253–275.

Arns, M., Peters, S., Breteler, R., & Verhoeven, L. (2007). Different brain activation patterns in dyslexic children: evidence from EEG power and coherence patterns for the double-deficit theory of dyslexia. *Journal of Integrative Neuroscience, 6*, 175–190.

Arrow, A. W., & Tunmer, W. E. (2012). Contemporary reading acquisition theory: The conceptual basis for differentiated reading instruction. In S. Suggate & E. Reese (Eds.), *Contemporary debates in childhood education and development* (pp. 241–249). London: Routledge.

Ashton, C. (1996). In defence of discrepancy definitions of specific learning difficulties. *Educational Psychology in Practice, 12*, 131–140.

Ashton, C. (1997). SpLD, discrepancies and dyslexia: A response to Solity and the Stanoviches. *Educational Psychology in Practice, 13*, 9–11.

Au, A., & Lovegrove, W. (2001). Temporal processing ability in above average and average readers. *Perception & Psychophysics, 63*(1), 148–155.

Avramopoulos, D. (2010). Genetics of psychiatric disorders methods: Molecular approaches. *Psychiatric Clinics of North America, 33*, 1–13.

Aylward, E., Richards, T., Berninger, V., Nagy, W., Field, K., Grimme, A., et al. (2003). Instructional treatment associated with changes in brain activation in children with dyslexia. *Neurology, 61*, 212–219.

Ayres, A. J. (1963). The development of perceptual-motor abilities: A theoretical basis for treatment of dysfunction. *American Journal of Occupational Therapy, 17*, 221–225.

Ayres, A. J. (1979). *Sensory integration and the child*. Los Angeles, CA: Western Psychological Services.

Bacon, A. M., Parmentier, F. B., & Barr, P. (2013). Visuospatial memory in dyslexia: Evidence for strategic deficits. *Memory, 21*(2), 189–209.

Badcock, N. A., Hogben, J. H., & Fletcher, J. F. (2008). No differential attentional blink in dyslexia after controlling for baseline sensitivity. *Vision Research, 48*, 1497–1502.

Baddeley, A. (2012). Working memory: Theories, models, and controversies. *Annual Review of Psychology, 63*, 1–29.

Baddeley, A. D. (1986). *Working memory*. London: Oxford University Press.

Baddeley, A. D. (1996). Exploring the central executive. *The Quarterly Journal of Experimental Psychology, 49A*, 5–28.

Baddeley, A. D. (2000). The episodic buffer: A new component of working memory? *Trends in Cognitive Sciences, 4*, 417–422.

Baddeley, A. D., & Hitch, G. (1974). Working memory. In G. Bower (Ed.), *The psychology of learning and motivation* (Vol. 8, pp. 47–90). New York: Academic Press.

Badian, N. A. (1997). Dyslexia and the double deficit hypothesis. *Annals of Dyslexia, 47*, 69–87.

Badzakova-Trajkov, G., Hamm, J. P., & Waldie, K. E. (2005). The effects of redundant stimuli on visuospatial processing in developmental dyslexia. *Neuropsychologia, 43*, 473–478.

Balow, B. (1996). Perceptual-motor activities in the treatment of severe reading disability. *The Reading Teacher, 50*, 88–97.

Banai, K., & Ahissar, M. (2004). Poor frequency discrimination probes dyslexics with particularly impaired working memory. *Audiology & Neuro-otology, 9*, 328–340.

Banai, K., & Ahissar, M. (2010). On the importance of anchoring and the consequences of its impairment in dyslexia. *Dyslexia, 16*, 240–257.

Barela, J. A., Dias, J. L., Godoi, D., Viana, A. R., & de Freitas, P. B. (2011). Postural control and automaticity in dyslexic children: The relationship between visual information and body sway. *Research in Developmental Disabilities, 32*, 1814–1821.

Barkovich, A. J., & Kuzniecky, R. I. (2000). Gray matter heterotopia. *Neurology, 55*, 1603–1608.

Barth, A. E., Denton, C. A., Stuebing, K. K., Fletcher, J. M., Cirino, P. T., Francis, D. J., et al. (2010). A test of the cerebellar hypothesis of dyslexia in adequate and inadequate responders to reading intervention. *Journal of International Neuropsychological Society, 16*, 526–536.

Bates, T. C., Luciano, M., Montgomery, G. W., Wright, M. J., & Martin, N. G. (2011). Genes for a component of the language acquisition mechanism: ROBO1 polymorphisms associated with phonological buffer deficit. *Behavior Genetics, 41*, 50–57.

Beach, K. D., & O'Connor, R. E. (in press). Early response-to-intervention measures and criteria as predictors of reading disability in the beginning of third grade. *Journal of Learning Disabilities*.

Beaton, A. A. (1997). The relation of planum temporale asymmetry and morphology of the corpus callosum to handedness, gender, and dyslexia: A review of the evidence. *Brain and Language, 60*, 255–322.

Beaton, A. A. (2004). *Dyslexia, reading and the brain: A sourcebook of psychological and biological research*. New York: Psychology Press.

Beattie, R. L., & Manis, F. R. (in press). The relationship between prosodic perception, phonological awareness and vocabulary in emergent literacy. *Journal of Research in Reading*.

Beattie, R. L., & Manis, F. R. (2012). Rise time perception in children with reading and combined reading and language difficulties. *Journal of Learning Disabilities, 46*(3), 200–209.

Beaulieu, C., Plewes, C., Paulson, L. A., Roy, D., Snook, L., Concha, L., et al. (2005). Imaging brain connectivity in children with diverse reading ability. *Neuroimage, 25*(4), 1266–1271.

Begeny, J. C., Mitchell, R. C., Whitehouse, M. H., Samuels, F. H., & Stage, S. A. (2011). Effects of the HELPS reading fluency program when implemented by classroom teachers with low-performing second-grade students. *Learning Disabilities Research & Practice, 26*, 122–133.

Bejerano, G., Lowe, C. B., Ahituv, N., King, B., Siepel, A., Salama, S. R., et al. (2006). A distal enhancer and an ultraconserved exon are derived from a novel retroposon. *Nature, 441*, 87–90.

Bell, T. K. (1990). Rapid sequential processing in dyslexic and ordinary readers. *Perceptual and Motor Skills, 71*, 1155–1159.

Bellocchi, S., Muneaux, M., Bastien-Toniazzo, M., & Ducrot, S. (2013). I can read it in your eyes: What eye movements tell us about visuo-attentional processes in developmental dyslexia. *Research in Developmental Disabilities, 34*, 452–460.

Benassi, M., Simonelli, L., Giovagnoli, S., & Bolzani, R. (2010). Coherence motion perception in developmental dyslexia: A meta-analysis of behavioral studies. *Dyslexia, 16*, 341–357.

Beneventi, H., Tønnessen, F. E., Ersland, L., & Hugdahl, K. (2010). Working memory deficit in dyslexia: Behavioral and fMRI evidence. *International Journal of Neuroscience, 120*, 51–59.

Benner, G. J., Nelson, J. R., Stage, S. A., & Ralston, N. C. (2011). The influence of fidelity of implementation on the reading outcomes of middle school students experiencing reading difficulties. *Remedial and Special Education, 32*, 79–88.

Ben-Shachar, M., Dougherty, R. F., & Wandell, B. A. (2007). White matter pathways in reading. *Current Opinion in Neurobiology, 17*, 258–270.

Ben-Yehudah, G., & Ahissar, M. (2004). Sequential spatial frequency discrimination is consistently impaired among adult dyslexics. *Vision Research, 44*, 1047–1063.

Berent, I, Vaknin-Nusbaum, V., Balaban, E., & Galaburda, A. M. (2012). Dyslexia impairs speech recognition but can spare phonological competence. *PLoS ONE, 7*, e44875.

Berkeley, S., Bender, W. N., Peaster, L. G., & Saunders, L. (2009). Implementation of response to intervention. A snapshot of progress. *Journal of Learning Disabilities, 42*, 85–95.

Berlin, R. (1887). Eine besondre Art der Wortblindheit.

Berninger, V. W., & Abbott, R. D. (1994). Redefining learning disabilities: Moving beyond aptitude–achievement discrepancies to failure to respond to validated treatment protocols. In G. R. Lyon (Ed.), *Frames of reference for the assessment of learning disabilities: New views on measurement issues* (pp. 163–183). Baltimore, MD: Paul H Brookes Publishing.

Berninger, V. W., Abbott, R. D., Nagy, W., & Carlisle, J. (2010). Growth in phonological, orthographic, and morphological awareness in grades 1 to 6. *Journal of Psycholinguistic Research, 39*, 141–163.

Berninger, V. W., Nielsen, K. H., Abbott, R. D., Wijsman, E., & Raskind, W. (2008). Gender differences in severity of writing and reading disabilities. *Journal of School Psychology, 46*, 151–172.

Berninger, V. W., Raskind, W., Richards, T., Abbott, R., & Stock, P. (2008). A multidisciplinary approach to understanding developmental dyslexia within working-memory architecture: Genotypes, phenotypes, brain, and instruction. *Developmental Neuropsychology, 33*, 707–744.

Betjemann, R. S., Willcutt, E. G., Olson, R. K., Keenan, J. M., DeFries, J. C., & Wadsworth, S. J. (2008). Word reading and reading comprehension: Stability, overlap and independence. *Reading and Writing, 21*, 539–558.

Biancarosa, G., & Snow, C. E. (2006). *Reading next: A vision for action and research in middle and high school literacy: A report to the Carnegie Corporation of New York* (2nd ed.). Washington, DC: Alliance for Excellent Education.

Bianco, M., Bressoux, P., Doyen, A., Lambert, E., Lima, L., Pellenq, C., et al. (2010). Early training in oral comprehension and phonological skills: Results of a three-year longitudinal study. *Scientific Studies of Reading, 14*, 211–246.

Bishop, D. V. (2006). Dyslexia: What's the problem? [Comment/Reply]. *Developmental science, 9*, 256–257.

Bishop, D. V. M. (1997). *Uncommon understanding.* Hove: Psychology Press.

Bishop, D. V. M. (2001). Genetic influences on language impairment and literacy problems in children: Same or different? *Journal of Child Psychology and Psychiatry, 42*, 189–198.

Bishop, D. V. M. (2002). Cerebellar abnormalities in developmental dyslexia: Cause, correlate or consequence? *Cortex, 38*, 491–498.

Bishop, D. V. M. (2007). Curing dyslexia and ADHD by training motor coordination: Miracle or myth? *Journal of Paediatrics and Child Health, 43,* 653–655.

Bishop, D. V. M. (2013). Research Review: Emanuel Miller Memorial Lecture 2012 – Neuroscientific studies of intervention for language impairment in children: interpretive and methodological problems. *Journal of Child Psychology & Psychiatry, 54*(3), 247–259.

Bishop, D. V. M., & Adams, C. (1990). A prospective study of the relationship between specific language impairment, phonological disorders, and reading retardation. *Journal of Child Psychology and Psychiatry, 31,* 1027–1050.

Bishop, D. V. M., Mcdonald, D., Bird, S., & Hayiou-Thomas, M. E. (2009). Children who read accurately despite language impairment: Who are they and how do they do it? *Child Development, 80,* 593–605.

Bishop, D. V. M., & Snowling, M. J. (2004). Developmental dyslexia and specific language impairment: same or different? *Psychological Bulletin, 130,* 858–886.

Blachman, B. A. (2000). Phonological awareness. In M. L. Kamil, P. B. Mosenthal, P. D. Pearson, & R. Barr (Eds.), *Handbook of word recognition research* (Vol. III, pp. 483–502). Mahwah, NJ: Erlbaum.

Blachman, B. A., Schatschneider, C., Fletcher, J. M., Francis, D., Clonan, S. M., Shaywitz, B. A., et al. (2004). Effects of intensive reading remediation for second and third graders and a 1-year follow-up. *Journal of Educational Psychology, 96,* 444–461.

Black, J., & Hoeft, F. (2012). Prediction of children's reading skills: Understanding the interplay among environment, brain, and behavior. In A. A. Benasich & R. H. Fitch (Eds.), *Developmental dyslexia: Early precursors, neurobehavioral markers, and biological substrates* (pp. 191–207). Baltimore, MD: Paul H. Brookes Publishing.

Black, J. M., Tanaka, H., Stanley, L., Nagamine, M., Zakerani, N., et al. (2012). Maternal history of reading difficulty is associated with reduced language-related gray matter in beginning readers. *Neuroimage, 59*(3), 3021–3032.

Blackmore, S. (1999). *The meme machine.* Oxford: Oxford University Press.

Blau, V., Reithler, J., van Atteveldt, N., Seitz, J., Gerretsen, P., Goebel, R., et al. (2010). Deviant processing of letters and speech sounds as proximate cause of reading failure: a functional magnetic resonance imaging study of dyslexic children. *Brain, 133,* 868–879.

Blau, V., van Atteveldt, N., Ekkebus, M., Goebel, R., & Blomert, L. (2009). Reduced neural integration of letters and speech sounds links phonological and reading deficits in adult dyslexia. *Current Biology, 19,* 503–508.

Blythe, P. (1992). *A physical approach to resolving specific learning difficulties.* Chester: Institute for Neuro-Physiological Psychology.

Boden, C., & Giaschi, D. (2007). M-Stream deficits and reading-related visual processes in developmental dyslexia. *Psychological Bulletin, 133,* 346–366.

Boets, B., De Smedt, B., Cleuren, L., Vandewalle, E., Wouters, J., & Ghesquire, P. (2010). Towards a further characterization of phonological and literacy problems in Dutch-speaking children with dyslexia. *British Journal of Developmental Psychology, 28,* 5–31.

Boets, B., Ghesquière, P., van Wieringen, A., & Wouters, J. (2007). Speech perception in preschoolers at family risk for dyslexia: Relations with low-level auditory processing and phonological ability. *Brain and Language, 101,* 19–30.

Boets, B., Vandermosten, M., Poelmans, H., Luts, H., Wouters, J., & Ghesquière, P. (2011). Preschool impairments in auditory processing and speech perception uniquely predict future reading problems. *Research in Developmental Disabilities*, *32*, 560–570.

Boets, B., Wouters, J., van Wieringen, A., & Ghesquière, P. (2007). Auditory processing, speech perception and phonological ability in preschool children at high-risk of dyslexia: A longitudinal study of the auditory temporal processing theory. *Neuropsychologia*, *45*, 1608–1620.

Bogliotti, C., Serniclaes, W., Messaoud-Galusi, S., & Sprenger-Charolles, L. (2008). Discrimination of speech sounds by children with dyslexia: Comparisons with chronological age and reading level. *Journal of Experimental Child Psychology*, *101*, 137–155.

Bonifacci, P., & Snowling, M. J. (2008). Speed of processing and reading disability: A cross-linguistic investigation of dyslexia and borderline intellectual functioning. *Cognition*, *107*, 999–1017.

Booth, J. R., Bebko, G., Burman, D. D., & Bitan, T. (2007). Children with reading disorder show modality independent brain abnormalities during semantic tasks. *Neuropsychologia*, *45*, 775–783.

Bosse, M. L., Tainturier, M. J., & Valdois, S. (2007). Developmental dyslexia: The visual attention span deficit hypothesis. *Cognition*, *104*, 198–230.

Bosse, M. L., & Valdois, S. (2009). Influence of the visual attention span on child reading performance: A cross-sectional study. *Journal of Research in Reading*, *32*, 230–253.

Bowers, P. G., Sunseth, K., & Golden, J. (1999). The route between rapid naming and reading progress. *Scientific Studies of Reading*, *3*, 31–53.

Bowers, P. G., & Wolf, M. (1993). Theoretical links among naming speed, precise timing mechanisms and orthographic skill in dyslexia. *Reading and Writing*, *5*, 69–85.

Bradley, L., & Bryant, P. E. (1983). Categorizing sounds and learning to read – A causal connection. *Nature*, *301*, 419–421.

Brambati, S. M., Termine, C., Ruffino, M., Danna, M., Lanzi, G., Stella, G., et al. (2006). Neuropsychological deficits and neural dysfunction in familial dyslexia. *Brain Research*, *1*, 174–185.

Brambati, S. M., Termine, C., Ruffino, M., Stella, G., Fazio, F., Cappa, S. F., et al. (2004). Regional reductions of gray matter volume in familial dyslexia. *Neurology*, *63*, 742–745.

Bramlett, R. K., Murphy, J. J., Johnson, J., & Wallingsford, L. (2002). Contemporary practices in school psychology: A national survey of roles and referral problems. *Psychology in the Schools*, *39*, 327–335.

Branum-Martin, L., Fletcher, J. M., & Stuebing, K. K. (2013). Classification and identification of reading and math disabilities: The special case of comorbidity. *Journal of Learning Disabilities*, *46*(6), 490–499.

Brem, S., Bach, S., Kucian, K., Guttorm, T. K., Martin, E., Lyytinen, H., et al. (2010). Brain sensitivity to print emerges when children learn letter–speech sound correspondences. *Proceedings of the National Academy of Sciences*, *107*, 7939–7944.

Breteler, M. H. M., Arns, M., Peters, S., Giepmans, I., & Verhoeven, J. (2010). Improvements in spelling after QEEG-based neurofeedback in dyslexia: A randomized controlled treatment study. *Applied Psychophysiological Biofeedback*, *35*, 5–11.

Breznitz, Z., & Misra, M. (2003). Speed of processing of the visual–orthographic and auditory–phonological systems in adult dyslexics: The contribution of "asynchrony" to word recognition deficits. *Brain & Language*, *85*, 486–502.

British Psychological Society. (1999). *Dyslexia, literacy and psychological assessment: Report by a Working Party of the Division of Educational and Child Psychology of the British Psychological Society*. Leicester: British Psychological Society.

Brkanac, Z., Chapman, N. H., Igo, R. P. J., Matsushita, M. M., Nielsen, K., Berninger, V. W., et al. (2008). Genome scan of a nonword repetition phenotype in families with dyslexia: Evidence for multiple loci. *Behavior Genetics*, *38*, 462–475.

Brooks, G. (1984). The teaching of silent reading to beginners. In G. Brooks & A. K. Pugh (Eds.), *Studies in the history of reading* (pp. 85–96). London and Reading: Centre for the Teaching of Reading, University of Reading and U.K. Reading Association.

Brooks, G. (2007). *What works for pupils with literacy difficulties? The effectiveness of intervention schemes*. London: Department for Education and Skills.

Brown, W. E., Eliez, S., Menon, V., Rumsey, J. M., White, C. D., & Reiss, A. L. (2001). Preliminary evidence of widespread morphological variations of the brain in dyslexia. *Neurology*, *56*, 781–783.

Brown Waesche, J. S., Schatschneider, C., Maner, J. K., Ahmed, Y., & Wagner, R. K. (2011). Examining agreement and longitudinal stability among traditional and RTI-based definitions of reading disability using the affected-status agreement statistic. *Journal of Learning Disabilities*, *44*, 296–307.

Bruder, J., Leppänen, P. H. T., Bartling, J., Csépe, V., Démonet, J., & Schulte-Körne, G. (2011). Children with dyslexia reveal abnormal native language representations: Evidence from a study of mismatch negativity. *Psychophysiology*, *48*, 1107–1118.

Bruno, J. L., Lu, Z. L., & Manis, F. R. (2013). Phonological processing is uniquely associated with neuro-metabolic concentration. *NeuroImage*, *67*, 175–181.

Brunswick, N., McCrory, E., Price, C. J., Frith, C. D., & Frith, U. (1999). Explicit and implicit processing of words and pseudowords by adult developmental dyslexics: A search for Wernicke's Wortschatz? *Brain*, *122*, 1901–1917.

Bryant, P. E., & Bradley, L. (1985). *Children's reading problems: Psychology and education*. Oxford: Blackwell.

Bryant, P. E., Maclean, L., Bradley, L., & Crossland, J. (1990). Rhyme and alliteration, phoneme detection, and learning to read. *Developmental Psychology*, *26*, 429–438.

Bull, L. (2009). Survey of complementary and alternative therapies used by children with specific learning difficulties (dyslexia). *International Journal of Language & Communication Disorders*, *44*(2), 224–235.

Buonincontri, R., Bache, I., Silahtaroglu, A., Elbro, C., Veber Nielsen, A.-M., Ullmann, R., et al. (2011). A cohort of balanced reciprocal translocations associated with dyslexia: identification of two putative candidate genes at DYX1. *Behavior Genetics*, *41*, 125–133.

Burden, R. (2008). Is dyslexia necessarily associated with negative feelings of self-worth? A review and implications for future research. *Dyslexia*, *14*, 188–196.

Burnett, J. R. (1998, October 19). Phonics controversy in Texas [Radio broadcast]. Washington, DC: National Public Radio.

Burt, C. (1937). *The backward child*. London: University of London Press.

Butterworth, B., & Kovas, Y. (2013). Understanding neurocognitive developmental disorders can improve education for all. *Science, 340*, 300–305.

Büttner, G., & Hasselhorn, M. (2011). Learning disabilities: Debates on definitions, causes, subtypes, and responses. *International Journal of Disability, Development and Education, 58*, 75–87.

Byrne, B. (2011). Evaluating the role of phonological factors in early literacy development: Insights from experimental and behavior-genetic studies. In S. A. Brady, D. Braze, & C. A. Fowler (Eds.), *Explaining individual differences in reading: Theory and evidence* (pp. 175–195). New York: Psychology Press.

Byrne, B., Coventry, W. L., Olson, R. K., Hulslander, J., Wadsworth, S., Defries, J., et al. (2008). A behaviour-genetic analysis of orthographic learning, spelling and decoding. *Journal of Research in Reading, 31*, 8–21.

Byrne, B., Coventry, W. L., Olson, R. K., Samuelsson, S., Corley, R., Willcutt, E. G., et al. (2009). Genetic and environmental influences on aspects of literacy and language in early childhood: Continuity and change from preschool to Grade 2. *Journal of Neurolinguistics, 22*, 219–236.

Byrne, B., Delaland, C., Fielding-Barnsley, R., & Quain, P. (2002). Longitudinal twins study of early reading development in three countries: Preliminary results. *Annals of Dyslexia, 52*, 49–73.

Calfee, R. C., & Drum, P. (1986). Research on teaching reading. In M. C. Whittock (Ed.), *Handbook of research on teaching* (pp. 804–849). New York: Macmillan.

Calfee, R. C., & Norman, K. A. (1998). Psychological perspectives on the early reading wars: The case of phonological awareness. *Teachers College Record, 100*, 242–274.

Callens, M., Tops, W., & Brysbaert, M. (2012). Cognitive profile of students who enter higher education with an indication of dyslexia. *PLoS One, 7*(6), e38081.

Callens, M., Whitney, C., Tops, W., & Brysbaert, M. (2013). No deficiency in left-to-right processing of words in dyslexia but evidence for enhanced visual crowding., *The Quarterly Journal of Experimental Psychology, 66*(9), 1803–1817.

Campbell, T. (2011). From aphasia to dyslexia, a fragment of a genealogy: An analysis of the formation of a "medical diagnosis". *Health Sociology Review, 20*, 450–461.

Campuzano, L., Dynarski, M., Agodini, R., & Rall, K. (2009). *Effectiveness of reading and mathematics software products: Findings from two student cohorts* (NCEE 2009–4041). Washington, DC: Institute of Education Sciences.

Canivez, G. L. (2013). Psychometric versus actuarial interpretation of intelligence and related aptitude batteries. In D. H. Saklofske, C. R. Reynolds, & V. L. Schwean (Eds.), *The Oxford handbook of child psychological assessment* (pp. 84–112). New York: Oxford University Press.

Cao, F., Bitan, T., Chou, T.-L., Burman, D. D., & Booth, J. R. (2006). Deficient orthographic and phonological representations in children with dyslexia revealed by brain activation patterns. *Journal of Child Psychology and Psychiatry, 47*, 1041–1050.

Cardona, G., Borràs, R., Peris, E., & Castañé, M. (2010). A placebo-controlled trial of tinted lenses in adolescents with good and poor academic performance: reading accuracy and speed. *Journal of Optometry, 3*(2), 94–101.

Carretti, B., Borella, E., Cornoldi, C., & De Beni, R. (2009). Role of working memory in explaining the performance of individuals with specific reading comprehension difficulties: A meta-analysis. *Learning and Individual Differences, 19*, 246–251.

Carroll, J. M., Snowling, M. J., Stevenson, J., & Hulme, C. (2003). The development of phonological awareness in preschool children. *Developmental Psychology, 39,* 913–923.

Casanova, M. F., Araque, J., Giedd, J., & Rumsey, J. M. (2004). Reduced brain size and gyrification in the brains of dyslexic patients. *Journal of Child Neurology, 19,* 275–281.

Cassar, M., Trieman, R., Moats, L., Pollo, T. C., & Kessler, B. (2005). How do the spellings of children with dyslexia compare with those of nondyslexic children? *Reading and Writing: An Interdisciplinary Journal, 18,* 27–49.

Castles, A., & Coltheart, M. (1996). Cognitive correlates of developmental surface dyslexia: A single case study. *Cognitive Neuropsychology, 13,* 25–50.

Castles, A., & Coltheart, M. (2004). Is there a causal link from phonological awareness to success in learning to read? *Cognition, 91,* 77–111.

Catts, H. W. (1991). Early identification of dyslexia: Evidence from a follow-up study of speech-language impaired children. *Annals of Dyslexia, 41,* 163–177.

Catts, H. W. (1993). The relationship between speech-language impairments and reading disabilities. *Journal of Speech, Language, and Hearing Research, 36,* 948–958.

Catts, H. W. (2012). Comments on the dyslexia and visual attention study. Retrieved May 18, *2012,* from http://www.interdys.org/VisualAttentionStudy.htm.

Catts, H. W., & Adlof, S. (2011). Phonological and other language deficits associated with dyslexia. In S. A. Brady, D. Braze, & C. A. Fowler (Eds.), *Explaining individual differences in reading: Theory and evidence* (pp. 137–151). New York: Psychology Press.

Catts, H. W., Adlof, S. M., Hogan, T. P., & Weismer, S. E. (2005). Are specific language impairment and dyslexia distinct disorders? *Journal of Speech Language and Hearing Research, 48,* 1378–1396.

Catts, H. W., Compton, D., Tomblin, J. B., & Bridges, M. S. (2012). Prevalence and nature of late-emerging poor readers. *Journal of Educational Psychology, 104*(1), 166–181.

Catts, H. W., Fey, M. E., Tomblin, J. B., & Zhang, X. (2002). A longitudinal investigation of reading outcomes in children with language impairments. *Journal of Speech, Language, and Hearing Research, 45,* 1142–1157.

Catts, H. W., Gillispie, M., Leonard, L., Kail, R. V., & Miller, C. A. (2002). The role of speed of processing, rapid naming, and phonological awareness in reading achievement. *Journal of Learning Disabilities, 35,* 509–524.

Catts, H. W., Hogan, T. P., & Fey, M. E. (2003). Subgrouping poor readers on the basis of individual differences in reading-related abilities. *Journal of Learning Disabilities, 36,* 151–164.

Catts, H. W., & Kamhi, A. (1999). *Language and reading disabilities.* Boston, MA: Allyn and Bacon.

Catts, H. W., & Kamhi, A. G. (Eds.). (2005). *Language and reading disabilities.* Boston, MA: Allyn & Bacon.

Catts, H. W., Petscher, Y., Schatschneider, C., Bridges, M. S., & Mendoza, K. (2009). Floor effects associated with universal screening and their impact on the early identification of reading disabilities. *Journal of Learning Disabilities, 42,* 163–176.

Chacko, A., Bedard, A. C., Marks, D. J., Feirsen, N., Uderman, J. Z., et al. (in press). A randomized clinical trial of Cogmed Working Memory Training in school-age children with ADHD: A replication in a diverse sample using a control condition. *Journal of Child Psychology and Psychiatry*.

Chaix, Y., Albaret, J., Brassard, C., Cheuret, E., DeCastelnau, P., Benesteau, J., et al. (2007). Motor impairment in dyslexia: The influence of attention disorders. *European Journal of Paediatric Neurology, 11*, 368–374.

Chall, J. S. (1996). *Learning to read: The great debate* (3rd ed.). Orlando, FL: Harcourt Brace.

Chall, J. S. (2000). *The academic achievement challenge*. New York: Guilford Press.

Chan, D. W., Ho, C. S. H., Tsang, S. M., Lee, S. H., & Chung, K. K. H. (2007). Prevalence, gender ratio and gender differences in reading-related cognitive abilities among Chinese children with dyslexia in Hong Kong. *Educational Studies, 33*, 249–255.

Cheung, A. C. K., & Slavin, R. E. (2012). How features of educational technology applications affect student reading outcomes: A meta-analysis. *Educational Research Review, 7*, 198–215.

Cheung, C. H., Wood, A. C., Paloyelis, Y., Arias-Vasquez, A., Buitelaar, J. K., et al. (2012). Aetiology for the covariation between combined type ADHD and reading difficulties in a family study: The role of IQ. *Journal of Child Psychology and Psychiatry, 53*(8), 864–873.

Chhabildas, N., Pennington, B. F., & Wilcutt, E. G. (2001). A comparison of the neuropsychological profiles of the DSM-IV subtypes of ADHD. *Journal of Abnormal Child Psychology, 29*, 529–540.

Chiappe, P., Stringer, R., Siegel, L. S., & Stanovich, K. E. (2002). Why the timing deficit hypothesis does not explain reading disability in adults. *Reading and Writing, 15*, 73–107.

Chiarello, C., Lombardino, L. J., Kacinik, N. A., Otto, R., & Leonard, C. M. (2006). Neuroanatomical and behavioral asymmetry in an adult compensated dyslexic. *Brain & Language, 98*, 169–181.

Chirkina, G. V., & Grigorenko, E. L. (in press). Tracking citations: A science detective story. *Journal of Learning Disabilities*.

Chiu, M. M., & McBride-Chang, C. (2006). Gender, context, and reading: A comparison of students in 43 countries. *Scientific Studies of Reading, 10*, 331–362.

Cho, E., Compton, D. L., Fuchs, D., Fuchs, L. S., & Bouton, B. (in press). Examining the predictive validity of a dynamic assessment of decoding to forecast response to Tier 2 intervention. *Journal of Learning Disabilities*.

Christo, C., Davis, J. M., & Brock, S. E. (2009). *Identifying, assessing, and treating dyslexia at school*. New York: Springer.

Christopher, M. E., Miyake, A., Keenan, J. M., Pennington, B., DeFries, J. C., Wadsworth, S. J., Willcutt, E., & Olson, R. K. (2012). Predicting word reading and comprehension with executive function and speed measures across development: A latent variable analysis. *Journal of Experimental Psychology: General, 141*(3), 470–488.

Cirino, P. T., Pollard-Durodola, S. D., Foorman, B. R., Carlson, C. D., & Francis, D. J. (2007). Teacher characteristics, classroom instruction, and student literacy and language outcomes in bilingual kindergartners. *The Elementary School Journal, 107,* 341–364.

Clamp, M., Fry, B., Kamal, M., Xie, X., Cuff, J., Lin, M. F., et al. (2007). Distinguishing protein-coding and noncoding genes in the human genome. *PNAS, 104,* 19428–19433.

Clark, D. B., & Uhry, J. K. (1955). *Dyslexia: Theory and practice of remedial instruction* (Vol. Ba). Baltimore, MD: York.

Clay, M. M. (1985). *The early detection of reading difficulties* (3rd ed.). Portsmouth, NH: Heinemann.

Clemens, N. H., Shapiro, E. S., Wu, J., Taylor, A. B., & Caskie, G. L. (in press). Monitoring early first-grade reading progress: A comparison of two measures. *Journal of Learning Disabilities.*

Coffield, M., Riddick, B., Barmby, P., & O'Neill, J. (2008). Dyslexia friendly primary schools: What can we learn from asking the pupils? In G. Reid, A. Fawcett, F. Manis, & L. Siegel (Eds.), *Sage handbook of dyslexia* (pp. 356–368). London: Sage.

Cohen-Mimran, R., & Sapir, S. (2007). Deficits in working memory in young adults with reading disabilities. *Journal of Communication Disorders, 40*(2), 168–183.

Coles, G. (1998). *Reading lessons: The debate over literacy.* New York: Hill and Wang.

Collis, N. L., Kohnen, S., & Kinoshita, S. (2013). The role of visual spatial attention in adult developmental dyslexia. *The Quarterly Journal of Experimental Psychology, 66*(2), 245–260.

Coltheart, M. (1981). Disorders of reading and their implications for models of normal reading. *Visible Language, 15,* 245–286.

Compton, D. L. (2003). Modeling the relationship between growth in rapid naming speed and growth in decoding skill in first-grade children. *Journal of Educational Psychology, 95,* 225–239.

Compton, D. L., & Carlisle, J. F. (1994). Speed of word recognition as a distinguishing characteristic of reading disabilities. *Educational Psychology Review, 6,* 115–139.

Compton, D. L., DeFries, J. C., & Olson, R. K. (2001). Are RAN and phonological awareness deficits additive in children with reading disabilities? *Dyslexia: An International Journal of Research & Practice, 7,* 125–149.

Compton, D. L., Fuchs, D., Fuchs, L. S., Bouton, B., Gilbert, J. K., Barquero, L. A., et al. (2010). Selecting at-risk first-grade readers for early intervention: eliminating false positives and exploring the promise of a two-stage gated screening process. *Journal of Educational Psychology, 102,* 327–340.

Compton, D. L., Fuchs, D., Fuchs, L. S., & Bryant, J. D. (2006). Selecting at-risk readers in first grade for early intervention: A two-year longitudinal study of decision rules and procedures. *Journal of Educational Psychology, 98,* 394–409.

Compton, D. L., Fuchs, D., Fuchs, L. S., Elleman, A. M., & Gilbert, J. K. (2008). Tracking children who fly below the radar screen: Latent transition modeling of students with late-emerging reading disability. *Learning and Individual Differences, 18,* 329–337.

Compton, D. L., Fuchs, L. S., Fuchs, D., Lambert, W., & Hamlett, C. (2012). The cognitive and academic profiles of reading and mathematics learning disabilities. *Journal of Learning Disabilities, 45,* 79–95.

Compton, D. L., Gilbert, J. K., Jenkins, J. R., Fuchs, D., Fuchs, L. S., Cho, E., Barquero, L. A., & Bouton, B. D. (2012). Accelerating chronically unresponsive children to Tier 3 instruction: What level of data is necessary to ensure selection accuracy? *Journal of Learning Disabilities, 45,* 204–216.

Conlon, E. G. (2012). Visual discomfort and reading. In J. Stein & Z. Kapoula (Eds.), *Visual aspects of dyslexia* (pp. 79–90). Oxford: Oxford University Press.

Conlon, E. G., Lilleskaret, G., Wright, C. M., & Power, G. F. (2012). The influence of contrast on coherent motion processing in dyslexia. *Neuropsychologia*, *50*, 1672–1681.

Conlon, E. G., Lovegrove, W., Chekaluk, E., & Pattison, P. (1999). Measuring visual discomfort. *Visual Cognition*, *6*, 637–663.

Conlon, E. G., Sanders, M. A., & Wright, C. M. (2009). Relationships between global motion and global form processing, practice, cognitive and visual processing in adults with dyslexia or visual discomfort. *Neuropsychologia*, *47*, 907–915.

Conlon, E. G., Wright, C. M., Norris, K., & Chekaluk, E. (2011). Does a sensory processing deficit explain counting accuracy on rapid visual sequencing tasks in adults with and without dyslexia? *Brain and Cognition*, *76*, 197–205.

Conners, F. A., Atwell, J. A., Rosenquist, C. J., & Sligh, A. C. (2001). Abilities underlying decoding differences in children with intellectual disability. *Journal of Intellectual Disability Research*, *45*, 292–299.

Connor, C. M. (2010). Child characteristics-instruction interactions: Implications for students' literacy skills development in the early grades. In S. B. Neuman & D. K. Dickinson (Eds.), *Handbook of early literacy* (3rd ed., pp. 256–278). New York: Guilford.

Connor, C. M., Morrison, F. J., Fishman, B., Crowe., E., Al Otaiba, S., & Schatschneider, C. (2013). A longitudinal cluster-randomized controlled study on the accumulating effects of individualized literacy instruction on students' reading from first through third grade. *Psychological Science*, *24*(8), 1408–1419.

Connor, C. M., Morrison, F. J., & Katch, E. L. (2004). Beyond the reading wars: Exploring the effect of child–instruction interaction on growth in early reading. *Scientific Studies of Reading*, *8*, 305–336.

Connor, C. M., Morrison, F. J., Fishman, B. J., Schatschneider, C., & Underwood, P. (2007). Algorithm-guided individualized reading instruction. *Science*, *315*, 464–465.

Connor, C. M., Piasta, S. B., Fishman, B., Glasney, S., Schatschneider, C., Crowe, E., et al. (2009). Individualizing student instruction precisely: Effects of child by instruction interactions on first graders' literacy development. *Child Development*, *80*, 77–100.

Cooke, A. (2001). Critical response to "Dyslexia, Literacy and Psychological Assessment (Report by a Working Party of the Division of Educational and Child Psychology of the British Psychological Society)": A view from the chalk face. *Dyslexia*, *7*, 47–52.

Cooper, G. M., Coe, B. P., Girirajan, S., Rosenfeld, J. A., Vu, T. H., Baker, C., et al. (2011). A copy number variation morbidity map of developmental delay. *Nature Genetics*, *43*, 838–846.

Corina, D. P., Richards, T. L., Serafini, S., Richards, A. L., Steury, K., Abbott, R. D., et al. (2001). fMRI auditory language differences between dyslexic and able reading children. *Neuroreport*, *12*, 1195–1201.

Cornelissen, P. L., Richardson, A., Mason, A., Fowler, S., & Stein, J. F. (1995). Contrast sensitivity and coherent motion detection measured at photopic luminance levels in dyslexics and controls. *Vision Research*, *35*, 1483–1494.

Corriveau, K. H., Goswami, U., & Thomson, J. M. (2010). Auditory processing and early literacy skills in a preschool and kindergarten population. *Journal of Learning Disabilities*, *43*, 369–382.

Coventry, W. L., Byrne, B., Olson, R. K., Corley, R., & Samuelsson, S. (2011). Dynamic and static assessment of phonological awareness in preschool: a behavior-genetic study. *Journal of Learning Disabilities, 44*, 322–329.

Covington, M. V. (1992). *Making the grade: A self-worth perspective on motivation and school reform.* New York: Cambridge University Press.

Cowan, N., & Alloway, T. P. (2008). The development of working memory. In N. Cowan (Ed.), *Development of memory in childhood* (pp. 303–342). New York: Psychology Press.

Crisfield, J. (1996). *The dyslexia handbook.* London: British Dyslexia Association.

Crombie, M., & Reid, G. (2009). The role of early identification research: Models from research and practice. In G. Reid (Ed.), *The Routledge companion to dyslexia* (pp. 71–79). London: Routledge.

Cronbach, L. J. (1975). Beyond the two disciplines of scientific psychology. *American Psychologist, 30*, 116–127.

Cronbach, L. J., & Snow, R. E. (1977). *Aptitudes and instructional methods: A handbook for research on interactions.* Irvington: Oxford University Press.

Cunningham, A. E., & Stanovich, K. E. (1998). The impact of print exposure on word recognition. In J. L. Metsala & L. C. Ehri (Eds.), *Word recognition in beginning literacy* (pp. 235–262). Mahwah, NJ: Erlbaum.

Curtis, M. (2004). Adolescents who struggle with word identification: Research and practice. In T. L. Jetton & J. A. Dole (Eds.), *Adolescent literacy research and practice* (pp. 119–134). New York: Guilford.

Cutting, L. E., & Denckla, M. B. (2001). The relationship of rapid serial naming and word reading in normally developing readers: An exploratory model. *Reading and Writing, 14*, 673–705.

Cyhlarova, E., Bell, J. G., Dick, J. R., Mackinley, E. E., Stein, J. F., & Richardson, A. J. (2007). Membrane fatty acids, reading and spelling in dyslexic and non-dyslexic adults. *European Neuropsychopharmacology, 17*, 116–121.

Dahlin, K. (2011). Effects of working memory training on reading in children with special needs. *Reading and Writing, 24*, 479–491.

Davey Smith, G., Ebrahim, S., Lewis, S., Hansell, A. L., Palmer, L. J., & Burton, P. R. (2005). Genetic epidemiology and public health: hope, hype, and future prospects. *Lancet, 366*, 1484–1498.

Davis, R. D. (1997). *The gift of dyslexia.* London: Souvenir Press.

Dawkins, R. (1976). *The selfish gene.* Oxford: Oxford University Press.

de Bree, E., Snowling, M. J., Gerrits, E., van Alphen, P., van der Leij, A., & Wijnen, F. (2012). Phonology and literacy. In A. A. Benasich & R. H. Fitch (Eds.), *Developmental dyslexia: Early precursors, neurobehavioral markers, and biological substrates* (pp. 133–150). Baltimore, MD: Paul H. Brookes Publishing.

De Clercq-Quaegebeur, M., Casalis, S., Lemaitre, M., Bourgois, B., Getto, M., & Vallée, L. (2010). Neuropsychological profile on the WISC-IV of French children with dyslexia. *Journal of Learning Disabilities, 43*, 563–574.

de Graaff, S. E. H., Bosman, A. M. T., Hasselman, F., & Verhoeven, L. (2009). Benefits of systematic phonics instruction. *Scientific Studies of Reading, 13*, 318–333.

de Kovel, C. G. F., Hol, F. A., Heister, J., Willemen, J., Sandkuijl, L. A., Franke, B., et al. (2004). Genomewide scan identifies susceptibility locus for dyslexia on Xq27 in an extended Dutch family. *Journal of Medical Genetics, 41*, 652–657.

De Weerdt, F., Desoete, A., & Roeyers, H. (2013). Working memory in children with reading disabilities and/or mathematical disabilities. *Journal of Learning Disabilities, 46*(5), 461–472.

Deffenbacher, K. E., Kenyon, J. B., Hoover, D. M., Olson, R. K., Pennington, B. F., DeFries, J. C., et al. (2004). Refinement of the 6p21.3 quantitative trait locus influencing dyslexia: linkage and association analyses. *Human Genetics, 115*, 128–138.

Dehaene, S. (2009). *Reading in the brain*. New York: Viking.

Delacato, C. H. (1959). *The treatment and prevention of reading problems*. Springfield, IL: Charles C. Thomas.

Demb, J. B., Boynton, G. M., Best, M., & Heeger, D. J. (1998). Psychophysical evidence for a magnocellular pathway deficit in dyslexia. *Vision Research, 38*, 1555–1559.

Demb, J. B., Boynton, G. M., & Heeger, D. J. (1998). Functional magnetic resonance imaging of early visual pathways in dyslexia. *Journal of Neuroscience, 18*, 6939–6951.

Démonet, J.-F., Taylor, M. J., & Chaix, Y. (2004). Developmental dyslexia. *Lancet, 363*, 1451–1460.

Denckla, M., & Rudel, R. (1974). Rapid "automatized" naming of pictured objects, colors, letters and numbers by normal children. *Cortex, 10*, 186–202.

Denckla, M., & Rudel, R. (1976a). Naming of object-drawings by dyslexic and other learning disabled children. *Brain and Language, 3*, 1–15.

Denckla, M., & Rudel, R. (1976b). Rapid "automatized' naming (R.A.N.): Dyslexia differentiated from other learning disabilities. *Neuropsychologia, 14*, 471–479.

Denckla, M. B. (1972). Color-naming deficits in dyslexic boys. *Cortex, 8*(2), 164–176.

Denton, C. A. (2012). Response to intervention for reading difficulties in the primary grades: Some answers and lingering questions. *Journal of Learning Disabilities, 45*(3), 232–243.

Denton, C. A., Cirino, P. T., Barth, A. E., Romain, M., Vaughn, S., Wexler, J., et al. (2011). An experimental study of scheduling and duration of "Tier 2" first-grade reading intervention. *Journal of Research on Educational Effectiveness, 4*, 208–230.

Denton, C. A., & Hocker, J. L. (2006). *Responsive reading instruction: Flexible intervention for struggling readers in the early grades*. Longmont, CO: Sopris West.

Denton, C. A., Nimon, K., Mathes, P. G., Swanson, E. A., Kethley, C., Kurz, T. B., & Shih, M. (2010). Effectiveness of a supplemental early reading intervention scaled up in multiple schools. *Exceptional Children, 76*, 394–416.

Denton, C. A., Tolar, T. D., Fletcher, J. M., Barth, A. E., Vaughn, S., & Francis, D. J. (2013). Effects of Tier 3 Intervention for Students with Persistent Reading Difficulties and Characteristics of Inadequate Responders. *Journal of Educational Psychology, 105*(3), 633–648.

Denton, C. A., & Vaughn, S. (2008). Reading and writing intervention for older students with disabilities: Possibilities and challenges. *Learning Disabilities Research & Practice, 23*, 61–62.

Denton, C. A., Wexler, J., Vaughn, S., & Bryan, D. (2008). Intervention provided to linguistically diverse middle school students with severe reading difficulties. *Learning Disabilities Research & Practice, 23*, 79–89.

Department of Education and Science. (1975). *A language for life (The Bullock Report)*. London: Her Majesty's Stationery Office.

Deutsch, G. K., Dougherty, R. F., Bammer, R., Siok, W. T., Gabrieli, J. D., & Wandell, B. (2005). Children's reading performance is correlated with white matter structure measured by diffusion tensor imaging. *Cortex, 41*, 354–363.

Diehl, J. J., Frost, S. J., Mencl, W. E., & Pugh, K. R. (2011). Neuroimaging and the phonlogical deficit hypothesis. In S. A. Brady, D. Braze, & C. A. Fowler (Eds.), *Explaining individual differences in reading: Theory and evidence* (pp. 217–237). New York: Psychology Press.

Dirks, E., Spyer, G., van Lieshout, E. C. D. M., & de Sonneville, L. (2008). Prevalence of combined reading and arithmetic disabilities. *Journal of Learning Disabilities, 41*(5), 460–473.

Doman, G., & Delacato, C. H. (1968). Doman-Delacato philosophy. *Human Potential, 1*, 113–116.

Dore, W., & Brookes, D. (2006). *Dyslexia: The miracle cure*. London: Blake.

Dorsaint-Pierre, R., Penhune, V. B., Watkins, K. E., Neelin, P., Lerch, J. P., Bouffard, M., et al. (2006). Asymmetries of the planum temporale and Heschl's gyrus: relationship to language lateralization. *Brain, 129*, 1164–1176.

Dougherty, R. F., Ben-Shachar, M., Deutsch, G. K., Hernandez, A., Fox, G. R., & Wandell, B. A. (2007). Temporal-callosal pathway diffusivity predicts phonological skills in children. *Proceedings of the National Academy of Sciences of the United States of America, 104*, 8556–8561.

Doyon, J., Song, A. W., Karni, A., Lalonde, F., Adams, M. M., & Ungerleider, L. G. (2002). Experience-dependent changes in cerebellar contributions to motor sequence learning. *Proceedings of the National Academy of Sciences of the United States of America, 99*, 1017–1022.

Drake, W. E. (1968). Clinical and pathological finding in a child with a developmental learning disability. *Journal of Learning Disabilities, 1*, 486–502.

Dresher, B. E. (2011). The phoneme. In M. v. Oostendorp, C. J. Ewen, E. Hume, & K. Rice (Eds.), *The Blackwell companion to phonology* (Vol. 1, pp. 241–266). Oxford: Wiley-Blackwell.

Duara, R., Kushch, A., Gross-Glenn, K., et al. (1991). Neuroanatomic differences between dyslexic and normal readers on magnetic resonance imaging scans. *Archives of Neurology, 48*, 410–416.

Dubois, M., Kyllingsboek, S., Prado, C., Musca, S. C., Peiffer, E., Lassus-Sangosse, D., et al. (2010). Fractionating the multi-character processing deficit in developmental dyslexia: Evidence from two case studies. *Cortex, 46*, 717–738.

Duff, F. J., & Clarke, P. J. (2011). Practitioner review: Reading disorders – What are effective interventions and how should they be implemented and evaluated? *Journal of Child Psychology & Psychiatry, 52*, 3–12.

Duff, F. J., Hayiou-Thomas, M. E., & Hulme, C. (2012). Evaluating the effectiveness of a phonologically based reading intervention for struggling readers with varying language profiles. *Reading and Writing, 25*, 621–640.

Dufor, O., Serniclaes, W., Sprenger-Charolles, L., & Démonet, J. F. (2007). Top-down processes during auditory phoneme categorization in dyslexia: A PET study. *Neuroimage, 34*, 1692–1707.

Duncan, C. C., Rumsey, J. M., Wilkniss, S. M., Denckla, M. B., Hamburger, S. D., & Odou-Potkin, M. (1994). Developmental dyslexia and attention dysfunction in adults: brain potential indices of information processing. *Psychophysiology, 31*, 386–401.

Dunning, D. L., Holmes, J., & Gathercole, S. E. (2013). Does working memory train-ing lead to generalized improvements in children with low working memory? A randomized controlled trial. *Developmental Science, 16*(6), 915–925.

Dynarski, M., Agodini, R., Heaviside, S., Novak, T., Carey, N., Campuzano, L., et al. (2007). *Effectiveness of reading and mathematics software products: Findings from the first student cohort*. Washington, DC: U.S. Department of Education.

Dyslexia Action. (2005). *The incidence of hidden disabilities in the prison population*. Egham, UK: Dyslexia Action.

Dyslexia Foundation of New Zealand. (2008). *Dealing with dyslexia: The way forward for New Zealand educators*. Christchurch, New Zealand: Author.

Eckert, M. A. (2004). Neuroanatomical markers for dyslexia: A review of dyslexia structural imaging studies. *Neuroscientist, 10*, 362–371.

Eckert, M. A., Leonard, C. M., Richards, T. L., Aylward, E. H., Thomson, J., & Berninger, V. W. (2003). Anatomical correlates of dyslexia: Frontal and cerebellar findings. *Brain, 126*, 482–494.

Eckert, M. A., Leonard, C. M., Wilke, M., Eckert, M., Richards, T., Richards, A., et al. (2005). Anatomical signatures of dyslexia in children: Unique information from manual and voxel based morphometry brain measures. *Cortex, 41*, 304–315.

Eden, G. F., VanMeter, J. W., Rumsey, J. M., Maisog, J. M., Woods, R. P., & Zeffiro, T. A. (1996). Abnormal processing of visual motion in dyslexia revealed by functional brain imaging. *Nature, 382*, 66–69.

Egeland, J., Aarlien, A. K., & Saunes, B. K. (2013). Few effects of far transfer of working memory training in ADHD: A randomized controlled trial. *PLOS ONE, 8*(10), e75660.

Ehri, L. C. (1999). Phases of development in learning to read words. In J. Oakhill & R. Beard (Eds.), *Reading development and the teaching of reading: A psychological perspective* (pp. 79–108). Oxford: Blackwell.

Ehri, L. C. (2002). Phases of acquisition in learning to read words and implications for teaching. *British Journal of Educational Psychology: Monograph Series, 1*, 7–28.

Ehri, L. C., Nunes, S. R., Stahl, S. A., & Willows, D. M. (2001). Systematic phonics instruction helps students learn to read: Evidence from the National Reading Panel's meta-analysis. *Review of Educational Research, 71*, 393–447.

Ehri, L. C., Nunes, S. R., Willows, D. M., Schuster, B. V., Yaghoub-Zadeh, Z., & Shana-han, T. (2001). Phonemic awareness instruction helps children learn to read: Evidence from the National Reading Panel's meta-analysis. *Reading Research Quarterly, 36*, 250–287.

Eichler, E. E., Flint, J., Gibson, G., Kong, A., Leal, S. M., Moore, J. H., et al. (2010). Missing heritability and strategies for finding the underlying causes of complex disease. *Nature Reviews Genetics, 11*, 446–450.

Eicher, J. D., Powers, N. R., Miller, L. L., Akshoomoff, N., Amaral, D. G., et al. (2013). Genome-wide association study of shared components of reading disability and language impairment. *Genes, Brain and Behavior, 12*(8), 792–801.

Eide, B. L., & Eide, F. F. (2011). *The dyslexic advantage: Unlocking the hidden potential of the dyslexic brain*. New York: Hudson Street Press.

Eissa, M. (2010). Behavioral and emotional problems associated with dyslexia in ado-lescence. *Current Psychiatry, 17*(1), 17–25.

Eklund, K. M., Torppa, M., & Lyytinen, H. (2013). Predicting reading disability: Early cognitive risk and protective factors. *Dyslexia, 19*(1), 1–10.

Elbeheri, G., & Everatt, J. (2009). Dyslexia and IQ: From research to practice. In G. Reid (Ed.), *The Routledge companion to dyslexia* (pp. 22–32). London: Routledge.

Elliott, J. G. (2003). Dynamic Assessment in educational settings: Realising potential, *Educational Review, 55*, 15–32.

Elliott, J. G. (2005). The dyslexia debate continues. *The Psychologist, 18*, 728–729.

Elliott, J. G. (2008). The dyslexia myth. *Learning Difficulties Australia Bulletin, 40*, 10–14.

Elliott, J. G., Gathercole, S. E., Alloway, T. P., Kirkwood, H., & Holmes, J. (2010). An evaluation of a classroom-based intervention to help overcome working memory difficulties. *Journal of Cognitive Education and Psychology, 9*, 227–250.

Elliott, J. G., & Gibbs, S. (2008). Does dyslexia exist? *Journal of Philosophy of Education, 42*, 475–491.

Elliott, J. G., & Place, M. (2012). *Children in difficulty: A guide to understanding and helping* (3rd ed.). London: Routledge.

Ellis, A. W., Flude, B. M., & Young, A. W. (1987). "Neglect dyslexia" and the early visual processing of letters in words and nonwords. *Cognitive Neuropsychology, 4*, 439–463.

Elston, R. C., & Johnson, W. D. (2008). *Basic biostatistics for geneticists and epidemiologists*. New York: Wiley.

Ercan-Sencicek, A. G., Davis Wright, N. R., Sanders, S. S., Oakman, N., Valdes, L., Bakkaloglu, B., et al. (2012). A balanced t(10;15) translocation in a male patient with developmental language disorder. *European Journal of Medical Genetics, 55*, 128–131.

Essex, M. J., Boyce, W. T., Hertzman, C., Lam, L. L., Armstrong, J. M., Neumann, S. M. A., et al. (2013). Epigenetic vestiges of early developmental adversity: Childhood stress exposure and DNA methylation in adolescence. *Child Development, 84*(1), 58–75.

Everatt, J., & Reid, G. (2009). Dyslexia: An overview of recent research. In G. Reid (Ed.), *The Routledge companion to dyslexia* (pp. 3–21). New York: Routledge.

Fabbro, F., Pesenti, S., Facoetti, A., Bonanomi, M., Libera, L., & Lorusso, M. L. (2001). Callosal transfer in different subtypes of developmental dyslexia. *Cortex, 37*, 65–73.

Facoetti, A., Lorusso, M. L., Cattaneo, C., Galli, R., & Molteni, M. (2005). Visual and auditory attentional capture are both sluggish in children with developmental dyslexia. *Acta Neurobiologiae Experimentalis, 65*, 61–72.

Facoetti, A., Lorusso, M. L., Paganoni, P., Umiltà, C., & Mascetti, G. C. (2003). The role of visuospatial attention in developmental dyslexia: Evidence from a rehabilitation study. *Cognitive Brain Research, 15*, 154–164.

Facoetti, A., Trussardi, A. N., Ruffino, M., Lorusso, M. L., Cattaneo, C., Galli, R., et al. (2009). Multisensory spatial attention deficits are predictive of phonological decoding skills in developmental dyslexia. *Journal of Cognitive Neuroscience, 22*, 1011–1025.

Fagerheim, T., Raeymaekers, P., Tonnessen, F. E., Pedersen, M., Tranebjaerg, L., & Lubs, H. A. (1999). A new gene (DYX3) for dyslexia is located on chromosome 2. *Journal of Medical Genetics, 35*, 664–669.

Fälth, L. Gustafson, S., Tjus, T., Heimann, M., & Svensson, I. (2013). Computer-assisted interventions targeting reading skills of children with reading disabilities – A longitudinal study. *Dyslexia, 19*, 37–53.

Farmer, M. E., & Klein, R. M. (1995). The evidence for a temporal processing deficit linked to dyslexia: A Review. *Psychonomic Bulletin & Review, 2*, 460–493.

Favell, J. E. (2005). Sifting sound practice from snake oil. In J. W. Jacobson, R. M. Foxx, & J. A. Mulick (Eds.), *Controversial therapies for developmental disabilities: Fad, fashion and science in professional practice* (pp. 19–30). Mahwah, NJ: Lawrence Erlbaum.

Fawcett, A. J., Nicolson, R., & Maclagan, F. (2001). Cerebellar tests differentiate between groups of poor readers with and without IQ discrepancy. *Journal of Learning Disabilities, 34*(2), 119–135.

Fawcett, A. J., & Nicolson, R. I. (1999). Performance of dyslexic children on cerebellar and cognitive tests. *Journal of Motor Behavior, 31*, 68–78.

Fawcett, A. J., Nicolson, R. I., & Lee, R. (2004). *Ready to learn*. San Antonio, TX: Harcourt Assessment.

Fawcett, A. J., & Reid, G. (2009). Dyslexia and alternative interventions for dyslexia: A critical commentary. In G. Reid (Ed.), *The Routledge companion to dyslexia* (pp. 157–174). New York: Routledge.

Feldman, H. M., Yeatman, J. D., Lee, E. S., Barde, L. H., & Gaman-Bean, S. (2010). Diffusion tensor imaging: A review for pediatric researchers and clinicians. *Journal of Developmental & Behavioral Pediatrics, 31*, 346–356.

Fernald, G. M., & Keller, H. (1921). The effect of kinaesthetic factors in the development of word recognition in the case of non-readers. *The Journal of Educational Research, 4*, 355–377.

Ferrer, E., Shaywitz, B. A., Holahan, J. M., Marchione, K., & Shaywitz, S. E. (2010). Uncoupling of reading and IQ over time: Empirical evidence for a definition of dyslexia. *Psychological Science, 21*, 93–101.

Field, L. L., Shumansky, K., Ryan, J., Truong, D., Swiergala, E. & Kaplan, B. J. (2013). Dense-map genome scan for dyslexia supports loci at 4q13, 16p12, 17q22, suggests novel locus at 7q36. *Genes, Brain and Behavior, 12*(6), 56–69.

Fields, R. D. (2008). White matter matters. *Scientific American, 298*, 42–49.

Fiez, J. A., Tranel, D., Seager-Frerichs, D., & Damasio, H. (2006). Specific reading and phonological processing deficits are associated with damage to the left frontal operculum. *Cortex, 42*(4), 624–643.

Finch, A. J., Nicolson, R. I., & Fawcett, A. J. (2002). Evidence for a neuroanatomical difference within the olivo-cerebellar pathway of adults with dyslexia. *Cortex, 38*, 529 539.

Finnucci, J. M., & Childs, B. (1981). Are there really more dyslexic boys than girls? In A. Ansora, N. Geschwind, A. Galaburda, M. Albert, & N. Gartrell (Eds.), *Sex differences in dyslexia* (pp. 1–9). Towson, MD: Orton Dyslexia Society.

Fisher, S. E., Francks, C., Marlow, A. J., MacPhie, I. L., Newbury, D. F., Cardon, L. R., et al. (2002). Independent genome-wide scans identify a chromosome 18 quantitative-trait locus influencing dyslexia. *Nature Genetics, 30*, 86–91.

Flannery, K. A., Liederman, J., Daly, L., & Schultz, J. (2000). Male prevalence for reading disability is found in a large sample of black and white children free from ascertainment bias. *Journal of the International Neuropsychological Society*, *6*, 433–442.

Flesch, R. (1955). *Why Johnny can't read and what you can do about it*. New York: Harper & Row.

Fletcher, J. M. (2009). Dyslexia: The evolution of a scientific concept. *Journal of the International Neuropsychological Society*, *15*, 501–508.

Fletcher, J. M., Foorman, B. R., Boudousquie, A., Barnes, M. A., Schatschneider, C., & Francis, D. J. (2002). Assessment of reading and learning disabilities, a research-based intervention-oriented approach. *Journal of School Psychology*, *40*, 27–63.

Fletcher, J. M., Lyon, G. R., Fuchs, L. S., & Barnes, M. A. (2007). *Learning disabilities*. New York: Guilford.

Fletcher, J. M., Morris, R.D., & Lyon, G. R. (2003). Classification and definition of learning disabilities: An integrative perspective. In H. L. Swanson, K. R. Harris, & S. Graham (Eds.), *Handbook of learning disabilities* (pp. 30–56). New York: Guilford Press.

Fletcher, J. M., Shaywitz, S. E., Shankweiler, D. P., Katz, L., Liberman, I. Y., Stuebing, K. K., et al. (1994). Cognitive profiles of reading disability: Comparisons of discrepancy and low achievement definitions. *Journal of Educational Psychology*, *86*, 6–23.

Fletcher, J. M., Stuebing, K. K., Barth, A. E., Denton, C. A., Cirino, P. T., Francis, D. J., et al. (2011). Cognitive correlates of inadequate response to reading intervention. *School Psychology Review*, *40*, 3–22.

Fletcher, J. M., Stuebing, K. K., Morris, R.D., & Lyon, G. R. (2013). Classification and definition of learning disabilities: A hybrid model. In H. L. Swanson, K. R. Harris, & S. Graham (Eds.), *Handbook of learning disabilities, second edition* (pp. 33–50). New York: Guilford Press.

Fletcher, J. M., & Vaughn, S. (2009). Response to intervention: Preventing and remediating academic difficulties. *Child Development Perspectives*, *3*, 30–37.

Flowers, L., Meyer, M., Lovato, J., Wood, F., & Felton, R. (2001). Does third grade discrepancy status predict the course of reading development? *Annals of Dyslexia*, *51*, 49–71.

Flynn, J. M., & Rahbar, M. H. (1994). Prevalence of reading failure in boys compared with girls. *Psychology in the Schools*, *31*, 66–70.

Flynn, L. J., Zheng, X., & Swanson, H. L. (2012). Instructing struggling older readers: A selective meta-analysis of intervention research. *Learning Disabilities Research & Practice*, *27*(1), 21–32.

Foorman, B. R. (2003). *Preventing and remediating reading difficulties: Bringing science to scale*. Baltimore, MD: York Press.

Foorman, B. R., Anthony, J., Seals, L., & Mouzaki, A. (2002). Language development and emergent literacy in preschool. *Seminars in Pediatric Neurology*, *9*, 172–183.

Foorman, B. R., Fletcher, J. M., & Francis, D. J. (2004). *Texas Primary Reading Inventory*. New York: McGraw-Hill.

Foorman, B. R., Fletcher, J. M., Francis, D. J., Carlson, C. D., Chen, D., Mouzaki, A., et al. (1998). *Technical report: Texas Primary Reading Inventory (1998 Edition)*. Houston, TX: Center for Academic and Reading Skills, University of Houston.

Foorman, B. R., Petscher, Y., Lefsky, E. B., & Toste, J. R. (2010). Reading First in Florida: Five years of improvement. *Journal of Literacy Research*, *42*, 71–93.

Foorman, B. R., York, M., Santi, K. L., & Francis, D. (2008). Contextual effects on predicting risk for reading difficulties in first and second grade. *Reading and Writing*, *21*, 371–394.

Foster, L. M., Hynd, G. W., Morgan, A. E., & Hugdahl, K. (2002). Planum temporale asymmetry and ear advantage in dichotic listening in developmental dyslexia and attention-deficit/hyperactivity disorder (ADHD). *Journal of the International Neuropsychological Society*, *8*, 22–36.

Franceschini, S., Gori, S., Ruffino, M., Pedrolli, K., & Facoetti, A. (2012). A causal link between visual spatial attention and reading acquisition. *Current Biology*, *22*, 814–819.

Franceschini, S., Gori, S., Ruffino, M., Viola, S., Molteni, M., & Facoetti, A. (2013). Action video games make dyslexic children read better. *Current Biology*, *23*, 462–466.

Francis, D. J., Shaywitz, S. E., Stuebing, K. K., Shaywitz, B. A., & Fletcher, J. M. (1996). Developmental lag versus deficit models of reading disability: A longitudinal individual growth curves analysis. *Journal of Educational Psychology*, *88*, 3–17.

Francks, C., Paracchini, S., Smith, S. D., Richardson, A. J., Scerri, T. S., Cardon, L. R., et al. (2004). A 77-kilobase region on chromosome 6p22.2 is associated with dyslexia in families from the United Kingdom and from the United States. *American Journal of Human Genetics*, *75*, 1046–1058.

Frederickson, N. (1999). The ACID test – or is it? *Educational Psychology in Practice*, *15*, 2–8.

Frederickson, N., & Frith, U. (1998). Identifying dyslexia in bilingual children: a phonological approach with inner London Sylheti speakers. *Dyslexia*, *4*, 119–131.

Friedmann, N., Biran, M., & Gvion, A. (2012). Patterns of visual dyslexia. *Journal of Neuropsychology*, *6*, 1–30.

Friedmann, N., & Gvion, A. (2001). Letter position dyslexia. *Cognitive Neuropsychology*, *18*, 673–696.

Friedmann, N., Kerbel, N., & Shvimer, L. (2010). Developmental attentional dyslexia. *Cortex*, *46*, 1216–1237.

Friedmann, N., & Rahamim, E. (2007). Developmental letter position dyslexia. *Journal of Neuropsychology*, *1*, 201–236.

Friedmann, N., & Rahamim, E. (in press). What can reduce letter migrations in letter position dyslexia? *Journal of Research in Reading*.

Friend, A., DeFries, J. C., & Olson, R. K. (2008). Parental education moderates genetic influences on reading disability. *Psychological Science*, *19*, 1–7.

Frijjters, J. C., Lovett, M. W., Steinbach, K. A., Wolf, M., Sevcik, R. A., & Morris, R. (2011). Neurocognitive predictors of reading outcomes for children with reading disabilities. *Journal of Learning Disabilities*, *44*, 150–166.

Friso-van den Bos, I., van der Ven, S. H. G., Kroesbergen, E. H., & van Luit, J. E. H. (2013). Working memory and mathematics in primary school children: A meta-analysis. *Educational Research Review*, *10*, 29–44.

Frith, U. (1997). Brain, mind and behaviour in dyslexia. In C. Hulme & M. J. Snowling (Eds.), *Dyslexia: Biology, cognition, and intervention* (pp. 1–19). London: Whurr.

Frye, R. E., Liederman, J., Malmberg, B., McLean, J., Strickland, D., & Beauchamp, M. S. (2010). Surface area accounts for the relation of gray matter volume to reading-related skills and history of dyslexia. *Cerebral Cortex*, *20*, 2625–2635.

Fuchs, D., Compton, D. L., Fuchs, L. S., Bryant, J., & Davis, G. N. (2008). Making "secondary intervention" work in a three-tier responsiveness-to-intervention model: findings from the first-grade longitudinal reading study of the National Research Center on Learning Disabilities. *Reading and Writing, 21*, 413–436.

Fuchs, D., Compton, D. L., Fuchs, L. S., Bryant, J., Hamlett, C. L., & Lambert, W. (2012). First-grade cognitive abilities as long-term predictors of reading comprehension and disability status. *Journal of Learning Disabilities, 45*, 217–231.

Fuchs, D., & Deshler, D. K. (2007). What we need to know about responsiveness to intervention (and shouldn't be afraid to ask). *Learning Disabilities Research & Practice, 20*, 129–136.

Fuchs, D., Fuchs, L. S., & Compton, D. L. (2012). Smart RTI: A next generation approach to multilevel prevention. *Exceptional Children, 78*(3), 263–279.

Fuchs, D., Fuchs, L. S., Mathes, P. G., & Simmons, D. C. (1997). Peer-assisted learning strategies: Making classrooms more responsive to diversity. *American Educational Research Journal, 34*, 174–206.

Fuchs, D., McMaster, K. L., Fuchs, L.S., & Al Otaiba, S. (2013). Data-based individualization as a means of providing intensive instruction to students with serious learning disorders. In H. L. Swanson, K. R. Harris, & S. Graham (Eds.), *Handbook of learning disabilities* (pp. 526–544). New York: Guilford Press.

Fuchs, L. S., & Fuchs, D. (1998). Treatment validity: A unifying concept for reconceptualizing the identification of learning disabilities. *Learning Disabilities Research & Practice, 13*, 204–219.

Fuchs, L. S., & Fuchs, D. (2009). Creating opportunities for intensive intervention for students with learning disabilities. *Teaching Exceptional Children, 42*, 60–62.

Fuchs, L. S., Fuchs, D., & Compton, D. L. (2010). Commentary: Rethinking response to intervention at middle and high school. *School Psychology Review, 39*, 22–28.

Fuchs, L. S., Fuchs, D., & Compton, D. L. (2013). Intervention effects for students with comorbid forms of learning disability: Understanding the needs of nonresponders. *Journal of Learning Disabilities, 46*(6), 534–548.

Fuchs, L. S., & Vaughn, S. (2012). Responsiveness-to-intervention: A decade later. *Journal of Learning Disabilities, 45*(3), 195–203.

Furnes, B., & Samuelsson, S. (2010). Predicting reading and spelling difficulties in transparent and opaque orthographies: A comparison between Scandinavian and US/Australian children. *Dyslexia, 16*, 119–142.

Furnes, B., & Samuelsson, S. (2011). Phonological awareness and raid automatized naming predicting early development in reading and spelling: Results from a cross-linguistic longitudinal study. *Learning and Individual Differences, 21*, 85–95.

Gabrieli, J. D. E. (2009). Dyslexia: A new synergy between education and cognitive neuroscience. *Science, 325*, 280–283.

Gabrieli, J. D. E., & Norton, E. S. (2012). Reading abilities: Importance of visual-spatial attention. *Cortex, 22*, R298–R299.

Galaburda, A. M. (1993). Neuroanatomic basis of developmental dyslexia. *Neurology Clinics, 11*, 161–173.

Galaburda, A. M., & Kemper, T. L. (1979). Cytoarchitectonic abnormalities in developmental dyslexia: a case study. *Annals of Neurology, 6*, 94–100.

Galaburda, A. M., LoTurco, J. J., Ramus, F., Fitch, R. H., & Rosen, G. D. (2006). From genes to behavior in developmental dyslexia. *Nature Neuroscience, 9*, 1213–1217.

Galaburda, A. M., Menard, M. T., & Rosen, G. D. (1994). Evidence for aberrant auditory anatomy in developmental dyslexia. *PNAS*, *91*, 8010–8013.

Galaburda, A. M., Schrott, L. M., & Sherman, G. F. (1996). *Animal models of developmental dyslexia*. Baltimore, MD: York Press.

Galaburda, A. M., Sherman, G. F., Rosen, G. D., Aboitiz, F., & Gerschwin, N. (1985). Developmental dyslexia: four consecutive patients with cortical anomalies. *Annals of Neurology*, *18*, 222–233.

Gamse, B. C., Tepper-Jacob, R., Horst, M., Boulay, B., & Unlu, F. (2008). *Reading First impact study: Final Report*. Washington, DC: Institute for Education Sciences, U.S. Department of Education.

Garner, M. (2004, September 10). Universities exaggerate dyslexia epidemic for own gain, expert claims, Times Higher Education. Retrieved October 6, 2013 from http://www.timeshighereducation.co.uk/story.asp?storyCode=191053&sectioncode=26.

Gathercole, S. E., & Alloway, T. P. (2008). *Working memory and learning: A practical guide*. London: Sage.

Gathercole, S. E., Alloway, T. P., Willis, C., & Adams, A. M. (2006). Working memory in children with reading disabilities. *Journal of Experimental Child Psychology*, *93*, 265–281.

Gathercole, S. E., Pickering, S. J., Knight, C., & Stegmann, Z. (2004). Working memory skills and educational attainment: Evidence from national curriculum assessments and 7 and 14 years of age. *Applied Cognitive Psychology*, *18*, 1–16.

Gayán, J., & Olson, R. K. (2001). Genetic and environmental influences on orthographic and phonological skills in children with reading disabilities. *Developmental Neurology*, *20*, 483–507.

Gayán, J., & Olson, R. K. (2003). Genetic and environmental influences on individual differences in printed word recognition. *Journal of Experimental Child Psychology*, *84*, 97–123.

Gelzheiser, L. M., Scanlon, D., Vellutino, F., Halgren-Flynn, L., & Schatschneider, C. (2011). Effects of the interactive strategies approach-extended: A responsive and comprehensive intervention for struggling readers. *Elementary School Journal*, *112*, 280–306.

Georgiewa, P., Rzanny, R., Gaser, C., Gerhard, U. J., Vieweg, U., Freesmeyer, D., et al. (2002). Phonological processing in dyslexic children: A study combining functional imaging and event related potentials. *Neuroscience Letters*, *318*, 5–8.

Georgiewa, P., Rzanny, R., Hopf, J. M., Knab, R., Glauche, V., Kaiser, W. A., et al. (1999). fMRI during word processing in dyslexic and normal reading children. *Neuroreport*, *10*, 3459–3465.

Georgiou, G. K., Papadopoulos, T. C., Zarouna, E., & Parrila, R. (2012). Are auditory and visual processing deficits related to developmental dyslexia? *Dyslexia*, *18*(2), 110–129.

Georgiou, G. K., & Parrila, R., (2013). Rapid automatized naming and reading: A review. In H. L. Swanson, K. R. Harris, & S. Graham (Eds.), *Handbook of learning disabilities* (pp. 169–185). New York: Guilford Press.

Georgiou, G. K., Parrila, R., Cui, Y., & Papadopoulos, T. C. (2013). Why is rapid automatized naming related to reading? *Journal of Experimental Child Psychology*, *115*(1), 218–225.

Georgiou, G. K., Parrila, R., & Kirby, J. R. (2009). RAN components and reading development from grade 3 to grade 5: What underlies their relationship? *Scientific Studies of Reading, 13,* 508–534.

Georgiou, G. K., Protopapas, A., Papadopoulos, T. C., Skaloumbakas, C., & Parrila, R. (2010). Auditory temporal processing and dyslexia in an orthographically consistent language. *Cortex, 46,* 1330–1344.

Gersten, R., Compton, D., Connor, C. M., Dimino, J., Santoro, L., Linan-Thompson, S., et al. (2008). *Assisting students struggling with reading: Response to intervention and multi-tier intervention in the primary grades. A practice guide* (NCEE 2009–4045). Washington, DC: National Center for Education Evaluation and Regional Assistance, Institute of Education Sciences, U.S. Department of Education.

Geschwind, N. (1982). Why Orton was right. *Annals of Dyslexia, 32,* 13–30.

Geschwind, N., & Levitsky, W. (1968). Human brain: Left-right asymmetries in temporal speech region. *Science, 161,* 186–187.

Getchell, N., Pabreja, P., Neeld, K., & Carrio, V. (2007). Comparing children with and without dyslexia on the movement assessment battery for children and the test of gross motor development. *Perceptual and Motor Skills, 105,* 207–214.

Giedd, J. N., & Rapoport, J. L. (2010). Structural MRI of pediatric brain development: What have we learned and where are we going? *Neuron, 67,* 728–734.

Gilbert, J. K., Compton, D. L., & Kearns, D. M. (2011). Word and person effects on decoding accuracy: A new look at an old question. *Journal of Educational Psychology, 103*(2), 489–507.

Gilger, J. W., Pennington, B. F., & DeFries, J. C. (1992). A twin study of the etiology of comorbidity: Attention deficit-hyperactivity disorder and dyslexia. *Journal of the American Academy of Child and Adolescent Psychiatry, 31,* 343–348.

Gillam, R. B., Loeb, D. F., Hoffman, L. M., Bohman, T., Champlin, C. A., Thibodeau, L., et al. (2008). The efficacy of Fast ForWord language intervention in school-age children with language impairment: A randomized controlled trial. *Journal of Speech, Language, and Hearing Research, 51,* 97–119.

Gillingham, A., & Stillman, B.W. (1997). *The Gillingham manual: Remedial training for children with specific disability in reading, spelling, and penmanship* (8th ed.). Cambridge, MA: Educators Publishing Service.

Girirajan, S., Brkanac, Z., Coe, B. P., Baker, C., Vives, L., Vu, T. H., et al. (2011). Relative burden of large CNVs on a range of neurodevelopmental phenotypes. *PLOS Genetics, 7,* e1002334.

Goddard, R. (1991). Why LINC matters. *English in Education, 25,* 32–39.

Goddard Blythe, S. (2005). Releasing educational potential through movement: A summary of individual studies carried out using the INPP test battery and developmental exercise programme for use in schools with children with special needs. *Child Care in Practice, 11,* 415–432.

Goe, L. (2007). *The link between teacher quality and student outcomes: A research synthesis.* Retrieved February 16, 2012 from http://www.tqsource.org/publications/LinkBetweenTQandStudentOutcomes.pdf.

Goldston, D. B., Walsh, A., Mayfield-Arnold, E., et al. (2007). Reading problems, psychiatric disorders and functional impairment from mid- to late adolescence. *Journal of the American Academy of Child and Adolescent Psychiatry, 46*(1), 25–32.

Gonzaga-Jauregui, C., Lupski, J. R., & Gibbs, R. A. (2012). Human genome sequencing in health and disease. *Annual Review of Medicine, 63*, 35–61.

Gooch, D., Snowling, M., & Hulme, C. (2011). Time perception, phonological skills and executive function in children with dyslexia and/or ADHD symptoms. *Journal of Child Psychology and Psychiatry, 52*, 195–203.

Good, R. H., & Kaminski, R. A. (2003). *Dynamic indicators of basic early literacy skills*. Longmont, CO: Sopris West Educational Services.

Good, R. H., Kaminski, R. A., Shinn, M., Bratten, J., Shinn, M., Laimon, L., et al. (2004). *Technical adequacy and decision making utility of DIBELS (Technical Report No. 7)*. Eugene: University of Oregon Press.

Goodman, I., Libenson, A., & Wade-Woolley, L. (2010) Sensitivity to linguistic stress, phonological awareness and early reading ability in preschoolers. *Journal of Research in Reading, 33*(2), 113–127.

Goodman, K. S. (1965). A linguistic study of cues and miscues in reading. *Elementary English, 42*, 639–643.

Goodman, K. S. (1967). Reading: A psycholinguistic guessing game. *Journal of the Reading Specialist, 6*, 126–135.

Goodman, K. S. (1969). Analysis or oral reading miscues: Applied psycholinguistics. *Reading Research Quarterly, 5*, 9–30.

Goodman, K. S. (1970). Reading: A psycholinguistic guessing game. In H. Singer & R. B. Ruddell (Eds.), *Theoretical models and processes of reading* (pp. 259–272). Newark, DE: International Reading Association.

Goodman, K. S. (1986). *What's whole in whole language?* Portsmouth, NH: Heinemann.

Goodman, K. S. (1992). Why whole language is today's agenda in education. *Language Arts, 69*, 354–363.

Gormley, K. A., & McDermott, P. (2011). Traditions of diagnosis: Learning from the past, moving past traditions. In R. Allington & A. McGill-Franzen (Eds.), *Handbook of research on reading disabilities* (pp. 162–172). New York: Routledge.

Goswami, U. (2002). Phonology, reading development and dyslexia: A cross-linguistic perspective. *Annals of Dyslexia, 52*, 1–23.

Goswami, U. (2012). Neuroscience and education: Can we go from basic research to translation? A possible framework from dyslexia research. *Educational Neuroscience, B.J.E.P. Monograph Series, 11*, 129–142.

Goswami, U., Gerson, D., & Astruc, L. (2010). Amplitude envelope perception, phonology and prosodic sensitivity in children with developmental dyslexia. *Reading & Writing, 23*, 995–1019.

Goswami, U., Huss, M., Mead, N., Fosker, T., & Verney, J. P. (2013). Perception of patterns of musical beat distribution in phonological developmental dyslexia: Significant longitudinal relations with word reading and reading comprehension. *Cortex, 49*(5), 1363–1376.

Goswami, U., Mead, N., Fosker, T., Huss, M., Barnes, L., & Leong, V. (2013). Impaired perception of syllable stress in children with dyslexia: A longitudinal study. *Journal of Memory and Language 69*, 1–17.

Goswami, U., & Szucs, D. (2011). Educational neuroscience, developmental mechanisms: Towards a conceptual framework. *Neuroimage, 57*, 651–658.

Goswami, U., Thomson, J., Richardson, U., Stainthorp, R., Hughes, D., Rosen, S., et al. (2002). Amplitude envelope onsets and developmental dyslexia: A new hypothesis. *Proceedings of the National Academy of Sciences*, *99*(16), 10911–10916.

Goswami, U., Wang, H. L., Cruz, A., Fosker, T., Mead, N., & Huss, M. (2011). Language-universal sensory deficits in developmental dyslexia: English, Spanish, and Chinese. *Journal of Cognitive Neuroscience*, *23*(2), 325–337.

Gough, P. B. (1983). Context, form and interaction. In K. Rayner (Ed.), *Eye movements in reading: Perceptual and language processes* (pp. 203–211). San Diego, CA: Academic Press.

Gough, P. B., & Tunmer, W. E. (1986). Decoding, reading, and reading disability. *Remedial and Special Education*, *7*, 6–10.

Grant, P. E. (2012). Evolution of pediatric neuroimaging and application of cutting-edge techniques. In A. A. Benasich & R. H. Fitch (Eds.), *Developmental dyslexia: Early precursors, neurobehavioral markers, and biological substrates* (pp. 227–240). Baltimore, MD: Paul H. Brookes Publishing.

Gray, S. A., Chaban, P., Martinussen, R., Goldberg, R., Gotlieb, H., Kronitz, R., Hockenberry, M. and Tannock, R. (2012). Effects of a computerized working memory training program on working memory, attention, and academics in adolescents with severe LD and comorbid ADHD: A randomized controlled trial. *Journal of Child Psychology and Psychiatry*, *53*, 1277–1284.

Greenspan, S. (2005). Credulity and gullibility among service providers: An attempt to understand why snake oil sells. In J. W. Jacobson, R. M. Foxx, & J. A. Mulick (Eds.), *Controversial therapies for developmental disabilities: Fad, fashion and science in professional practice* (pp. 129–138). Mahwah, NJ: Lawrence Erlbaum.

Gresham, F. M. (2009). Using response to intervention for identification of specific learning disabilities. In A. Akin-Little, S. G. Little, M. A. Bray, & T. J. Kehl (Eds.), *Behavioral interventions in schools: Evidence-based positive strategies* (pp. 205–220). Washington, DC: American Psychological Association.

Gresham, F. M., & Vellutino, F.R. (2010). What is the role of intelligence in the identification of specific learning disabilities? Issues and clarifications. *Learning Disabilities Research & Practice*, *25*(4), 194–206.

Griffiths, Y. M., Hill, N. I., Bailey, P. J., & Snowling, M. J. (2003). Auditory temporal order discrimination and backward recognition masking in adults with dyslexia. *Journal of Speech, Language, and Hearing Research*, *46*, 1352–1366.

Grigorenko, E. L. (2001). Developmental dyslexia: An update on genes, brains, and environments. *Journal of Child Psychology and Psychiatry*, *42*, 91–125.

Grigorenko, E. L. (2004). Genetic bases of developmental dyslexia: A capsule review of heritability estimates. *Enfance*, *3*, 273–287.

Grigorenko, E. L. (2005). A conservative meta-analysis of linkage and linkage-association studies of developmental dyslexia. *Scientific Studies of Reading*, *9*, 285–316.

Grigorenko, E. L. (2006). Learning disabilities in juvenile offenders. *Child and Adolescent Psychiatric Clinics of North America*, *15*, 353–371.

Grigorenko, E. L. (2007). Triangulating developmental dyslexia: Behavior, brain, and genes. In D. Coch, G. Dawson, & K. Fischer (Eds.), *Human behavior and the developing brain* (pp. 117–144). New York: Guilford Press.

Grigorenko, E. L. (2009). At the height of fashion: what genetics can teach us about neurodevelopmental disabilities. *Current Opinion in Neurology*, *22*, 126–130.

Grigorenko, E. L. (2011). Language-based learning disabilities. In N. Seel (Ed.), *Encyclopedia of the sciences of learning*. New York: Springer.

Grigorenko, E. L. (2012). Commentary: Translating quantitative genetics into molecular genetics: decoupling reading disorder and ADHD – reflections on Greven et al. and Rosenberg et al. *Journal of Child Psychology and Psychiatry*, *53*(3), 252–253.

Grigorenko, E. L., Klin, A., & Volkmar, F. (2003). Hyperlexia: Disability or superability? *Journal of Child Psychology and Psychiatry*, *44*, 1079–1091.

Grigorenko, E. L., & Naples, A. (Eds.). (2008). *Single-word reading: Biological and behavioral perspectives*. Mahwah, NJ: Lawrence Erlbaum Associates.

Grigorenko, E. L., & Naples, A. J. (2009). The devil is in the details: Decoding the genetics of reading. In P. McCardle & K. Pugh (Eds.), *Helping children learn to read: Current issues and new directions in the integration of cognition, neurobiology and genetics of reading and dyslexia* (pp. 133–148). New York: Psychological Press.

Grigorenko, E. L., & Sternberg, R. J. (1998). Dynamic testing. *Psychological Bulletin*, *124*, 111–132.

Grills-Taquechel, A. E., Fletcher, J. M., Vaughn, S. R., & Stuebing, K. K. (2012). Anxiety and reading difficulties in early elementary school: Evidence for unidirectional- or bi-directional relations? *Child Psychiatry & Human Development*, *43*, 35–47.

Gross-Glenn, K., Skottun, B. C., Glenn, W., Kushch, A., Lingua, R., Dunbar, M., et al. (1995). Contrast sensitivity in dyslexia. *Visual Neuroscience*, *12*, 153–163.

Grünling, C., Ligges, M., Huonker, R., Klingert, M., Mentzel, H. J., Rzanny, R., et al. (2004). Dyslexia: The possible benefit of multimodal integration of fMRI- and EEG-data. *Journal of Neural Transmission*, *111*, 951–969.

Gunn, B., Smolkowski, K., Biglan, A., Black, C., & Blair, J. (2005). Fostering the development of reading skill through supplemental instruction: Results for Hispanic and non-Hispanic students. *The Journal of Special Education*, *39*, 66–85.

Guthrie, J. T., & Davis, M. H. (2003). Motivating struggling readers in middle school through an engagement model of classroom practice. *Reading and Writing Quarterly*, *19*, 59–85.

Gwernan-Jones, R., & Burden, R. L. (2010). Are they just lazy? Student teachers' attitudes about dyslexia. *Dyslexia*, *16*, 66–86.

Habib, M. (2000). The neurological basis of developmental dyslexia. *Brain*, *123*, 2373–2399.

Habib, M., Robichon, F., Levrier, O., Khalil, R., & Salamon, G. (1995). Diverging asymmetries of temporo-parietal cortical areas: a reappraisal of Geschwind/Galaburda theory. *Brain and Language*, *48*, 238–258.

Hackman, D. A., & Farah, M. J. (2009). Socioeconomic status and the developing brain. *Trends in Cognitive Sciences*, *13*, 65–73.

Hackman, D. A., Farah, M. J., & Meaney, M. J. (2010). Socioeconomic status and the brain: mechanistic insights from human and animal research. *Nature Reviews Neuroscience*, *11*, 651–659.

Haddow, J. E., & Palomaki, G. E. (2003). ACCE: A model process for evaluating data on emerging genetic tests. In M. Khoury, J. Little, & W. Burke (Eds.), *Human genome epidemiology: A scientific foundation for using genetic information to improve health and prevent disease* (pp. 217–233). New York: Oxford University Press.

Hadzibeganovic, T., van den Noort, M., Bosch, P., Perc, M., van Kralingen, R., Mondt, K., et al. (2011). Cross-linguistic neuroimaging and dyslexia: A critical view. *Cortex*, *46*, 1312–1316.

Hagan-Burke, S., Coyne, M. D., Kwok, O., Simmons, D., Kim, M., Simmons, L., et al. (2013). The effects and interactions of student, teacher, and setting variables on reading outcomes for kindergarteners receiving supplemental reading intervention. *Journal of Learning Disabilities*, *46*(3), 260–277.

Hale, J. B., Alfonso, V., Berninger, V., Bracken, B., Christo, C., Clark, E., et al. (2010). Critical issues in response to intervention, comprehensive evaluation, and specific learning disabilities evaluation and intervention: An expert white paper consensus. *Learning Disability Quarterly*, *33*, 223–236.

Hale, J. B., Fiorello, C. A., Miller, J. A., Wenrich, K., Teodori, A. M., & Henzel, J. (2008). WISC-IV assessment and intervention strategies for children with specific learning difficulties. In A. Prifitera, D. H. Saklofske, & L. G. Weiss (Eds.), *WISC-IV clinical assessment and intervention* (pp. 109–171). New York: Elsevier.

Hale, J. B., Kaufman, A., Naglieri, J., & Kavale, K. (2006). Implementation of IDEA: Integrating response to intervention and cognitive assessment methods. *Psychology in the Schools*, *43*, 753–770.

Hallahan, D. P., & Mercer, C. D. (2001). *Learning disabilities: Historical perspectives*. Washington, DC: Department of Education, Office of Special Education Programs.

Hallahan, D. P., & Mock, D. R. (2003). A brief history of the field of learning disabilities. In H. L. Swanson, K. R. Harris, & S. Graham (Eds.), *Handbook of learning disabilities* (pp. 16–29). New York: Guilford Press.

Halliday, L. F., & Bishop, D. V. M. (2006). Is poor frequency modulation detection linked to literacy problems? A comparison of specific reading disability and mild to moderate sensorineural hearing loss. *Brain and Language*, *97*, 200–213.

Hämäläinen, J. A., Salminen, H. K., & Leppänen, P. H. T. (2013). Basic auditory processing deficits in dyslexia: review of the behavioural, event-related potential and magnetoencephalographic evidence. *Journal of Learning Disabilities*, *46*(5), 413–427.

Handler, S. M., Fierson, W. M., the Section of Ophthalmology and Council on Children with Disabilities, American Academy of Ophthalmology, American Association for Pediatric Ophthalmology and Strabismus, & and American Association of Certified Orthoptists. (2011). Joint technical report – Learning disabilities, dyslexia, and vision. *Pediatrics*, *127*, e818–e856.

Hannula-Jouppi, K., Kaminen-Ahola, N., Taipale, M., Eklund, R., Nopola-Hemmi, J., Kääriäinen, H., et al. (2005). The axon guidance receptor gene ROBO1 is a candidate dene for developmental dyslexia. *PLoS*, *1*, e50.

Hari, R., & Renvall, H. (2001). Impaired processing of rapid stimulus sequences in dyslexia. *Trends in Cognitive Sciences*, *5*, 525–532.

Harlaar, N., Dale, P. S., & Plomin, R. (2007). From learning to read to reading to learn: Substantial and stable genetic influence. *Child Development*, *78*, 116–131.

Harn, B., Parisi, D., & Stoolmiller, M. (2013). Balancing fidelity with flexibility and fit: What do we really know about fidelity of implementation in schools? *Exceptional Children*, *79*(2), 181–193.

Harn, B. A., Kame'enui, E., & Simmons, D. C. (2007). The nature and role of the third tier in a prevention model for kindergarten students. In D. Haager, J. Klingner, &

S. Vaughn (Eds.), *Evidence-based reading practices for responses to intervention* (pp. 161–184). Baltimore, MD: Paul Brookes.

Harn, B. A., Linan-Thompson, S., & Roberts, G. (2008). Intensifying instruction does additional instructional time make a difference for the most at-risk first graders? *Journal of Learning Disabilities, 41*(2), 115–125.

Hart, B., & Risley, T. (2003). The early catastrophe. *American Educator, 27*, 6–9.

Hart, S. A., Petrill, S. A., DeThorne, L. S., Deater-Deckard, K., Thompson, L. A., Schatschneider, C., et al. (2009). Environmental influences on the longitudinal covariance of expressive vocabulary: measuring the home literacy environment in a genetically sensitive design. *Journal of Child Psychology and Psychiatry, 50*, 911–919.

Hartas, D. (2011). Families' social backgrounds matter: Socioeconomic factors, home learning and young children's language, literacy and social outcomes. *British Educational Research Journal, 37*, 893–914.

Hasan, K. M., Molfese, D. L., Walimuni, I. S., Stuebing, K. K., Papanicolaou, A. C., Narayana, P. A., & Fletcher, J. M. (2012). Diffusion tensor quantification and cognitive correlates of the macrostructure and microstructure of the corpus callosum in typically developing and dyslexic children. *NMR in Biomedicine, 25*(11), 1263–1270.

Hasbrouck, J. E., Ihnot, C., & Rogers, G. (1999). "Read naturally": A strategy to increase oral reading fluency. *Reading Research and Instruction, 39*, 27–38.

Hatcher, P. J., Hulme, C., Miles, J. N., Carroll, J. M., Hatcher, J., Gibbs, S., et al. (2006). Efficacy of small group reading intervention for beginning readers with reading delay: A randomised controlled trial. *Journal of Child Psychology & Psychiatry, 47*, 820–827.

Hayiou-Thomas, M. E., Harlaar, N., Dale, P. S., & Plomin, R. (2010). Preschool speech, language skills, and reading at 7, *9*, and 10 Years: Etiology of the relationship *Journal of Speech, Language, and Hearing Research, 53*, 311–332.

Heath, S. M., Bishop, D. V. M., Hogben, J., & Roach, N. (2006). Psychophysical indices of perceptual functioning in dyslexia: A psychometric analysis. *Cognitive Neuropsychology, 23*(6), 905–929.

Heath, S. M., & Hogben, J. H. (2004). Cost-effective prediction of reading difficulties. *Journal of Speech, Language, and Hearing Research, 47*, 751–765.

Heaton, P., & Winterton, P. (1996). *Dealing with dyslexia* (2nd ed.). London: Whurr Publishers.

Heiervang, E., Hugdahl, K., Steinmetz, H., Inge Smievoll, A., Stevenson, J., Lund, A., et al. (2000). Planum temporale, planum parietale and dichotic listening in dyslexia. *Neuropsychologia, 38*, 1704–1713.

Heim, S., & Grande, M. (2012). Fingerprints of developmental dyslexia. *Trends in Neuroscience and Education, 1*(1), 10–14.

Heim, S., & Keil, A. (2004). Large-scale neural correlates of developmental dyslexia. *European Child & Adolescent Psychiatry, 13*, 125–140.

Helenius, P., Tarkiainen, A., Cornelissen, P., Hansen, P., & Salmelin, R. (1999). Dissociation of normal feature analysis and deficient processing of letter-strings in dyslexic adults. *Cerebral Cortex, 9*, 476–483.

Hemminki, K., Forsti, A., Houlston, R., & Bermejo, J. L. (2011). Searching for the missing heritability of complex diseases. *Human Mutation, 32*, 259–262.

Henderson, L. M., Tsogda, N., & Snowling, M. J. (2013). Questioning the benefits that coloured overlays can have for reading in students with and without dyslexia. *Journal of Research in Special Educational Needs, 13*(1), 57–65.

Herbers, J. E., Cutuli, J. J., Supkoff, L. M., Heistad, D., Chan, C., Hinz, E., & Masten, A. S. (2012). Early reading skills and academic achievement trajectories of students facing poverty, homelessness, and high residential mobility. *Educational Researcher, 41*(9), 366–374.

Herrington, M., & Hunter-Carsch, M. (2001). A social interactive model of specific learning difficulties. In M. Hunter-Carsch (Ed.), *Dyslexia: A psycho-social perspective* (pp. 107–133). London: Whurr.

Hinshelwood, J. (1895). Word-blindness and visual memory. *Lancet, 146*, 1564–1570.

Hinshelwood, J. (1902). Congenital word-blindness, with reports of two cases. *Ophthalmology Review, 21*, 91–99.

Hinshelwood, J. (1907). Four cases of congenital word-blindness occurring in the same family. *British Medical Journal, 1*, 608–609.

Hinshelwood, J. (1917). *Congenital word blindness*. London: H. K. Lewis & Co.

Ho, A. (2004). To be labelled, or not to be labelled: That is the question. *British Journal of Learning Disabilities, 32*, 86–92.

Hoeft, F., Hernandez, A., McMillon, G., Taylor-Hill, H., Martindale, J. L., Meyler, A., et al. (2006). Neural basis of dyslexia: A comparison between dyslexic and nondyslexic children equated for reading ability. *Journal of Neuroscience, 26*, 10700–10708.

Hoeft, F., McCandliss, B. D., Black, J. M., Gantman, A., Zakerani, N., Hulme, C., et al. (2011). Neural systems predicting long-term outcome in dyslexia. *Proceedings of the National Academy of Sciences of the United States of America, 108*, 361–366.

Hoeft, F., Meyler, A., Hernandez, A., Juel, C., Taylor-Hill, H., Martindale, J. L., et al. (2007). Functional and morphometric brain dissociation between dyslexia and reading ability. *Proceedings of the National Academy of Sciences of the United States of America, 104*, 4234–4239.

Hogan, T. P., & Thomson, J. M. (2010). Epilogue to *Journal of Learning Disabilities* special edition "Advances in the early detection of reading risk": Future advances in the early detection of reading risk: Subgroups, dynamic relations, and advanced methods. *Journal of Learning Disabilities, 43*, 383–386.

Holliman, A. J., Wood, C., & Sheehy, K. (2010). Does speech rhythm sensitivity predict children's reading ability one year later? *Journal of Educational Psychology, 102*, 356–366.

Holm, V. A. (1983). A western version of the Doman-Delacato eatment of patterning for developmental disabilities. *The Western Journal of Medicine, 139*, 553–556.

Holmes, J., & Gathercole, S. E. (in press). Taking working memory training from the laboratory into schools, *Educational Psychology*.

Holmes, J., Gathercole, S. E., & Dunning, D. L. (2009). Adaptive training leads to sustained enhancement of poor working memory in children. *Developmental Science, 12*, 9–15.

Hoogeven, J., Smeets, P., & Lancioni, G. (1989). Teaching moderately mentally retarded children. *Research in Developmental Disabilities, 10*, 1–18.

Hornickel, J., & Kraus, N. (2013). Unstable representation of sound: A biological marker of dyslexia. *The Journal of Neuroscience, 33*(8), 3500–3504.

Hornickel, J., Zecker, S. G., Bradlow, A.R., & Kraus, N. (2012). Assistive listening devices drive neuroplasticity in children with dyslexia. *Proceedings of the National Academy of Sciences of the United States of America, 109*, 16731–16736.

Horwitz, B., Rumsey, J. M., & Donohue, B. C. (1998). Functional connectivity of the angular gyrus in normal reading and dyslexia. *Proceedings of the National Academy of Sciences of the United States of America, 95*, 8939–8944.

Hoskyn, M., & Swanson, H. L. (2000). Cognitive processing of low achievers and children with reading disabilities: A selective meta-analytic review of the published literature. *School Psychology Review 29*, 102–119.

House of Commons. Science and Technology Committee. (2009). *Evidence check 1: Early literacy interventions*. London: The Stationery Office.

Howard, D., & Best, W. (1996). Developmental phonological dyslexia: Word reading can be completely normal. *Cognitive Neuropsychology, 13*, 887–934.

Howard-Jones, P. A. (2007). *Neuroscience and education: Issues and opportunities. Commentary by the Teaching and Learning Research Programme*. London: TLRP.

Hu, W., Lee, H. L., Zhang, Q., Liu, T., Geng, L. B., Seghier, M. L., et al. (2010). Developmental dyslexia in Chinese and English populations: Dissociating the effect of dyslexia from language differences. *Brain, 133*, 1694–1706.

Huemer, S., Aro, M., Landerl, K., & Lyytinen, H. (2010). Repeated reading of syllables among Finnish-speaking children with poor reading skills. *Scientific Studies of Reading, 14*, 317–340.

Hugdahl, K., Heiervang, E., Ersland, L., Lundervold, A., Steinmetz, H., & Smievoll, A. I. (2003). Significant relation between MR measures of planum temporale area and dichotic processing of syllables in dyslexic children. *Neuropsychologia, 41*, 666–675.

Hulme, C., & Snowling, M. J. (1992). Deficits in output phonology: An explanation of reading failure? *Cognitive Neuropsychology, 9*, 47–72.

Hulme, C., & Snowling, M. J. (2009). *Developmental disorders of language learning and cognition*. Oxford: Wiley-Blackwell.

Hulslander, J., Olson, R. K., Willcutt, E. G., & Wadsworth, S. J. (2010). Longitudinal stability of reading-related skills and their prediction of reading development. *Scientific Studies of Reading, 14*, 111–136.

Humphreys, P., Kaufmann, W. E., & Galaburda, A. M. (1990). Developmental dyslexia in women: Neuropathological findings in three patients. *Annals of Neurology, 28*, 727–738.

Hurford, D. P., Potter, T. S., & Hart, G. S. (2002). Examination of three techniques for identifying first-grade children at risk for difficulty in word identification with an emphasis on reducing the false negative error rate. *Reading Psychology, 23*, 159–180.

Hutton, U. M. Z., & Towse, J. N. (2001). Short-term memory and working memory as indices of children's cognitive skills. *Memory, 9*, 383–394.

Hutzler, F., Kronbichler, M., Jacobs, A. M., & Wimmer, H. (2006). Perhaps correlational but not causal: No effect of dyslexic readers' magnocellular system on their eye movements during reading. *Neuropsychologia, 44*, 637–648.

Hyatt, K. J. (2007). Brain Gym®: Building stronger brains or wishful thinking? *Remedial and Special Education, 28*, 117–124.

Hyatt, K. J., Stephenson, J., & Carter, M. (2009). A review of three controversial educational practices: Perceptual motor programs, sensory integration, and tinted lenses. *Education and Treatment of Children, 32*, 313–342.

Hynd, G. W., Hall, J., Novey, E. S., Eliopulos, D., Black, K., Gonzalez, J. J., et al. (1995). Dyslexia and corpus callosum morphology. *Archives of Neurology, 52*, 32–38.

Hynd, G. W., Semrud-Clikeman, M., Lorys, A. R., Novey, E. S., & Eliopulos, D. (1990). Brain morphology in developmental dyslexia and attention deficit disorder/hyperactivity. *Archives of Neurology, 47*, 919–926.

Igo, R. P. J., Chapman, N. H., Berninger, V. W., Matsushita, M., Brkanac, Z., Rothstein, J. H., et al. (2006). Genomewide scan for real-word reading subphenotypes of dyslexia: novel chromosome 13 locus and genetic complexity. *American Journal of Medical Genetics (Neuropsychiatric Genetics), 141*, 15–27.

Ihnot, C., Mastoff, J., Gavin, J., & Hendrickson, L. (2001). *Read naturally* [Curriculum program]. St. Paul, MN: Read Naturally.

Individuals with Disabilities Education Improvement Act, H.R. 1350, 108th Congress (2004).

Ingvar, M., af Trampe, P., Greitz, T., Eriksson, L., Stone-Elander, S., & von Euler, C. (2002). Residual differences in language processing in compensated dyslexics revealed in simple word reading tasks. *Brain & Language, 83*, 249–267.

International Dyslexia Association Scientific Advisory Board (2012). Diagnosis and treatment of dyslexia: Comments on proposed DSM-5 criteria for learning disabilities (disorders) (May 29). Retrieved March 30, 2013 from http://www.interdys.org/EWEBEDITPRO5/UPLOAD/IDAPOSITIONDSM5(4).PDF

Irlen, H. (1991). *Reading by the colors: Overcoming dyslexia and other reading disabilities through the Irlen method*. New York: Avery.

Jacobson, J. W., Foxx, R. M., & Mulick, J. A. (2005). *Controversial therapies for developmental disabilities: Fad, fashion and science in professional practice*. Mahwah, NJ: Lawrence Erlbaum.

Jainta, S., & Kapoula, Z. (2011). Dyslexic children are confronted with unstable binocular fixation while reading. *PlosOne, 6*, 1–10.

Jalal, S. M., Harwood, A. R., Sekhon, G. S., Lorentz, C. P., Ketterling, R. P., Babovic-Vuksanovic, D., et al. (2003). Utility of subtelomeric fluorescent DNA probes for detection of chromosome anomalies in 425 patients. *Genetics in Medicine, 5*, 28–34.

Jeanes, R., Busby, A., Martin, J., Lewis, E., Stevenson, N., Pointon, D., et al. (1997). Prolonged use of coloured overlays for classroom reading. *British Journal of Psychology, 88*, 531–548.

Jednoróg, K., Altarelli, I., Monzalvo, K., Fluss, J., Dubois, J., Billard, C., Dehaene-Lambertz, G., & Ramus, F. (2012). The influence of socioeconomic status on children's brain structure. *PLoS ONE, 7*(8), e42486.

Jeffries, S., & Everatt, J. (2004). Working memory: Its role in dyslexia and other specific learning difficulties. *Dyslexia, 10*, 196–214.

Jenkins, J. R., Hudson, R. F., & Johnson, E. S. (2007). Screening for at-risk readers in a response-to-intervention (RTI) framework. *School Psychology Review, 36*, 582–600.

Jenkins, J. R., & O'Connor, R. E. (2002). Early identification and intervention for young children with reading/learning disabilities. In R. Bradley, L. Danielson, & D. P. Hallahan (Eds.), *Identification of learning disabilities: Research to practice* (pp. 99–149). Mahwah, NJ: Erlbaum.

Jenner, A. R., Rosen, G. D., & Galaburda, A. M. (1999). Neuronal asymmetries in primary visual cortex of dyslexic and nondyslexic brains. *Annals of Neurology, 46*, 189–196.

Jiménez, J. E., de la Cadena, C., Siegel, L., O'Shanahan, I., García, E., & Rodríguez, C. (2011). Gender ratio and cognitive profiles in dyslexia: A cross-national study. *Reading and Writing*, *24*, 729–747.

Jiménez, J. E., & Garcia de la Cadena, C. (2007). Learning disabilities in Guatemala and Spain: A cross-national study of the prevalence and cognitive processes associated with reading and spelling disabilities. *Learning Disabilities Research & Practice*, *22*, 161–169.

Jobard, G., Crivello, F., & Tzourio-Mazoyer, N. (2003). Evaluation of the dual route theory of reading: A metanalysis of 35 neuroimaging studies. *Neuroimage*, *20*, 693–712.

Johannes, S., Kussmaul, C. L., Munte, T. F., & Mangun, G. R. (1996). Developmental dyslexia: Passive visual stimulation provides no evidence for a magnocellular processing deficit. *Neuropsychologia*, *34*, 1123–1127.

Johnson, A., Bruno, A., Watanabe, J., Quansah, B., Patel, N., Dakin, S., et al. (2008). Visually-based temporal distortion in dyslexia. *Vision Research*, *48*, 1852–1858.

Johnson, E. P., Pennington, B. F., Lee, N. R., & Boada, R. (2009). Directional effects between rapid auditory processing and phonological awareness in children. *Journal of Child Psychology and Psychiatry*, *50*, 902–910.

Johnson, E. P., Pennington, B. F., Lowenstein, J. H., & Nittrouer, S. (2011). Sensitivity to structure in the speech signal by children with speech sound disorder and reading disability. *Journal of Communication Disorders*, *44*, 294–314.

Johnson, E. S., Humphrey, M., Mellard, D. F., Woods, K., & Swanson, H. L. (2010). Cognitive processing deficits and students with specific learning disabilities: A selective meta-analysis of the literature. *Learning Disability Quarterly*, *33*, 3–18.

Johnson, E. S., Jenkins, J. R., Petscher, Y., & Catts, H. W. (2009). How can we improve the accuracy of screening instruments? *Learning Disabilities Research & Practice*, *24*, 174–185.

Jones, M. W., Branigan, H. P., Hatzidaki, A., & Obregón, A. (2010). Is the "naming" deficit in dyslexia a misnomer? *Cognition*, *116*, 56–70.

Juel, C., & Minden-Cupp, C. (2000). Learning to read words: Linguistic units and instructional strategies. *Reading Research Quarterly*, *35*, 458–492.

Kail, R., & Hall, L. K. (1994). Processing speed, naming speed, and reading. *Developmental Psychology*, *30*, 949–954.

Kairaluoma, L., Närhi, V., Ahonen, T., Westerholm, J., & Aro, M. (2008). Do fatty acids help in overcoming reading difficulties? A double-blind, placebo-controlled study of the effects of eicosapentaenoic acid and carnosine supplementation on children with dyslexia. *Child: Care, Health and Development*, *35*, 112–119.

Kamerow, D. (2008). Waiting for the genetic revolution. *British Medical Journal*, *336*, 22.

Kamhi, A. G. (2004). A meme's eye view of speech-language pathology. *Language, Speech, and Hearing Services in Schools*, *35*, 105–111.

Kamhi, A. G. (2009). Solving the reading crisis – Take 2: The case for differentiated assessment. *Language, Speech and Hearing Services in Schools*, *40*, 212–215.

Kaminen, N., Hannula-Jouppi, K., Kestila, M., Lahermo, P., Muller, K., Kaaranen, M., et al. (2003). A genome scan for developmental dyslexia confirms linkage to chromosome 2p11 and suggests a new locus on 7q32. *Journal of Medical Genetics*, *40*, 340–345.

Kamps, D., Abbott, M., Greenwood, C., Wills, H., Veerkamp, M., & Kaufman, J. (2008). Effects of small group reading instruction and curriculum differences for students most at risk in kindergarten: Two-year results for secondary- and tertiary-level interventions. *Journal of Learning Disabilities, 41*, 101–114.

Kaplan, B. J., Wilson, N. B., Dewey, D., & Crawford, S. G. (1998). DCD may not be a discrete disorder. *Human Movement Science, 17*, 471–490.

Kapoula, Z., Ganem, R., Poncet, S., Gintautas, D., Eggert, T., Brémond-Gignac, D., & Bucci, M.P. (2008). Free exploration of painting uncovers particularly loose yoking of saccades in dyslexics. *Dyslexia, 15*(3), 243–259.

Katusic, S. K., Colligan, R. C., Barbaresi, W. J., Schaid, D. J., & Jacobsen, S. J. (2001). Incidence of reading disability in a population-based birth cohort, 1976–1982, Rochester, Minnesota. *Mayo Clinic Proceedings, 76*, 1081–1092.

Katzir, T., Misra, M., & Poldrack, R. A. (2005). Imaging phonology without print: assessing the neural correlates of phonemic awareness using fMRI. *Neuroimage, 27*, 106–115.

Kauffman, J. M., Hallahan, D. P., & Lloyd, J. W. (1998). Politics, science, and the future of learning disabilities. *Learning Disability Quarterly, 21*, 276–280.

Kaufman, A. S. (1994). *Intelligent Testing with the WISC-III*. New York: Wiley.

Kavale, K. A., & Forness, S. R. (1984). A meta-analysis of the validity of Wechsler scale profiles and recategorisations: Patterns or parodies? *Learning Disability Quarterly, 7*, 136–156.

Kavale, K. A., & Forness, S. R. (1995). *The nature of learning disabilities*. Mahwah, NJ: Lawrence Erlbaum.

Kavale, K. A., & Forness, S. R. (2003). Learning disability as a disciple. In H. L. Swanson, K. R. Harris, & S. Graham (Eds.), *Handbook of learning disabilities* (pp. 76–93). New York: Guilford Press.

Kavale, K. A., & Mattson, P. D. (1983). "One jumped off the balance beam": Meta-analysis of perceptual-motor training. *Journal of Learning Disabilities, 16*, 165–173.

Kavale, K. A., & Mostert, M. P. (2004). *The positive side of special education: Minimizing its fads, fancies, and follies*. Lanham, MD: Scarecrow Education.

Kavale, K. A., & Spaulding, L. S. (2008). Is response to intervention good policy for specific learning disability? *Learning Disabilities Research and Practice, 23*, 169–179.

Kavale, K. A., Spaulding, L. S., & Beam, A. P. (2009). A time to define: Making the specific learning disability definition prescribe specific learning disability. *Learning Disability Quarterly, 32*, 39–48.

Kearns, D., & Fuchs, D. (2013). Does cognitively focused instruction improve the academic performance of low-achieving students? *Exceptional Children, 79*(3), 263–290.

Keenan, J. M., Betjemann, R., Wadsworth, S., DeFries, J., & Olson, R. (2006). Genetic and environmental influences on reading and listening comprehension. *Journal of Research In Reading, 29*, 75–91.

Keller, T. A., & Just, M. A. (2009). Altering cortical connectivity: Remediation-induced changes in the white matter of poor readers. *Neuron, 64*, 624–631.

Kelly, K., & Phillips, S. (2011). *Teaching literacy to learners with dyslexia: A multisensory approach*. London: Sage.

Kendell, R. E. (1975). *The role of diagnosis in psychiatry*. Oxford: Blackwell.

Kersting, K. (2004, October). Debating learning-disability identification. *APA Monitor*, 54–55.

Khoury, M. J., Bowen, S., Bradley, L. A., Coates, R., Dowling, N. F., Gwinn, M., et al. (2008). A decade of public health genomics in the United States: Centers for Disease Control and Prevention 1997–2007. *Public Health Genomics, 12*, 20–29.

Khoury, M. J., Gwinn, M., Yoon, P. W., Dowling, N., Moore, C. A., & Bradley, L. (2007). The continuum of translation research in genomic medicine: How can we accelerate the appropriate integration of human genome discoveries into health care and disease prevention? *Genetics in Medicine, 9*, 665–674.

Khoury, M. J., Little, J., Gwinn, M., & Ioannidis, J. P. (2007). On the synthesis and interpretation of consistent but weak gene-disease associations in the era of genome-wide association studies. *International Journal of Epidemiology, 36*, 439–445.

Khoury, M. J., Valdez, R., & Albright, A. (2008). Public health genomics approach to type 2 diabetes. *Diabetes, 57*, 2911–2914.

Kibby, M. Y., Fancher, J. B., Markanen, R., & Hynd, G. W. (2008). A quantitative magnetic resonance imaging analysis of the cerebellar deficit hypothesis of dyslexia. *Journal of Child Neurology, 23*, 368–380.

Kibby, M. Y., Marks, W., Morgan, S., & Long, C. J. (2004). Specific impairment in developmental reading disabilities: A working memory approach. *Journal of Learning Disabilities, 37*, 349–363.

Kieffer, M. J. (2012). Before and after third grade: Longitudinal evidence for the shifting role of socioeconomic status in reading growth. *Reading and Writing, 25*(7), 1725–1746.

Kipp, K. H., & Mohr, G. (2008). Remediation of developmental dyslexia: Tackling a basic memory deficit. *Cognitive Neuropsychology, 25*, 38–55.

Kirby, A., Woodward, A., Jackson, S., Wang, Y., & Crawford, M. A. (2010). A double-blind, placebo-controlled study investigating the effects of omega-3 supplementation in children aged 8–10 years from a mainstream school population. *Research in Developmental Disabilities, 31*, 718–730.

Kirby, J. R., Georgiou, G. K., Martinussen, R., Parrila, R., Bowers, P., & Landerl, K. (2010). Naming speed and reading: From prediction to instruction. *Reading Research Quarterly, 45*, 341–362.

Kirk, J., & Reid, G. (2001). An examination of the relationship between dyslexia and offending in young people and the implications for the training system. *Dyslexia, 7*, 77–84.

Kirk, S. A. (1962). *Educating exceptional children*. Boston: Houghton Mifflin.

Kiuru, N., Haverinen, K., Salmela-Aro, K., Nurmi, J. E., Savolainen, H., & Holopainen, L. (2011). Students with reading and spelling disabilities: Peer groups and educational attainment in secondary education. *Journal of Learning Disabilities, 44*, 556–569.

Klein, R. M., & Farmer, M. E. (1995). Dyslexia and a temporal processing deficit: A reply to the commentaries. *Psychonomic Bulletin & Review, 2*, 515–526.

Klicpera, C., & Schabmann, A. (1993). Do German-speaking children have a chance to overcome reading and spelling difficulties? A longitudinal survey from the second until the eighth grade. *European Journal of Psychology of Education, 8*, 307–323.

Klingberg, T. (2010). Training and plasticity of working memory. *Trends in Cognitive Sciences, 14*, 317–324.

Klingberg, T., Hedehus, M., Temple, E., Salz, T., Gabrieli, J. D., Moseley, M. E., et al. (2000). Microstructure of temporo-parietal white matter as a basis for reading ability: evidence from diffusion tensor magnetic resonance imaging. *Neuron, 25*, 493–500.

Klingberg, T., Vaidya, C. J., Gabrieli, J. D., Moseley, M. E., & Hedehus, M. (1999). Myelination and organization of the frontal white matter in children: a diffusion tensor MRI study. *Neuroreport, 10*, 2817–2821.

Kochunov, P., Fox, P., Lancaster, J., Tan, L. H., Amunts, K., Zilles, K., et al. (2003). Localized morphological brain differences between English-speaking Caucasians and Chinese-speaking Asians: New evidence of anatomical plasticity. *Neuroreport, 14*, 961–964.

Koponen, T., Salmi, P., Eklund, K., & Aro, T. (2013). Counting and RAN: Predictors of arithmetic calculation and reading fluency. *Journal of Learning Disabilities, 105*(1), 162–175.

Kortteinen, H., Närhi, V., & Ahonen, T. (2009). Does IQ matter in adolescents' reading disability? *Learning and Individual Differences, 19*, 257–261.

Kramer, J. J., Henning-Stout, M., Ullman, D. P., & Schellenberg, R. P. (1987). The viability of scatter analysis on the WISC-R and the SBIS: Examining a vestige. *Journal of Psychoeducational Assessment, 5*, 37–47.

Kriss, I., & Evans, B. J. W. (2005). The relationship between dyslexia and Meares-Irlen syndrome. *Journal of Research in Reading, 28*, 350–364.

Kronbichler, M., Hutzler, F., Staffen, W., Mair, A., Ladurner, G., & Wimmer, H. (2006). Evidence for a dysfunction of left posterior reading areas in German dyslexic readers. *Neuropsychologia, 44*, 1822–1832.

Kronbichler, M., Hutzler, F., & Wimmer, H. (2002). Dyslexia: Verbal impairments in the absence of magnocellular impairments. *Cognitive Neuroscience and Neuropsychology, 13*, 617–620.

Kronbichler, M., Wimmer, H., Staffen, W., Hutzler, F., Mair, A., & Ladurner, G. (2008). Developmental dyslexia: Gray matter abnormalities in the occipitotemporal cortex. *Human Brain Mapping, 29*, 613–625.

Kujala, T., Karma, K., Ceponiene, R., Belitz, S., Turkkila, P., Tervaniemi, M., et al. (2001). Plastic neural changes and reading improvement caused by audiovisual training in reading-impaired children. *Proceedings of the National Academy of Sciences of the United States of America, 98*, 10509–10514.

Kushch, A., Gross-Glenn, K., Jallad, B., Lubs, H., Rabin, M., Feldman, E., et al. (1993). Temporal lobe surface area measurements on MRI in normal and dyslexic readers. *Neuropsychologia, 31*, 811–821.

Kussmaul, L. A. (1877). Disturbances of speech. In H. von Ziemssen (Ed.), *Cyclopedia of the Practice of Medicine, Vol. 14*. New York: William Wood and Co.

Laasonen, M., Service, E., & Virsu, V. (2001). Temporal order and processing acuity of visual, auditory, and tactile perception in developmentally dyslexic young adults. *Cognitive, Affective, & Behavioral Neuroscience, 1*, 394–410.

Laasonen, M., Virsu, V., Oinonen, S., Sandbacka, M., Salakari, A., & Service, E. (2012), Phonological and sensory short-term memory are correlates and both affected in developmental dyslexia. *Reading and Writing, 25*, 2247–2273.

Lachmann, T., & van Leeuwen, C. (2007). Paradoxical enhancement of letter recognition in developmental dyslexia. *Developmental Neuropsychology, 31*, 61–77.

Lack, D. (2010). Another joint statement regarding learning disabilities, dyslexia, and vision – A rebuttal. *Optometry, 81,* 533–543.

Lackaye, T. D., & Margalit, M. (2006). Comparisons of achievement, effort, and self-perceptions among students with learning disabilities and their peers from different achievement groups. *Journal of Learning Disabilities, 39,* 432–446.

Lallier, M., Donnadieu, S., Berger, C., & Valdois, S. (2010). A case study of developmental phonological dyslexia: Is the attentional deficit in the perception of rapid stimuli sequences amodal? *Cortex, 46,* 231–241.

Lallier, M., Tainturier, M., Dering, B., Donnadieu, S., Valdois, S., & Thierry, G. (2010). Behavioral and ERP evidence for amodal sluggish attentional shifting in developmental dyslexia. *Neuropsychologia, 48,* 4125–4135.

Lallier, M., Thierry, G., Tainturier, M., Donnadieu, S., Peyrin, C., Billard, C., et al. (2009). Auditory and visual stream segregation in children and adults: An assessment of the amodality assumption of the sluggish attentional shifting theory. *Brain Research, 1302,* 132–147.

Lander, E. S. (2011). Initial impact of the sequencing of the human genome. *Nature, 470,* 187–197.

Landerl, K., & Moll, K. (2010). Comorbidity of learning disorders: Prevalence and familial transmission. *Journal of Child Psychology and Psychiatry, 51,* 287–294.

Landerl, K., Ramus, F., Moll, K., Lyytinen, H., Leppänen, P., et al. (2013). Predictors of developmental dyslexia in European orthographies with varying complexity. *Journal of Child Psychology and Psychiatry, 54*(6), 686–694.

Landerl, K., & Willburger, E. (2010). Temporal processing, attention, and learning disorders. *Learning and Individual Differences, 20,* 393–401.

Landerl, K., & Wimmer, H. (2000). Deficits in phoneme segmentation are not the core problem in dyslexia: Evidence from German and English children. *Applied Psycholinguistics, 21,* 243–262.

Larsen, J. P., Hoien, T., Lundberg, I., & Odegaard, H. (1990). MRI evaluation of the size and symmetry of the planum temporale in adolescents with developmental dyslexia. *Brain and Language, 39,* 289–301.

Larsen, J. P., Hoien, T., & Odegaard, H. (1992). Magnetic resonance imaging of the corpus callosum in developmental dyslexia. *Cognitive Neuropsychology, 9,* 123–134.

Laycock, R., Crewther, D. P., & Crewther, S. G. (2012). Abrupt and ramped flicker-defined form shows evidence for a large magnocellular impairment in dyslexia. *Neuropsychologia, 50,* 2107–2113.

Laycock, S. K., Wilkinson, I. D., Wallis, L. I., Darwent, G., Wonders, S. H., Fawcett, A. J., et al. (2008). Cerebellar volume and cerebellar metabolic characteristics in adults with dyslexia. *Annals of the New York Academy of Sciences, 1145,* 222–236.

Lebel, C., Shaywitz, B., Holahan, J., Shaywitz, S. E., & Machione, K. (2013). Diffusion tensor imaging correlates of reading ability in dysfluent and non-impaired readers. *Brain & Language, 125*(2), 215–222.

Le Jan, G., R., L. B.-J., Costet, N., Trolès, N., Scalart, P., Pichancourt, D., et al. (2011). Multivariate predictive model for dyslexia diagnosis. *Annals of Dyslexia, 61,* 1–20.

Leach, J. M., Scarborough, H. S., & Rescorla, L. (2003). Late-emerging reading disabilities. *Journal of Educational Psychology, 95,* 211–224.

Lee, R., Nicolson, R. I., & Fawcett, A. J. (2001). *Pre-School Screening Test (PREST)*. Oxford: Pearson Assessment.

Leonard, C. M., & Eckert, M. A. (2008). Asymmetry and dyslexia. *Developmental Neuropsychology*, *33*(6), 663–681.

Leonard, C. M., Eckert, M. A., Lombardino, L. J., Oakland, T., Kranzler, J., Mohr, C. M., et al. (2001). Anatomical risk factors for phonological dyslexia. *Cerebral Cortex*, *11*, 148–157.

Leppanen, P. H., & Lyytinen, H. (1997). Auditory event-related potentials in the study of developmental language-related disorders. *Audiology & Neuro Otology*, *2*, 308–340.

Leppänen, P. H. T., Hämäläinen, J. A., Salminen, H. K., Eklund, K. M., Guttorm, T. K., Lohvansuu, K., et al. (2010). Newborn brain event-related potentials revealing atypical processing of sound frequency and the subsequent association with later literacy skills in children with familial dyslexia. *Cortex*, *46*, 1362–1376.

Lervåg, A., Bråten, I., & Hulme, C. (2009). The cognitive and linguistic foundations of early reading development: A Norwegian latent variable longitudinal study. *Developmental Psychology*, *45*, 764–781.

Liao, C. H., Georgiou, G. K., & Parrila, R. (2008). Rapid naming speed and Chinese character recognition. *Reading and Writing*, *21*, 231–253.

Liberman, A. M. (1999). The reading researcher and the reading teacher need the right theory of speech. *Scientific Studies of Reading*, *3*, 95–111.

Liberman, I. Y., & Shankweiler, D. P. (1985). Phonology and the problems of learning to read and write. *Remedial and Special Education*, *6*, 8–17.

Liddle, E., Jackson, G., & Jackson, S. (2005). An evaluation of a visual biofeedback intervention in dyslexic adults. *Dyslexia*, *11*, 61–77.

Lidz, C. S., & Elliott, J. G. (Eds.). (2000). *Dynamic assessment: Prevailing models and applications*. London: Elsevier.

Liederman, J., Kantrowitz, L., & Flannery, K. (2005). Male vulnerability to reading disability is not likely to be a myth: A call for new data. *Journal of Learning Disabilities*, *38*, 109–129.

Ligges, C., & Blanz, B. (2007). [Survey of fMRI results regarding a phonological deficit in children and adults with dyslexia: Fundamental deficit or indication of compensation?]. *Zeitschrift fur Kinder und Jugendpsychiatrie und Psychotherapie*, *35*, 107–115.

Ligges, C., Ungureanu, M., Ligges, M., Blanz, B., & Witte, H. (2010). Understanding the time variant connectivity of the language network in developmental dyslexia: New insights using Granger causality. *Journal of Neural Transmission*, *117*, 529–543.

Lim, K. O., & Helpern, J. A. (2002). Neuropsychiatric applications of DTI – a review. *NMR Biomed*, *15*, 587–593.

Lindmark, L., & Clough, P. (2007). A 5-month open study with long-chain polyunsaturated fatty acids in dyslexia. *Journal of Medicinal Food*, *10*, 662–666.

Lionel, A. C., Crosbie, J., Barbosa, N., Goodale, T., Thiruvahindrapuram, B., Rickaby, J., et al. (2011). Rare copy number variation discovery and cross-disorder comparisons identify risk genes for ADHD. *Science Translational Medicine*, *3*, 95–75.

Lipka, O., Lesaux, N. K., & Siegel, L. (2006). Retrospective analyses of the reading development of grade 4 students with reading disabilities: Risk status and profiles over 5 years. *Journal of Learning Disabilities*, *39*, 364–378.

Liu, L., Wang, W., You, W., Li, Y., Awati, N., et al. (2012). Similar alterations in brain function for phonological and semantic processing to visual characters in Chinese dyslexia. *Neuropsychologia*, *50*, 2224–2232.

Livingstone, M. S., Rosen, G. D., Drislane, F. W., & Galaburda, A. M. (1991). Physiological and anatomical evidence for a magnocellular defect in developmental dyslexia. *Proceedings of the National Academy of Sciences of the United States of America*, *88*, 7943–7947.

Lloyd, J. W., Hallahan, D. P., & Kauffman, J. M. (1980). Learning disabilities: Selected topics. In L. Mann & D. Sabatino (Eds.), *The fourth review of special education* (pp. 35–60). New York: Grune & Stratton.

Lobier, M., Zoubrinetzky, R., & Valdois, S. (2012). The visual attention span deficit in dyslexia is visual and not verbal. *Cortex*, *48*(6), 768–773.

Łockiewicz, M., Bogdanowicz, K.M., & Bogdanowicz, M. (in press). Psychological resources of adults with developmental dyslexia. *Journal of Learning Disabilities*.

Logan, J. (2009). Dyslexic entrepreneurs: The incidence, their coping strategies and their business skills. *Dyslexia*, *15*, 328–346.

Loosli, S. V., Buschkuehl, M., Perrig, W. J., & Jaeggi, S. M. (2012). Working memory training improves reading processes in typically developing children. *Child Neuropsychology*, *18*(1), 62–78.

Lopes, J. (2012). Biologising reading problems: The specific case of dyslexia. *Contemporary Social Science*, *7*(2), 215–229.

Lovegrove, W. J., Bowling, A., Badcock, D., & Blackwood, M. (1980). Specific reading disability: differences in contrast sensitivity as a function of spatial frequency. *Science*, *210*, 439–440.

Lovett, M. W., Barron, R. W., & Frijters, J. C. (2013). Word identification difficulties in children and adolescents with reading dusabilities. In H. L. Swanson, K.R. Harris, and S. Graham (Eds.), *Handbook of learning disabilities* (pp. 329–360). New York: Guilford Press.

Lu, X., Shaw, C. A., Patel, A., Li, J., Cooper, M. L., Wells, W. R., et al. (2007). Clinical implementation of chromosomal microarray analysis: Summary of 2513 postnatal cases. *PLoS ONE*, *2*(3), e327. doi: 10.1371/journal.pone.0000327.

Luciano, M., Evans, D. M., Hansell, N. K., Medland, S. E., Montgomery, G. W., et al. (2013). A genome-wide association study for reading and language abilities in two population cohorts. *Genes, Brain and Behavior*.

Lundberg, I., Larsman, P., & Strid, A. (2012). Development of phonological awareness during the preschool year: The influence of gender and socio-economic status. *Reading and Writing*, *25*, 305–320.

Lyon, G. R. (1995). Towards a definition of dyslexia. *Annals of Dyslexia*, *45*, 3–27.

Lyon, G. R., & Moats, L. C. (1997). Critical conceptual and methodological considerations in reading intervention research. *Journal of Learning Disabilities*, *30*, 578–588.

Lyon, G. R., Shaywitz, S. E., & Shaywitz, B. A. (2003). A definition of dyslexia. *Annals of Dyslexia*, *53*, 1–14.

Lyon, G. R., & Weiser, B. (2013). The state of the science in learning disabilities: Research impact on the field from 2001 to 2011. In H. L. Swanson, K. R. Harris, & S. Graham (Eds.), *Handbook of learning disabilities* (pp. 118–151). New York: Guilford Press.

Lyytinen, H., Erskine, J., Tolvanen, A., Torppa, M., Poikkeus, A., & Lyytinen, P. (2006). Trajectories of reading development: A follow-up from birth to school age of children with and without risk for dyslexia. *Merrill-Palmer Quarterly: Journal of Developmental Psychology*, *52*, 514–546.

MacArthur, C. A. (2013). Technology applications for improving literacy. In H. L. Swanson, K. R. Harris, & S. Graham (Eds.), *Handbook of learning disabilities* (pp. 565–590). New York: Guilford Press.

Macaruso, P., Locke, J., Smith, S. T., & Powers, S. (1995). Short-term memory and phonological coding in developmental dyslexia. *Journal of Neurolinguistics, 9,* 135–146.

Macdonald, S. (2009). Towards a social reality of dyslexia. *British Journal of Learning Disabilities, 38,* 271–279.

Machek, G. R., & Nelson, J. M. (2007). How should reading disabilities be operationalized? A survey of practicing school psychologists. *Learning Disabilities Research & Practice, 22,* 147–157.

Machin, S., & Pekkarinen, T. (2008). Global sex differences in test score variability. *Science, 322,* 1331–1332.

Macmillan, D. L., & Siperstein, G. N. (2002). Learning disabilities as operationally defined by schools. In R. Bradley, L. Danielson, & D. P. Hallahan (Eds.), *Identification of learning disabilities: Research to policy* (pp. 287–333). Mahwah, NJ: Erlbaum.

Maehler, C., & Schuchardt, K. (2009). Working memory in children with learning disabilities: Does intelligence make a difference? *Journal of Intellectual Disability Research, 53,* 3–10.

Maehler, C., & Schuchardt, K. (2011). Working memory in children with learning disabilities: Rethinking the criterion of disability. *International Journal of Disability, Development and Education, 58*(1), 5–17.

Maisog, J. M., Einbinder, E. R., Flowers, D. L., Turkeltaub, P. E., & Eden, G. F. (2008). A meta-analysis of functional neuroimaging studies of dyslexia. In G. F. Eden & D. L. Flowers (Eds.), *Learning, skill acquisition, reading, and dyslexia* (pp. 237–259). New York: Wiley-Blackwell.

Manis, F. R., Doi, L. M., & Bhadha, B. (2000). Naming speed, phonological awareness, and orthographic knowledge in second graders. *Journal of Learning Disabilities, 33,* 325–333.

Mann, L. (1979). *On the trail of process.* New York: Grune & Stratton.

Marazzi, C. (2011). Dyslexia and the economy. *Angelaki: Journal of the Theoretical Humanities, 16*(3), 19–32.

Markham, R. (2002). Developmental dyslexia. *Focus: Occasional Update from the Royal College of Opthalmologists,* No 23.

Marshall, C. M., Snowling, M. J., & Bailey, P. J. (2001). Rapid auditory processing and phonological ability in normal readers and readers with dyslexia. *Journal of Speech, Language, and Hearing Research, 44,* 925–940.

Martelli, M., Di Filippo, G., Spinelli, D., & Zoccolotti, P. (2009). Crowding, reading, and developmental dyslexia. *Journal of Vision, 9,* 1–18.

Mather, N., & Wendling, B. J. (2012). *Essentials of dyslexia assessment and intervention.* Hoboken, NJ: Wiley.

Mathes, P. G., & Denton, C. A. (2002). The prevention and identification of reading disability. *Seminars in Pediatric Neurology, 9,* 185–191.

Mathes, P. G., Denton, C. A., Fletcher, J. M., Anthony, J. L., Francis, D. J., & Schatschneider, C. (2005). The effects of theoretically different instruction and student characteristics on the skills of struggling readers. *Reading Research Quarterly, 40,* 148–182.

Mattson, M. P. (2002). Neurogenetics: White matter matters. *Trends in Neurosciences*, *25*, 135–136.

Maurer, U., Brem, S., Bucher, K., Kranz, F., Benz, R., Steinhausen, H. C., et al. (2007). Impaired tuning of a fast occipito-temporal response for print in dyslexic children learning to read. *Brain*, *130*(12), 3200–3210.

Mayes, S. D., & Calhoun, S. L. (2006). Frequency of reading, math, and writing disabilities in children with clinical disorders. *Learning and Individual Differences*, *16*, 145–157.

Mazzocco, M. M., & Grimm, J. J. (2013). Growth in rapid automatized naming from Grades K to 8 in children with math or reading disabilities. *Journal of Learning Disabilities*, *46*(6), 517–533.

McArthur, G. (2007). Test-retest effects in treatment studies of reading disability: The devil is in the detail. *Dyslexia*, *13*, 240–252.

McArthur, G. M. (2009). Auditory processing disorders: Can they be treated? *Current Opinion in Neurology*, *22*, 137–143.

McArthur, G. M., & Bishop, D. V. M. (2001). Auditory perceptual processing in people with reading and oral language impairments: Current issues and recommendations. *Dyslexia*, *7*, 150–170.

McArthur, G. M., & Bishop, D. V. M. (2004). Frequency discrimination deficits in people with specific language impairment: Reliability, validity, and linguistic correlates. *Journal of Speech, Language, and Hearing Research*, *47*, 527–541.

McArthur, G. M., & Castles, A. (2013). Phonological processing deficits in specific reading disability and specific language impairment: Same or different? *Journal of Research in Reading*, *36*(3), 280–302.

McArthur, G. M., Castles, A., Kohnen, S., Larsen, L., Jones, K., et al. (in press). Sight word and phonics training in children with dyslexia. *Journal of Learning Disabilities*.

McArthur, G. M., Ellis, D., Atkinson, C. M., & Coltheart, M. (2008). Auditory processing deficits in children with reading and language impairments: Can they (and should they) be treated? *Cognition*, *107*, 946–977.

McArthur, G. M., & Hogben, J. H. (2012). Poor auditory task scores in children with specific reading and language difficulties: Some poor scores are more equal than others. *Scientific Studies of Reading*, *16*, 63–89.

McArthur, G. M., Hogben, J. H., Edwards, V. T., Heath, S. M., & Mengler, E. D. (2000). On the "specifics" of specific reading disability and specific language impairment. *Journal of Child Psychology and Psychiatry*, *41*(7), 869–874.

McCandliss, B. D., & Noble, K. G. (2003). The development of reading impairment: A cognitive neuroscience model. *Mental Retardation & Developmental Disabilities Research Reviews*, *9*, 196–204.

McCardle, P., & Chhabra, V. (2004). *The voice of evidence in reading research*. Baltimore: Brookes.

McCardle, P., & Miller, B. (2012). Conclusion/next steps: Critical research directions and priorities. In A. A. Benasich & R. Holly Fitch (Eds.), *Developmental dyslexia: Early precursors, neurobehavioral markers, and biological substrates* (pp. 329–337). Baltimore, MD: Paul H. Brookes Publishing.

McCrory, E. J., Mechelli, A., Frith, U., & Price, C. J. (2005). More than words: A common neural basis for reading and naming deficits in developmental dyslexia? *Brain*, *128*, 261–267.

McDermott, R., Goldman, S., & Varenne, H. (2006). The cultural work of learning disabilities. *Educational Researcher, 35*, 12–17.

McGee, R., Williams, S., Share, D. L., Anderson, J., & Silva, P. A. (1986). The relationship between specific reading retardation, general reading backwardness and behavioral problems in a large sample of Dunedin boys: A longitudinal study from five to eleven years. *Journal of Child Psychology and Psychiatry, 27*, 597–610.

McGrath, L. M., Pennington, B. P., Shanahan, M. A., Santerre-Lemmon, L. E., Barnard, H. D., Willcutt, E. G., et al. (2011). A multiple deficit model of reading disability and attention-deficit/hyperactivity disorder: Searching for shared cognitive deficits. *Journal of Child Psychology and Psychiatry, 52*, 547–557.

McIntosh, R. D., & Ritchie, S. J. (2012). Rose-tinted? The use of coloured overlays to treat reading difficulties. In S. D. Sala & M. Anderson (Eds.), *Neuroscience in education: The good, the bad and the ugly* (pp. 230–243). Oxford: Oxford University Press.

McKenzie, R. G. (2009). Obscuring vital distinctions: The oversimplification of learning disabilities within RTI. *Learning Disability Quarterly, 32*, 203–215.

McLean, G. M. T., Castles, A., Coltheart, V., & Stuart, G. W. (2010). No evidence for a prolonged attentional blink in developmental dyslexia. *Cortex, 46*, 1317–1329.

McLean, G. M. T., Stuart, G. W., Coltheart, V., & Castles, A. (2011). Visual temporal processing in dyslexia and the magnocellular deficit theory: The need for speed? *Journal of Experimental Psychology: Human Perception and Performance, 37*(6), 1957–1975.

McLeskey, J., & Waldron, N. L. (2002). Inclusion and school change: Teacher perceptions of curricular and instructional adaptations. *Teacher Education and Special Education, 25*, 41–54.

McLeskey, J., & Waldron, N. L. (2011). Educational programs for elementary students with learning disabilities: Can they be both effective and inclusive? *Learning Disabilities Research & Practice, 26*(1), 48–57.

McLoughlin, D., & Leather, C. (2009). Dyslexia: Meeting the needs of employers and employees in the workplace. In G. Reid (Ed.), *The Routledge companion to dyslexia* (pp. 286–294). London: Routledge.

McPhillips, M., Hepper, P. G., & Mulhern, G. (2000). Effects of replicating primary-reflex movements on specific reading difficulties in children: A randomised, double-blind, controlled trial. *Lancet, 355*, 537–541.

McPhillips, M., & Jordan-Black, J. A. (2007). Primary reflex persistence in children with reading difficulties (dyslexia): A cross-sectional study. *Neuropsychologia, 45*, 748–754.

Meaburn, E., Harlaar, N., Craig, I., Schalkwyk, L., & Plomin, R. (2008). Quantitative trait locus association scan of early reading disability and ability using pooled DNA and 100K SNP microarrays in a sample of 5760 children. *Molecular Psychiatry, 13*, 729–740.

Mechelli, A., Price, C. J., Friston, K. J., et al., (2005). Voxel-based morphometry of the human brain: methods and applications. *Current Methods in Imaging, 1*, 105–113.

Melby-Lervåg, M., & Hulme, C. (2013). Is working memory training effective? A meta-analytic review. *Developmental Psychology, 49*(2), 270–291.

Melby-Lervåg, M., Lyster, S., & Hulme, C. (2012). Phonological skills and their role in learning to read: A meta-analytic review. *Psychological Bulletin, 138*, 322–352.

Mellard, D. F., Deshler, D. D., & Barth, A. (2004). LD identification: It's not simply a matter of building a better mousetrap. *Learning Disability Quarterly, 27*, 229–242.

Menghini, D., Carlesimo, G. A., Marotta, L., Finzi, A., & Vicari, S. (2010). Developmental dyslexia and explicit long-term memory. *Dyslexia, 16*, 213–225.

Menghini, D., Finzi, A., Carlesimo, G. A., & Vicari, S. (2011). Working memory impairment in children with developmental dyslexia: Is it just a phonological deficit? *Developmental Neuropsychology, 36*, 199–213.

Menghini, D., Hagberg, G. E., Petrosini, L., Bozzali, M., Macaluso, E., Caltagirone, C., et al. (2008). Structural correlates of implicit learning deficits in subjects with developmental dyslexia. *Annals of the New York Academy of Sciences, 1145*, 212–221.

Merzenich, M. M., Jenkins, W. M., Johnston, P., Schreiner, C., Miller, S. L., & Tallal, P. (1996). Temporal processing deficits of language-learning impaired children ameliorated by training. *Science, 271*, 77–81.

Meyer, M. S., Wood, F. B., Hart, L. A., & Felton, R. H. (1998). Longitudinal course of rapid naming in disabled and nondisabled readers. *Annals of Dyslexia, 48*, 91–114.

Meyler, A., Keller, T. A., Cherkassky, V. L., Lee, D., Hoeft, F., Whitfield-Gabrieli, S., et al. (2007). Brain activation during sentence comprehension among good and poor readers. *Cerebral Cortex, 17*, 2780–2787.

Middleton, F. A., & Strick, P. L. (1997). Cerebellar output channels. *International Review of Neurobiology, 41*, 61–82.

Miles, T. R., Haslum, M. N., & Wheeler, T. J. (1998). Gender ratio in dyslexia. *Annals of Dyslexia, 48*, 27–55.

Miller, D. T., Adam, M. P., Aradhya, S., Biesecker, L. G., Brothman, A. R., Carter, N. P., et al. (2010). Consensus statement: Chromosomal microarray is a first-tier clinical diagnostic test for individuals with developmental disabilities or congenital anomalies. *American Journal of Human Genetics, 86*, 749–764.

Moats, L. C., & Farrell, M. L. (1999). Multi-sensory instruction. In J. Birsh (Ed.), *Multi-sensory teaching of basic language skills* (pp. 1–18). Baltimore, MD: Brookes.

Moats, L. C., & Farrell, M. L. (2005). Multisensory structured language education. In J. Birsh (Ed.), *Multi-sensory teaching of basic language skills* (2nd ed., pp. 23–37). Baltimore, MD: Brookes.

Moats, L. C., & Foorman, B. (1997). Introduction to special issue of SSR: Components of effective reading instruction. *Scientific Studies of Reading, 1*, 187–189.

Mody, M., Studdert-Kennedy, M., & Brady, S. (1997). Speech perception deficits in poor readers: Auditory processing or phonological coding? *Journal of Experimental Child Psychology, 64*, 199–231.

Mol, S. E., & Bus, A. G. (2011). To read or not to read: A meta-analysis of print exposure from infancy to early childhood. *Psychological Bulletin, 137*, 267–296.

Molfese, D. L., Molfese, V. J., Barnes, M. E., Warren, C. G., & Molfese, P. J. (2008). Familial predictors of dyslexia: Evidence from preschool children with and without familial dyslexia risk. In G. Reid, A. J. Fawcett, F. Manis, & L. S. Siegel (Eds.), *The Sage handbook of dyslexia* (pp. 99–121). London: Sage Publications.

Moll, K., Fussenegger, B., Willburger, E., & Landerl, K. (2009). RAN is not a measure of orthographic processing. Evidence from the asymmetric German orthography. *Scientific Studies of Reading, 13*, 1–25.

Moll, K., Loff, A., & Snowling, M. J. (2013). Cognitive endophenotypes of dyslexia. *Scientific Studies of Reading, 17*(6), 385–397.

Monzalvo, K., Fluss, J., Billard, C., Dehaene, S., & Dehaene-Lambertz, G. (2012). Cortical networks for vision and language in dyslexic and normal children of variable socio-economic status. *Neuroimage*, *61*, 258–274.

Moody, S., Vaughn, S., Hughes, M., & Fischer, M. (2000). Reading instruction in the resource room: Set up for failure. *Exceptional Children*, *53*, 391–316.

Moonesinghe, R., Khoury, M. J., Liu, T., & Ioannidis, J. P. (2008). Required sample size and nonreplicability thresholds for heterogeneous genetic associations. *Proceedings of the National Academy of Sciences of the United States of America*, *105*, 617–622.

Moores, E., Cassim, R., & Talcott, J. B. (2011). Adults with dyslexia exhibit large effects of crowding, increased dependence on cues, and detrimental effects of distractors in visual search tasks. *Neuropsychologia*, *49*, 3881–3890.

Morgan, P. L., Farkas, G., Tufis, P. A., & Sperling, R. A. (2008). Are reading and behaviour problems risk factors for each other? *Journal of Learning Disabilities*, *41*, 417–436.

Morgan, P. L., & Fuchs, D. (2007). Is there a bidirectional relationship between children's reading skills and reading motivation? *Exceptional Children*, *73*, 165–183.

Morgan, P. L., Fuchs, D., Compton, D. L., Cordray, D. S., & Fuchs, L. S. (2008). Does early reading failure decrease children's reading motivation? *Journal of Learning Disabilities*, *41*, 387–404.

Morgan, W. P. (1896). A case of congenital word-blindness (inability to learn to read). *British Medical Journal*, *2*, 1543–1544.

Morris, R. D., Lovett, M. W., Wolf, M., Sevcik, R. A., Steinbach, K. A., Frijters, J. C., et al. (2012). Multiple-component remediation for developmental reading disabilities: I.Q., socioeconomic status, and race as factors in remedial outcome. *Journal of Learning Disabilities*, *45*(2), 99–127.

Morris, R. D., Steubing, K. K., Fletcher, J. M., Shaywitz, S. E., Lyon, G. R., Shankweiler, D. P., et al. (1998). Subtypes of reading disability: Variability around a phonological core. *Journal of Educational Psychology*, *90*, 347–373.

Moss, M., Fountain, A. R., Boulay, B., Horst, M., Rodger, C., & Brown-Lyons, M. (2008). *Reading First implementation evaluation: Final Report*. Cambridge, MA: ABT Associates.

Mugnaini, D., Lassi, S., La Malfa, G., & Albertini, G. (2009). Internalizing correlates of dyslexia. *World Journal of Pediatrics*, *5*, 255–264.

Mundy, I. R., & Carroll, J. M. (2012). Speech prosofy and developmental dyslexia: Reduced phonological awareness in the context of intact phonological representations. *Journal of Cognitive Psychology*, *24*, 560–581.

Nandakumar, K., & Leat, S. J. (2008). Dyslexia: A review of two theories. *Clinical and Experimental Optometry*, *91*, 333–340.

Naples, A. J., Chang, J. T., Katz, L., & Grigorenko, E. L. (2009). Same or different? Insights into the etiology of phonological awareness and rapid naming. *Biological Psychology*, *80*, 226–239.

Naples, A. J., Katz, L., & Grigorenko, E. L. (2012). Reading and a diffusion model analysis of reaction time. *Developmental Neuropsychology*, *37*(4), 299–316.

Nash, H. M., Hulme, C., Gooch, D., & Snowling, M. J. (2013). Preschool language profiles of children at family risk of dyslexia: continuities with specific language impairment. *Journal of Child Psychology and Psychiatry*, *54*(9), 958–968.

National Early Literacy Panel. (2008). *Developing early literacy: Report of the National Early Literacy Panel*. Washington, DC: National Institute for Literacy.

National Institute of Child Health and Development. (2007). Learning disabilities: What are learning disabilities? Retrieved August 29, 2010 from http://www.nichd.nih.gov/health/topics/learning_disabilities.cfm.

National Reading Panel. (2000). *Teaching children to read: An evidence-based assessment of the scientific literature on reading and its implications for reading instruction*. Bethesda, MD: National Institute of Child Health and Human Development.

Naumova, O., Lee, M., Koposov, R., Szyf, M., Dozier, M., & Grigorenko, E. L. (2012). Differential patterns of whole-genome DNA methylation in institutionalized children and children raised by their biological parents. *Development and Psychopathology, 24*, 143–155.

Nelson, J. R., Benner, G. J., & Gonzalez, J. (2003). Learner characteristics that influence the treatment of effectiveness of early literacy interventions: A meta-analytic review. *Learning Disabilities Research and Practice, 18*, 255–267.

Nevo, E., & Breznitz, Z. (2011). Assessment of working memory components at 6 years of age as predictors of reading achievements a year later. *Journal of Experimental Child Psychology, 109*, 73–90.

Newbury, D. F., Paracchini, S., Scerri, T. S., Winchester, L., Addis, L., Richardson, A. J., Walter, J., et al. (2011). Investigation of dyslexia and SLI risk-variants in reading- and language-impaired subjects. *Behavior Genetics, 41*, 90–104.

Nicolson, R. (2005). Dyslexia: Beyond the myth. *The Psychologist, 18*, 658–659.

Nicolson, R. I., & Fawcett, A. J. (1990). Automaticity: A new framework for dyslexia research? *Cognition, 35*, 159–182.

Nicolson, R. I., & Fawcett, A. J. (2004). *Dyslexia Early Screening Test (DEST)*. Oxford: Pearson Education.

Nicolson, R. I., & Fawcett, A. J. (2006). Do cerebellar deficits underlie phonological problems in dyslexia? *Developmental Science, 9*, 259–262.

Nicolson, R. I., & Fawcett, A. J. (2007). Procedural learning difficulties: Reuniting the developmental disorders? *Trends in Neurosciences, 30*, 135–141.

Nicolson, R. I., & Fawcett, A. J. (2008). *Dyslexia, learning, and the brain*. Cambridge, MA: MIT Press.

Nicolson, R. I., Fawcett, A. J., & Dean, P. (2001a). Developmental dyslexia: The cerebellar deficit hypothesis. *Trends in Neurosciences, 24*, 508–511.

Nicolson, R. I., Fawcett, A. J., & Dean, P. (2001b). Dyslexia, development and the cerebellum. *Trends in Neurosciences, 24*, 515–516.

Nicolson, R. I., & Reynolds, D. (2007). Sound design and balanced analyses: Response to Rack and colleagues. *Dyslexia, 13*, 105–109.

Niogi, S. N., & McCandliss, B. D. (2006). Left lateralized white matter microstructure accounts for individual differences in reading ability and disability. *Neuropsychologia, 44*, 2178–2188.

Nittrouer, S. (1999). Do temporal processing deficits cause phonological processing problems? *Journal of Speech, Language, and Hearing Research, 42*, 925–942.

Noble, K. G., Farah, M. J., & McCandliss, B. D. (2006). Socioeconomic background modulates cognition-achievement relationships in reading. *Cognitive Development, 21*, 349–368.

Nopola-Hemmi, J., Myllyluoma, B., Voutilainen, A., Leinonen, S., Kere, J., & Ahonen, T. (2002). Familial dyslexia: Neurocognitive and genetic correlation in a large Finnish family. *Developmental Medicine and Child Neurology, 44*, 580–586.

Norton, E. S., & Wolf, M. (2012). Rapid automatized naming (RAN) and reading fluency: Implications for understanding and treatment of reading disabilities. *Annual Review of Psychology, 63*, 427–452.

Norwich, B. (2010). Book review of *Developmental disorders of language, learning and cognition* by C. Hulme and M. J. Snowling. *Journal of Research in Special Educational Needs, 10*, 133–135.

O'Connor, R. E., Bocian, K. M., Sanchez, V., & Beach, K. D. (in press). Access to a responsiveness to intervention model: Does beginning intervention in kindergarten matter? *Journal of Learning Disabilities*.

O'Connor, R. E., Fulmer, D., Harty, K. R., & Bell, K. M. (2005). Layers of reading intervention in kindergarten through third grade: Changes in teaching and student outcomes. *Journal of Learning Disabilities, 38*, 440–455.

O'Connor, R. E., White, A., & Swanson, H. L. (2007). Repeated reading versus continuous reading: Influences on reading fluency and comprehension. *Exceptional Children, 74*, 31–46.

O'Donnell, P. S., & Miller, D. N. (2011). Identifying students with specific learning disabilities: School psychologists' acceptability of the discrepancy model versus response to intervention. *Journal of Disability Policy Studies, 22*, 83–94.

Office of Inspector General of the U.S. Department of Education. (2007). *The department's administration of selected aspects of the Reading First program: Final audit report (ED-OIG/A03G0006)*. Washington, DC: U.S. Department of Education.

Oganian, Y., & Ahissar, M. (2012). Poor anchoring limits dyslexics' perceptual, memory, and reading skills. *Neuropsychologia, 50*, 1895–1905.

Olson, R. K. (1985). Disabled reading processes and cognitive profiles. In D. B. Gray & J. F. Kavanagh (Eds.), *Biobehavioral measures of dyslexia* (pp. 215–244). Parkton, MD: York Press.

Olson, R. K. (2011). Genetic and environmental influences on phonological abilities and reading achievement. In S. A. Brady, D. Braze, & C. A. Fowler (Eds.), *Explaining individual differences in reading: Theory and evidence* (pp. 197–216). New York: Psychology Press.

Olson, R. K., & Datta, H. (2002). Visual-temporal processing in reading-disabled and normal twins. *Reading and Writing: An Interdisciplinary Journal, 15*(15), 127–149.

Olulade, O. A., Napoliello, E. M., & Eden, G. F. (2013). Abnormal visual motion processing is not a cause of dyslexia. *Neuron, 79*, 180–190.

O'Roak, B. J., Deriziotis, P., Lee, C., Vives, L., Schwartz, J. J., Girirajan, S., et al. (2011). Exome sequencing in sporadic autism spectrum disorders identifies severe de novo mutations. *Nature Genetics, 43*, 585–589.

Orton, S. T. (1937). *Reading, writing, and speech problems in children*. New York: W. W. Norton & Company.

Orton, S. T. (1939). A neurological explanation of the reading disability. *Education Record, 12*, 58–68.

Pammer, K. (2012). The role of the dorsal pathway in word recognition. In J. Stein & Z. Kapoula (Eds.), *Visual aspects of dyslexia* (pp. 137–149). Oxford: Oxford University Press.

Paracchini, S., Steer, C. D., Buckingham, L. L., Morris, A. P., Ring, S., Scerri, T., et al. (2008). Association of the KIAA0319 dyslexia susceptibility gene with reading skills in the general population. *The American Journal of Psychiatry, 165*, 1576–1584.

Park, R. L. (2003). The seven warning signs of bogus science. *Chronicle of Higher Education, 49*, 20–21.

Parker, R. M. (1990). Power, control, and validity in research. *Journal of Learning Disabilities, 23*, 613–620.

Pashler, H., McDaniel, M., Rohrer, D., & Bjork, R. (2008). Learning styles: Concepts and evidence. *Psychological Science in the Public Interest, 9*, 106–119.

Paul, I., Bott, C., Heim, S., Eulitz, C., & Elbert, T. (2006). Reduced hemispheric asymmetry of the auditory N260m in dyslexia. *Neuropsychologia, 44*, 785–794.

Paulesu, E., Demonet, J.-F., Fazio, F., McCrory, E., Chanoine, V., Brunswick, N., et al. (2001). Dyslexia: Cultural diversity and biological unity. *Science, 291*, 2165–2167.

Paulesu, E., Frith, U., Snowling, M., Gallagher, A., Morton, J., Frackowiak, R. S., et al. (1996). Is developmental dyslexia a disconnection syndrome? Evidence from PET scanning. *Brain, 119*, 143–157.

Pearson, P. D. (2004). The reading wars. *Education Policy, 18*, 216–252.

Pellicano, E., & Gibson, L.Y. (2008). Investigating the functional integrity of the dorsal visual pathway in autism and dyslexia. *Neuropsychologia, 46*(10), 2593–2596.

Pennington, B. F. (2006). From single to multiple deficit models of developmental disorders. *Cognition, 101*, 385–413.

Pennington, B. F. (2009). *Diagnosing learning disorders: A neuropsychological framework* (2nd ed.). New York: Guilford Press.

Pennington, B. F., & Bishop, D. V. M. (2009). Relations among speech, language, and reading disorders. *Annual Review of Psychology, 60*, 283–306.

Pennington, B. F., Cardoso-Martins, C., Green, P. A., & Lefly, D. L. (2001). Comparing the phonological and double deficit hypotheses for developmental dyslexia. *Reading and Writing, 14*, 707–755.

Pennington, B. F., & Olson, R. K. (2005). Genetics of dyslexia. In M. Snowling & C. Hulme (Eds.), *The science of reading: A handbook* (pp. 453–472). Oxford: Blackwell.

Pennington, B. F., Santerre-Lemmon, L., Rosenberg, J., MacDonald, B., Boada, R., et al. (2012). Individual prediction of dyslexia by single versus multiple deficit models. *Journal of Abnormal Psychology, 121*(1), 212–224.

Pennington, B. F., van Orden, G. C., Smith, S. D., Green, P. A., & Haith, M. M. (1990). Phonological processing skills and deficits in adult dyslexics. *Child Development, 61*, 1753–1778.

Penolazzi, B., Spironelli, C., & Angrilli, A. (2008). Delta EEG activity as a marker of dysfunctional linguistic processing in developmental dyslexia. *Psychophysiology, 45*, 1025–1033.

Penolazzi, B., Spironelli, C., Vio, C., & Angrilli, A. (2006). Altered hemispheric asymmetry during word processing in dyslexic children: An event-related potential study. *Neuroreport, 17*, 429–433.

Penolazzi, B., Spironelli, C., Vio, C., & Angrilli, A. (2010). Brain plasticity in developmental dyslexia after phonological treatment: A beta EEG band study. *Behavioural Brain Research, 209*, 179–182.

Perea, M., Panadero, V., Moret-Tatay, C., & Gómez, P. (2012). The effects of inter-letter spacing in visual-word recognition: Evidence with young normal readers and developmental dyslexics. *Learning and Instruction, 22,* 420–430.

Perceptual Development Corporation (1998). Irlen Institute Website: Who we help. Retrieved July 14, 2012 from http://irlen.com/index.php?s=who.

Perfetti, C. A. (1991). The psychology, pedagogy and politics of reading. *Psychological Science, 2,* 70–76.

Perfetti, C. A., Liu, Y., & Tan, L. H. (2005). The lexical constituency model: Some implications of research on Chinese for general theories of reading. *Psychological Review, 112,* 43–59.

Pernet, C. R., Andersson, J., Paulesu, E., & Demonet, J. F. (2009). When all hypotheses are right: A multifocal account of dyslexia. *Human Brain Mapping, 30,* 2278–2292.

Perrachione, T. K., Del Tufo, S. N., & Gabrieli, J. D. (2011). Human voice recognition depends on language ability. *Science, 333*(6042), 595.

Peterson, R. L., & Pennington, B. F. (2012). Developmental dyslexia. *The Lancet, 379,* 1997–2007.

Peterson, R. L., Pennington, B. F., Shriberg, L. D., & Boada, R. (2009). What influences literacy outcome in children with speech sound disorder? *Journal of Speech, Language, and Hearing Research, 52,* 1175–1188.

Petrill, S. A., Deater-Deckard, K., Thompson, L. A., Schatschneider, C., Dethorne, L. S., & Vandenbergh, D. J. (2007). Longitudinal genetic analysis of early reading: The Western Reserve Reading Project. *Reading and Writing, 20,* 127–146.

Petrill, S. A., Hart, S. A., Harlaar, N., Logan, J., Justice, L. M., Schatschneider, C., et al. (2010). Genetic and environmental influences on the growth of early reading skills. *Journal of Child Psychology & Psychiatry, 51*(6), 660–667.

Peyrin, C., Démonet, J. F., N'guyen-Morel, M. A., Le Bas, J. F., & Valdois, S. (2011). Superior parietal lobe dysfunction in a homogeneous group of dyslexic children with a visual attention span disorder. *Brain & Language, 118,* 128–138.

Peyrin, C., Lallier, M., Démonet, J. F., Pernet, C., Baciu, M., Le Bas, J. F., et al. (2012). Neural dissociation of phonological and visual attention span disorders in developmental dyslexia: FMRI evidence from two case reports. *Brain & Language, 120,* 381–394.

Pfost, M., Dörfler, T., & Artelt, C. (2012). Reading competence development of poor readers in a German elementary school sample: An empirical examination of the Matthew effect model. *Journal of Research in Reading, 35*(4), 411–426.

Piasta, S. B., & Wagner, R. K. (2010). Learning letter names and sounds: Effects of instruction, letter type, and phonological processing skill. *Journal of Experimental Child Psychology, 105,* 324–344.

Pierrehumbert, J. (2003). Phonetic diversity, statistical learning and acquisition of phonology. *Language & Speech, 46,* 115–154.

Pine, D. (2011). Commentary: Diagnosis and classification: There must be something left about which to argue – reflections on Rutter (2011). *Journal of Child Psychology and Psychiatry, 52*(6), 663–664.

Pinker, S. (1998). Foreword. In D. McGuinness (Ed.), *Why children can't read: And what can we do about it.* London: Penguin Books.

Plakas, A., van Zuijen, T., van Leevwen, T., Thomson, J. M., & van der Leij, A. (2003). Impaired non-speech auditory processing at a pre-reading age is a risk factor for dyslexia but not a predictor: An ERP study. *Cortex, 49*(4), 1034–1045.

Plante, E. (2012). Windows into receptive processing. In A. A. Benasich & R. H. Fitch (Eds.), *Developmental dyslexia: Early precursors, neurobehavioral markers, and biological substrates* (pp. 257–274). Baltimore, MD: Paul H. Brookes Publishing.

Plomin, R., & Kovas, Y. (2005). Generalist genes and learning disabilities. *Psychological Bulletin, 131*, 592–617.

Pokorni, J. L., Worthington, C. K., & Jamison, P. J. (2004). Phonological awareness intervention: Comparison of Fast ForWord, Earobics, and LiPS. *Journal of Educational Research, 97*, 147–157.

Poulsen, M., Juul, H., & Elbro, C. (in press). Multiple mediation analysis of the relationship between rapid naming and reading. *Journal of Research in Reading.*

Powell, D., Stuart, M., Garwood, H., Quinlan, P., & Stainthorp, R. (2007). An experimental comparison between rival theories of Rapid Automatised Naming (RAN) performance and its relationship to reading. *Journal of Experimental Child Psychology, 98*, 46–68.

Prado, C., Dubois, M., & Valdois, S. (2007). Eye movements in reading aloud and visual search in developmental dyslexia: Impact of the VA span. *Vision Research, 47*, 2521–2530.

Pressley, M. (2006). *Reading instruction that works: The case for balanced teaching.* New York: The Guilford Press.

Pressley, M., & Wharton-McDonald, R. (1997). Skilled comprehension and its development through instruction. *School Psychology Review, 26*, 448–466.

Price, C. J., & Mechelli, A. (2005). Reading and reading disturbance. *Current Opinion in Neurobiology, 15*, 231–238.

Priebe, S. J., Keenan, J. M., & Miller, A. C. (2012). How prior knowledge affects word identification and comprehension. *Reading and Writing, 25*, 131–149.

Prifitera, A., & Dersch, J. (1993). Base rates of WISC-III diagnostic subtest patterns among normal, learning disabled and ADHD samples. *Journal of Psychoeducational Assessment, WISC-III Monograph,* 43–55.

Pringle-Morgan, W. (1896). A case of congenital word blindness. *British Medical Journal, 2*, 178.

Pugh, K. R., Landi, N., Preston, J. L., Mencl, W. E., Austin, A. C., Sibley, D., et al. (2013). The relationship between phonological and auditory processing and brain organization in beginning readers. *Brain & Language, 125*(2), 173–183.

Pugh, K. R., & McCardle, P. (Eds.). (2009). *How children learn to read: Current issues and new directions in the integration of cognition, neurobiology and genetics of reading and dyslexia research and practice.* New York: Psychology Press.

Pugh, K. R., Mencl, W. E., Jenner, A. R., Katz, L., Frost, S. J., Lee, J. R., et al. (2000). Functional neuroimaging studies of reading and reading disability (developmental dyslexia). *Mental Retardation & Developmental Disabilities Research Reviews, 6*, 207–213.

Puolakanaho, A., Ahonen, T., Aro, M., Eklund, K., Leppanen, P. H. T., Poikkeus, A.-M., Tolvanen, A., Torppa, M., & Lyytinen, H. (2007). Very early phonological and language skills: Estimating individual risk of reading disability. *Journal of Child Psychology and Psychiatry, 48*(9), 923–931.

Quercia, P., Demougeot, L., Dos Santos, M. Bonnetblanc, F. (2011). Integration of proprioceptive signals and attentional capacity during postural control are impaired but subject to improvement in dyslexic children. *Experimental Brain Research, 209*(4), 599–608.

Quercia, P., Feiss, L., & Michel, C. (2013). Developmental dyslexia and vision. *Clinical Opthalmology*, *7*, 869–881.

Quinn, J. M., & Wagner, R. K. (in press). Gender differences in reading impairment and in the identification of impaired readers: results from a large-scale study of at-risk readers. *Journal of Learning Disabilities*.

Rack, J. P. (2003). The who, what, why and how of intervention programmes: Comments on the DDAT evaluation. *Dyslexia*, *9*, 137–139.

Rack, J. P., Snowling, M. J., Hulme, C., & Gibbs, S. (2007). No evidence that an exercise-based treatment programme (DDAT) has specific benefits for children with reading difficulties. *Dyslexia*, *13*, 97–104.

Rack, J. P., Snowling, M. J., & Olson, R. K. (1992). The nonword reading deficit in developmental dyslexia – a review. *Reading Research Quarterly*, *27*, 28–53.

Rae, C., Lee, M. A., Dixon, R. M., Blamire, A. M., Thompson, C. H., Styles, P., et al. (1998). Metabolic abnormalities in developmental dyslexia detected by 1H magnetic resonance spectroscopy. *Lancet*, *351*, 1849–1852.

Raij, T., Uutela, K., & Hari, R. (2000). Audiovisual integration of letters in the human brain. *Neuron*, *28*, 617–625.

Ramsden, S., Richardson, F. M., Josse, M. S. C., Ellis, C., Shakeshaft, C., Seghier, M. L., et al. (2011). Verbal and non-verbal intelligence changes in the teenage brain. *Nature*, *479*, 113–116.

Ramus, F. (2003). Developmental dyslexia: Specific phonological deficits or general sensorimotor dysfunction? *Current Opinion in Neurology*, *13*, 212–218.

Ramus, F. (2004). Neurobiology of dyslexia: A reinterpretation of the data. *Trends in Neurosciences*, *27*, 720–726.

Ramus, F., & Ahissar, M. (2012). Developmental dyslexia: The difficulties of interpreting poor performance, and the importance of normal performance. *Cognitive Neuropsychology*, *29*(1–2), 104–122.

Ramus, F., Marshall, C. R., Rosen, S., & van der Lely, H. K. J. (2013). Phonological deficits in specific language impairment and developmental dyslexia: Towards a multidimensional model. *Brain*, *136*, 630–645.

Ramus, F., Pidgeon, E., & Frith, U. (2003). The relationship between motor control and phonology in dyslexic children. *Journal of Child Psychology and Psychiatry and Allied Disciplines*, *44*, 712–722.

Ramus, F., Rosen, S., Dakin, S. C., Day, B. L., Castellote, J. M., White, S., et al. (2003). Theories of developmental dyslexia: Insights from a multiple case study of dyslexic adults. *Brain*, *126*, 841–865.

Ramus, F., & Szenkovits, G. (2008). What phonological deficit? *The Quarterly Journal of Experimental Psychology*, *61*, 129–141.

Raschle, N. M., Stering, P. L., Meissner, S. N., & Gaab, N. (in press). Altered neuronal response during rapid auditory processing and its relation to phonological processing in prereading children at familial risk for dyslexia. *Cerebral Cortex*.

Rashotte, C. A., MacPhee, K., & Torgesen, J. K. (2001). The effectiveness of a group reading instruction program with poor readers in multiple grades. *Learning Disability Quarterly*, *24*, 119–134.

Rasinski, T., Rikli, A., & Johnston, S. (2009). Reading fluency: More than automaticity? More than a concern for the primary grades? *Literacy Research and Instruction*, *48*, 350–351.

Raskind, W. H., Igo, R. P. J., Chapman, N. H., Berninger, V. W., Thomson, J. B., Matsushita, M., et al. (2005). A genome scan in multigenerational families with dyslexia: Identification of a novel locus on chromosome 2q that contributes to phonological decoding efficiency. *Molecular Psychiatry*, *10*, 699–711.

Reason, R. (2001). Letter to the Editor. *Dyslexia*, *7*, 174.

Reason, R., & Stothard, J. (2013). Is there a place for dyslexia in educational psychology practice? *Debate*, *146*, 8–13.

Redick, T. S., Shipstead, Z., Harrison, T. L., Hicks, K. L., Fried, D. E., Hambrick, D. Z., Kane, M. J., & Engle, R. W. (2013). No evidence of intelligence improvement after working memory training: A randomized, placebo-controlled study. *Journal of Experimental Psychology: General*, *142*(2), 359–379.

Regan, T., & Woods, K. (2000). Teachers' understandings of dyslexia: Implications for educational psychology practice. *Educational Psychology in Practice*, *16*, 333–347.

Reid, D. K., & Valle, J. W. (2004). The discursive practice of learning disability: Implications for instruction and parent-school relations. *Journal of Learning Disabilities*, *37*, 466–481.

Renvall, A., & Hari, R. (2002). Auditory cortical responses to speech-like stimuli in dyslexic adults. *Journal of Cognitive Neuroscience*, *14*, 757–768.

Reschly, D. (2005). Learning disabilities identification: Primary intervention, secondary intervention, and then what? *Journal of Learning Disabilities*, *38*, 510–515.

Reschly, D. J., & Tilley, W. D. (1999). Reform trends and system design alternatives. In D. J. Reschly, W. D. Tilley, & J. P. Grimes (Eds.), *Special education in transition: Functional assessment and noncategorical programming* (pp. 19–48). Longmont, CO: Sopris West.

Reynolds, C. R., & Shaywitz, S. E. (2009a). Response to intervention: Prevention and remediation, perhaps. Diagnosis, no. *Child Development Perspectives*, *3*, 44–47.

Reynolds, C. R., & Shaywitz, S. E. (2009b). Response to intervention: Ready or not? Or, from wait-to-fail to watch-them-fail. *School Psychology Quarterly*, *24*, 130–145.

Reynolds, D., & Nicolson, R. I. (2007). Follow-up of an exercise-based treatment for children with reading difficulties. *Dyslexia*, *13*, 78–96.

Reynolds, D., Nicolson, R. I., & Hambly, H. (2003). Evaluation of an exercise-based treatment for children with reading difficulties. *Dyslexia*, *9*, 48–71.

Rezaie, R., Simos, P. G., Fletcher, J. M., Cirino, P. T., Vaughn, S., & Papanicolaou, A. C. (2011). Temporo-parietal brain activity as a longitudinal predictor of response to educational interventions among middle school struggling readers. *Journal of the International Neuropsychological Society*, *17*, 875–885.

Riccio, C. A., Sullivan, J. R., & Cohen, M. J. (2010). *Neuropsychological assessment and intervention for childhood and adolescent disorders*. Trenton, NJ: John Wiley and Sons.

Rice, M. (1999). *Literacy and behaviour: The prison reading survey*. Cambridge: Cambridge University Press.

Rice, M., & Brooks, G. (2004). *Developmental dyslexia in adults: A research review*. London: National Research and Development Centre for Adult Literacy and Numeracy.

Richards, T. L., & Berninger, V. W. (2008). Abnormal fMRI connectivity in children with dyslexia during a phoneme task: before but not after treatment. *Journal of Neurolinguistics*, *21*, 294–304.

Richards, T. L., Corina, D. P., Serafini, S., Steury, K., Echelard, D. R., Dager, S. R., et al. (2000). Effects of a phonologically driven treatment for dyslexia on lactate levels measured by proton MR spectroscopic imaging. *American Journal of Neuroradiology*, *21*, 916–922.

Richards, T. L., Dager, S. R., Corina, D., Serafini, S., Heide, A. C., Steury, K., et al. (1999). Dyslexic children have abnormal brain lactate response to reading-related language tasks. *American Journal of Neuroradiology*, *20*, 1393–1398.

Richards, T. L., Stevenson, J., Crouch, J., Johnson, L. C., Maravilla, K., Stock, P., et al. (2008). Tract-based spatial statistics of diffusion tensor imaging in adults with dyslexia. *American Journal of Neuroradiology*, *29*, 1134–1139.

Richardson, A. J. (2006). Omega-3 fatty acids in ADHD and related neurodevelopmental disorders. *International Review of Psychiatry*, *18*, 155–172.

Richardson, A. J., Burton, J. R., Sewell, R. P., Spreckelsen, T. F., & Montgomery, P. (2012). Docosahexaenoic acid for reading, cognition and behavior in children aged 7–9 Years: A randomized, controlled trial (The DOLAB Study). *PLoS ONE*, *7*(9), e43909.

Richardson, A. J., Cox, I. J., Sargentoni, J., & Puri, B. K. (1997). Abnormal cerebral phospholipid metabolism in dyslexia indicated by phosphorus-31 magnetic resonance spectroscopy. *NMR in Biomedicine*, *10*, 309–314.

Richardson, A. J., & Montgomery, P. (2005). The Oxford-Durham study: A random-ized, controlled trial of dietary supplementation with fatty acids in children with developmental coordination disorder. *Pediatrics*, *115*, 1360–1366.

Richardson, U., Leppanen, P. H. T., Leiwo, M., & Lyytinen, H. (2003). Speech per-ception of infants with high familial risk for dyslexia differ at the age of 6 months. *Developmental Neuropsychology*, *23*, 385–397.

Richlan, F., Kronbichler, M., & Wimmer, H. (2009). Functional abnormalities in the dyslexic brain: A quantitative meta-analysis of neuroimaging studies. *Human Brain Mapping*, *30*, 3299–3308.

Richlan, F., Kronbichler, M., & Wimmer, H. (2011). Meta-analyzing brain dysfunctions in dyslexic children and adults. *Neuroimage*, *56*, 1735–1742.

Ricketts, J. (2011). Research review: Reading comprehension in developmental disor-ders of language and communication. *Journal of Child Psychology and Psychiatry*, *52*(11), 1111–1123.

Riddick, B. (2000). An examination of the relationship between labeling and stigma-tization with special reference to dyslexia. *Disability and Society*, *15*, 653–657.

Riddick, B. (2001). Dyslexia and inclusion: Time for a social model of disability? *International Studies in Sociology of Education*, *11*, 223–236.

Riddick, B. (2010). *Living with dyslexia: The social and emotional consequences of specific learning difficulties/disabilities*. Oxford: Routledge.

Riddick, B., Wolfe, J., & Lumsdon, D. (2002). *Dyslexia: A practical guide for teachers and parents*. London: David Fulton.

Rimkute, L., Torppa, M., Eklund, K., Nurmi, J. E., & Lyytinen, H. (2013). The impact of adolescents' dyslexia on parents' and their own educational expectations. *Reading and Writing*.

Ritchie, S. J., Della Sala, S., & McIntosh, R. D. (2011). Irlen colored overlays do not alleviate reading difficulties. *Pediatrics*, *128*, e932–e938.

Ritchie, S. J., Della Sala, S., & McIntosh, R. D. (2012). Irlen colored overlays in the classroom: A one-year follow-up. *Mind, Brain, and Education*, *6*, 74–80.

Roach, N., Edwards, V., & Hogben, J. (2004). The tale is in the tail: An alternative hypothesis for psychophysical performance variability in dyslexia. *Perception*, *33*(7), 817–830.

Roberts, A. E., Cox, G. F., Kimonis, V., Lamb, A., & Irons, M. (2004). Clinical presentation of 13 patients with subtelomeric rearrangements and a review of the literature. *American Journal of Medical Genetics*, *128A*, 352–363.

Roberts, G., Torgesen, J. K., Boardman, A., & Scammacca, N. (2008). Evidence-based strategies for reading instruction of older students with learning disabilities *Learning Disabilities Research and Practice*, *23*, 63–69.

Robertson, C., & Salter, W. (1997). *The Phonological Awareness Test*. East Moline, IL: LinguiSystems.

Rochelle, K. S., & Talcott, J. B. (2006). Impaired balance in developmental dyslexia? A meta-analysis of the contending evidence. *Journal of Child Psychology and Psychiatry*, *47*, 1159–1166.

Roeske, D., Ludwig, K. U., Neuhoff, N., Becker, J., Bartling, J., Bruder, J., et al. (2011). First genome-wide association scan on neurophysiological endophenotypes points to trans-regulation effects on SLC2A3 in dyslexic children. *Molecular Psychiatry*, *16*, 97–107.

Romani, C., Tsouknida, E., di Betta, A. M., & Olson, A. (2011). Reduced attentional capacity, but normal processing speed and shifting of attention in developmental dyslexia: Evidence from a serial task. *Cortex*, *47*, 715–733.

Rooney, K. J. (1995). Dyslexia revisited: History, educational philosophy, and clinical assessment applications. *Intervention in School and Clinic*, *31*, 6–15.

Rose, J. (2009). *Identifying and teaching children and young people with dyslexia and literacy difficulties. (The Rose Report)*. Nottingham, UK: DCSF Publications.

Rose, L. T., & Rouhani, P. (2012). Influence of verbal working memory depends on vocabulary: oral reading fluency in adolescents with dyslexia. *Mind, Brain, and Education*, *6*, 1–9.

Rosen, V., & Engle, R.W. (1997). Forward and backward serial recall. *Intelligence*, *25*, 37–47.

Rosenberg, J., Pennington, B. F., Willcutt, E. G., & Olson, R. K. (2012). Gene by environment interactions influencing reading disability and the inattentive symptom dimension of attention deficit/hyperactivity disorder. *Journal of Child Psychology and Psychiatry*, *53*(3), 243–251.

Rubenstein, K., Matsushita, M., Berninger, V. W., Raskind, W. H., & Wijsman, E. M. (2011). Genome scan for spelling deficits: Effects of verbal IQ on models of transmission and trait gene localization. *Behavior Genetics*, *41*, 31–42.

Rubie-Davies, C. M., Blatchford, P., Webster, R., Koutsoubou, M., & Bassett, P. (2010). Enhancing learning? A comparison of teacher and teaching assistant interactions with pupils. *School Effectiveness and School Improvement*, *21*, 429–449.

Ruffino, M., Trussardi, A. N., Gori, S., Finzi, A., Giovagnoli, S., Menghini, D., et al. (2010). Attentional engagement deficits in dyslexic children. *Neuropsychologia*, *48*, 3793–3801.

Rumsey, J. M., Andreason, P., Zametkin, A. J., Aquino, T., King, A. C., Hamburger, S. D., et al. (1992). Failure to activate the left temporoparietal cortex in dyslexia. An oxygen 15 positron emission tomographic study. *Archives of Neurology, 49*, 527–534.

Rumsey, J. M., Casanova, M., Mannheim, G. B., Patronas, N., De Vaughn, N., Hamburger, S. D., et al. (1996). Corpus callosum morphology, as measured with MRI, in dyslexic men. *Biological Psychiatry, 39*, 769–775.

Rumsey, J. M., Donohue, B. C., Brady, D. R., Nace, K., Giedd, J. N., & Andreason, P. (1997). A magnetic resonance imaging study of planum temporale asymmetry in men with developmental dyslexia. *Archives of Neurology, 54*, 1481–1489.

Rumsey, J. M., Nace, K., Donohue, B., Wise, D., Maisog, J. M., & Andreason, P. (1997). A positron emission tomographic study of impaired word recognition and phonological processing in dyslexic men. *Archives of Neurology, 54*, 562–573.

Rumsey, J. M., Zametkin, A. J., Andreason, P., Hanahan, A. P., Hamburger, S. D., Aquino, T., et al. (1994). Normal activation of frontotemporal language cortex in dyslexia, as measured with oxygen 15 positron emission tomography. *Archives of Neurology, 51*, 27–38.

Rutter, M. (1978). Prevalence and types of dyslexia. In A. Benton & D. Pearl (Eds.), *Dyslexia: An appraisal of current knowledge* (pp. 5–28). New York: Oxford University Press.

Rutter, M. (2011). Child psychiatric diagnosis and classification: Concepts, findings, challenges and potential. *Journal of Child Psychology and Psychiatry, 52*(6), 647–660.

Rutter, M., Caspi, A., Fergusson, D., Horwood, L. J., Goodman, R., Maughan, B., et al. (2004). Sex differences in developmental reading disability: New findings from 4 epidemiological studies. *Journal of the American Medical Association, 291*, 2007–2012.

Rutter, M., Kim-Cohen, J., & Maughan, B. (2006). Continuities and discontinuities in psychopathology between childhood and adult life. *Journal of Child Psychology and Psychiatry, 47*, 276–295.

Rutter, M., & Maughan, B. (2005). Dyslexia: 1965–2005. *Behavioural and Cognitive Psychotherapy, 33*, 389–402.

Ryder, J. F., Tunmer, W. E., & Greaney, K. T. (2008). Explicit instruction in phonemic awareness and phonemically based decoding skills as an intervention strategy for struggling readers in whole language classrooms. *Reading and Writing, 21*, 299–316.

Saine, N. L., Lerkkanen, M. K., Ahonen, T., Tolvanen, A., & Lyytinen, H. (2011). Computer assisted remedial reading intervention for school beginners at risk for reading disability. *Child Development, 82*(3), 1013–1028.

Salmelin, R., Service, E., Kiesilä, P., Uutela, K., & Salonen, O. (1996). Impaired visual word processing in dyslexia revealed with magnetoencephalography. *Annals of Neurology, 40*, 157–162.

Samuelsson, S., Byrne, B., Olson, R. K., Hulslander, Wadsworth, S., Corley, R., et al. (2008). Response to early literacy instruction in the United States, Australia, and Scandinavia: A behavioral-genetic analysis. *Learning and Individual Differences, 18*, 289–295.

Samuelsson, S., Herkner, B., & Lundberg, I. (2003). Reading and writing difficulties among prison inmates: A matter of experiential factors rather than dyslexic problems. *Scientific Studies of Reading, 7*, 53–73.

Sandak, R., Mencl, W. E., Frost, S. J., & Pugh, K. R. (2004). The neurobiological basis of skilled and impaired reading: Recent findings and new directions. *Scientific Studies of Reading, 8*, 273–292.

Sanders, S. J., Ercan-Sencicek, A. G., Hus, V., Luo, R., Murtha, M. T., Moreno-De-Luca, D., et al. (2011). Multiple recurrent de novo CNVs, including duplications of the 7q11.23 Williams Syndrome region, are strongly associated with autism. *Neuron, 70*, 863–885.

Sanders, S. J., Murtha, M. T., Gupta, A. R., Murdoch, J. D., Raubeson, M. J., Willsey, A. J., et al. (2012). De novo mutations revealed by whole-exome sequencing are strongly associated with autism. *Nature, 485*, 237–241.

Sandu, A. L., Specht, K., Beneventi, H., Lundervold, A., & Hugdahl, K. (2008). Sex-differences in grey-white matter structure in normal-reading and dyslexic adolescents. *Neuroscience Letters, 438*, 80–84.

Santi, K. L., York, M., Foorman, B., & Francis, D. J. (2009). The timing of early reading assessment in kindergarten. *Learning Disability Quarterly, 32*, 217–227.

Savage, R. S. (2004). Motor skills, automaticity and developmental dyslexia: A review of the research literature. *Reading and Writing, 17*, 301–324.

Savage, R. S., & Frederickson, N. (2005). Evidence of a highly specific relationship between rapid automatic naming of digits and text-reading speed. *Brain and Language, 93*, 152–159.

Savage, R. S., Frederickson, N., Goodwin, R., Patni, U., Smith, N., & Tuersley, L. (2005). Relationships among rapid digit naming, phonological processing, motor automaticity, and speech perception in poor, average, and good readers and spellers. *Journal of Learning Disabilities, 38*, 12–28.

Savage, R. S., Lavers, N., & Pillay, V. (2007). Working memory and reading difficulties: What we know and what we don't know about the relationship. *Educational Psychology Review, 19*, 185–221.

Saygin, Z. M., Norton, E. S., Osher, D. E., Beach, S. D., Cyr, A. B., et al. (2013). Tracking the roots of reading ability: White matter volume and integrity correlate with phonological awareness in prereading and early-reading kindergarten children. *The Journal of Neuroscience, 33*(33), 13251–13258.

Scammacca, N., Roberts, G., Vaughn, S., Edmonds, M., Wexler, J., Reutebuch, C. K., et al. (2007). *Reading interventions for adolescent struggling readers: A meta-analysis with implications for practice.* Portsmouth, NH: RMC Research Corporation Center on Instruction.

Scammacca, N., Roberts, G. Vaughn, S., & Stuebing, K. K. A. (in press). A meta-analysis of interventions for struggling readers in Grades 4–12: 1980–2011. *Journal of Learning Disabilities*

Scanlon, D. (2013). Specific learning disability and its newest definition: Which is comprehensive and which is insufficient? *Journal of Learning Disabilities, 46*(1), 26–33.

Scanlon, D. M. (2011). Response to intervention as an assessment approach. In A. McGill-Franzen & R. L. Allington (Eds.), *Handbook of reading disability research* (pp. 139–148). New York: Routledge.

Scanlon, D. M., Gelzheiser, L. M., Vellutino, F. R., Schatschneider, C., & Sweeney, J. M. (2008). Reducing the incidence of early reading difficulties: Professional development for classroom teachers versus direct interventions for children. *Learning and Individual Differences, 18*, 346–359.

Scanlon, D. M., Vellutino, F. R., Small, S. G., Fanuele, D., & Sweeney, J. M. (2005). Severe reading difficulties: Can they be prevented? A comparison of prevention and intervention approaches. *Exceptionality, 13*, 209–227.

Scarborough, H. S. (1998a). Early identification of children at risk for reading disabilities: Phonological awareness and some other promising predictors. In B. K. Shapiro, P. J. Accardo, & A. J. Capute (Eds.), *Specific reading disability: A view of the spectrum* (pp. 75–119). Timonium, MD: York Press.

Scarborough, H. S. (1998b). Predicting the future achievement of second graders with reading disabilities: Contributions of phonemic awareness, verbal memory, rapid naming, and IQ. *Annals of Dyslexia, 48*, 115–136.

Scarborough, H. S., & Brady, S. A. (2002). Toward a common terminology for talking about speech and reading: A glossary of the "phon" words and some related terms. *Journal of Literacy Research, 34*, 299–336.

Scerri, T. S., Paracchini, S., Morris, A., MacPhie, I. L., Talcott, J., Stein, J., et al. (2010). Identification of candidate genes for dyslexia susceptibility on chromosome 18. *PLoS ONE, 5*, e13712.

Schatschneider, C., Fletcher, J. M., Francis, D. J., Carlson, C. D., & Foorman, B. R. (2004). Kindergarten prediction of reading skills: A longitudinal comparative analysis. *Journal of Educational Psychology, 96*, 265–282.

Schatschneider, C., Wagner, R. K., & Crawford, E. (2008). The importance of measuring growth in response to intervention models: Testing a core assumption. *Learning and Individual Differences, 18*, 310–315.

Schlaggar, B. L., & McCandliss, B. D. (2007). Development of neural systems for reading. *Annual Review of Neuroscience, 30*, 475–503.

Schmahmann, J. D., & Pandya, D. N. (1997). The cerebrocerebellar system. *International Review of Neurobiology, 41*, 31–60.

Schneps, M. H., Thomson, J. M., Sonnert, G., Pomplun, M., Chen, C., & Heffner-Wong, A. (2013). Shorter lines facilitate reading in those who struggle. *PLoS One, 8*(8), e 71161.

Schuchardt, K., Maehler, C., & Hasselhorn, M. (2008). Working memory deficits in children with specific learning disorders. *Journal of Learning Disabilities, 41*, 514–523.

Schulte-Körne, G., & Bruder, J. (2010). Clinical neurophysiology of visual and auditory processing in dyslexia: A review. *Clinical Neurophysiology, 121*, 1794–1809.

Schulte-Körne, G., Deimel, W., Bartling, J., & Remschmidt, H. (1998). Auditory processing and dyslexia: Evidence for a specific speech processing deficit. *Neuroreport, 9*, 337–340.

Schulz, E., Maurer, U., van der Mark, S., Bucher, K., Brem, S., Martin, E., et al. (2008). Impaired semantic processing during sentence reading in children with dyslexia: Combined fMRI and ERP evidence. *Neuroimage, 41*, 153–168.

Schumacher, J., Hoffmann, P., Schmal, C., Schulte-Korne, G., & Nothen, M. M. (2007). Genetics of dyslexia: The evolving landscape. *Journal of Medical Genetics, 44*, 289–297.

Sela, I. (2012). The relationships between motor learning, the visual system and dyslexia. Reading, Writing, Mathematics and the Developing Brain: Listening to Many Voices, *Literacy Studies, 6*, 177–189.

Selemon, L. D., & Goldman-Rakic, P. S. (1999). The reduced neuropil hypothesis: A circuit based model of schizophrenia. *Biological Psychiatry, 45*, 17–25.

Senco Forum. (2005). Points of view from the SENCo Forum: Is it dyslexia? *British Journal of Special Education, 32,* 165.

Sexton, C. C., Gelhorn, H. L., Bell, J. A., & Classi, P. M. (2012). The co-occurrence of reading disorder and ADHD: Epidemiology, treatment, psychosocial impact, and economic burden. *Journal of Learning Disabilities, 45*(6), 538–564.

Shallice, T., & Warrington, E. K. (1977). The possible role of selective attention in acquired dyslexia. *Neuropsychologia, 15,* 31–41.

Shalom, D. B., & Poeppel, D. (2008). Functional anatomic models of language: Assembling the pieces. *Neuroscientist, 14,* 119–127.

Shanahan, M. A., Pennington, B. F., Yerys, B. E., Scott, A., Boada, R., Willcutt, E. G., et al. (2006). Processing speed deficits in attention deficit/hyperactivity disorder and reading disability. *Journal of Abnormal Child Psychology, 34,* 585–602.

Shankweiler, D., & Crain, S. (1986). Language mechanisms and reading disorders: A modular approach. *Cognition, 24,* 139–168.

Shankweiler, D., & Fowler, A. E. (2004). Questions people ask about the role of phonological processes in learning to read. *Reading and Writing: An Interdisciplinary Journal, 17,* 483–515.

Shapleske, J., Rossell, S. L., & Woodruff, P. W. (1999). The planum temporale: A systematic, quantitative review of its structural, functional and clinical significance. *Brain Research Review, 29,* 26–49.

Share, D. L. (1995). Phonological recoding and self-teaching: Sine qua non of reading acquisition. *Cognition, 55,* 151–218.

Share, D. L. (1999). Phonological recoding and orthographic learning: A direct test of the self-teaching hypothesis. *Journal of Experimental Child Psychology, 72,* 95–129.

Share, D. L. (2004). Orthographic learning at a glance: On the time course and developmental onset of self-teaching. *Journal of Experimental Child Psychology, 87,* 267–298.

Share, D. L. (2008). On the anglocentricities of current reading research and practice: The perils of overreliance on an "outlier" orthography. *Psychological Bulletin, 134,* 584–615.

Share, D. L., Jorm, A. F., Maclean, R., & Matthews, R. (2002). Temporal processing and reading disability. *Reading and Writing: An Interdisciplinary Journal, 15,* 151–178.

Share, D. L., & Silva, P. A. (2003). Gender bias in IQ-discrepancy and post-discrepancy definitions of reading disability. *Journal of Learning Disabilities, 36,* 4–14.

Share, D. L., & Stanovich, K. E. (1995). Cognitive processes in early reading development: Accommodating individual differences into a model of acquisition. *Issues in Education, 1,* 1–57.

Shaywitz, S., Morris, R., & Shaywitz, B. (2008). The education of dyslexic children from childhood to young adulthood. *Annual Review of Psychology, 59,* 451–475.

Shaywitz, B. A., Shaywitz, S. E., Blachman, B. A., & Pugh, K. R., et al. (2004a). Development of left occipitotemporal systems for skilled reading in children after a phonologically-based intervention. *Biological Psychiatry, 55*(9), 926–933.

Shaywitz, B. A., Shaywitz, S. E., Blachman, B. A., Pugh, K. R., Fulbright, R. K., Skudlarski, P., et al. (2004b). Development of left occipitotemporal systems for skilled reading in children after a phonologically-based intervention. *Biological Psychiatry, 55,* 926–933.

Shaywitz, B. A., Shaywitz, S. E., Pugh, K. R., Mencl, W. E., Fulbright, R. K., Skudlarski, P., et al. (2002). Disruption of posterior brain systems for reading in children with developmental dyslexia. *Biological Psychiatry, 52*, 101–110.

Shaywitz, B. A., Skudlarski, P., Holahan, J. M., Marchione, K. E., Constable, R. T., Fulbright, R. K., et al. (2007). Age-related changes in reading systems of dyslexic children. *Annals of Neurology, 61*, 363–370.

Shaywitz, S. E. (1996). Dyslexia. *Scientific American, 275*(5), 98–104.

Shaywitz, S. E. (2005). *Overcoming dyslexia.* New York: Alfred Knopf.

Shaywitz, S. E., Morris, R., & Shaywitz, B. A. (2008). The education of dyslexic children from childhood to young adulthood. *Annual Review of Psychology, 59*, 451–475.

Shaywitz, S. E., & Shaywitz, B. A. (2005). Dyslexia (specific reading disability). *Biological Psychiatry, 57*, 1301–1309.

Shaywitz, S. E., & Shaywitz, B. A. (2008). Paying attention to reading: The neurobiology of reading and dyslexia. *Development and Psychopathology, 20*, 1329–1349.

Shaywitz, S. E., & Shaywitz, B. A. (2013). Making a hidden disability visible: What has been learned from neurobiological studies of dyslexia. In H. L. Swanson, K. R. Harris, & S. Graham (Eds.), *Handbook of learning disabilities* (pp. 643–657). New York: Guilford Press.

Shaywitz, S. E., Shaywitz, B. A., Pugh, K. R., Fulbright, R. K., Constable, R. T., Mencl, W. E., et al. (1998). Functional disruption in the organization of the brain for reading in dyslexia. *Proceedings of the National Academy of Sciences, 95*, 2636–2641.

Shen, H., Liu, Y., Liu, P., Recker, R. R., & Deng, H. W. (2005). Nonreplication in genetic studies of complex diseases – lessons learned from studies of osteoporosis and tentative remedies. *Journal of Bone & Mineral Research, 20*, 365–376.

Shipstead, Z., Hicks, K. L., & Engle, R. W. (2012). CogMed working memory training: Does the evidence support the claims? *Journal of Applied Research in Memory and Cognition, 1*, 85–193.

Shipstead, Z., Redick, T. S., & Engle, R. W. (2012). Is working memory training effective? *Psychological Bulletin, 138*, 628–654.

Shiran, A., & Breznitz, Z. (2011). The effect of cognitive training on recall range and speed of information processing in the working memory of dyslexic and skilled readers. *Journal of Neurolinguistics, 24*, 524–537.

Shovman, M. M., & Ahissar, M. (2006). Isolating the impact of visual perception on dyslexics' reading ability. *Vision Research, 46*, 3514–3525.

Siegel, L. S., & Lipka, O. (2008). The definition of learning disabilities: Who is the individual with learning disabilities? In G. Reid, A. Fawcett, F. Manis, & L. Siegel (Eds.), *The Sage handbook of dyslexia* (pp. 290–307). London: Sage.

Siegel, L. S., & Mazabel, S. (2013). Basic cognitive processes and reading disabilities. In H. L. Swanson, K. R. Harris, & S. Graham (Eds.), *Handbook of learning disabilities* (pp. 186–213). New York: Guilford Press.

Siegel, L. S., & Ryan, E. B. (1989). The development of working memory in normally achieving and subtypes of learning disabled children. *Child Development, 60*, 973–980.

Silani, G., Frith, U., Demonet, J. F., Fazio, F., Perani, D., Price, C., et al. (2005). Brain abnormalities underlying altered activation in dyslexia: A voxel based morphometry study. *Brain, 128*, 2453–2461.

Silver, L. B. (1987). A review of the current controversial approaches for treating learning disabilities. *Journal of Learning Disabilities, 20*, 498–504.

Simmers, A. J., Bex, P. J., Smith, F. K. H., & Wilkins, A. J. (2001). Spatiotemporal visual function in tinted lens wearers. *Investigative Ophthalmology & Visual Science, 42*, 879–884.

Simos, P. G., Breier, J. I., Fletcher, J. M., Foorman, B. R., Bergman, E., Fishbeck, K., et al. (2000). Brain activation profiles in dyslexic children during non-word reading: a magnetic source imaging study. *Neuroscience Letters, 290*, 61–65.

Simos, P. G., Breier, J. I., Wheless, J. W., Maggio, W. W., Fletcher, J. M., Castillo, E. M., et al. (2000). Brain mechanisms for reading: The role of the superior temporal gyrus in word and pseudoword naming. *Neuroreport, 11*, 2443–2447.

Simos, P. G., Fletcher, J. M., Bergman, E., Breier, J. I., Foorman, B. R., Castillo, E. M., et al. (2002). Dyslexia-specific brain activation profile becomes normal following successful remedial training. *Neurology, 58*, 1203–1213.

Simos, P. G., Rezaie, R., Fletcher, J. M., Juranek, J., Passaro, A. D., Li, Z., et al. (2011). Functional disruption of the brain mechanism for reading: Effects of comorbidity and task difficulty among children with developmental learning problems. *Neuropsychology, 25*, 520–534.

Simpson, J., & Everatt, J. (2001). *Phonological skills and naming speed as predictors of future literacy deficits.* Paper presented at the British Dyslexia Association International Conference, Dyslexia: Dawn of the New Century, University of York. Reading.

Simpson, J., & Everatt, J. (2005). Reception class predictors of literacy skills. *British Journal of Educational Psychology, 75*, 171–188.

Singleton, C. H. (2009a). Visual stress and dyslexia. In G. Reid (Ed.), *The Routledge companion to dyslexia* (pp. 43–57). New York: Routledge.

Singleton, C. H. (2009b). *Intervention for dyslexia: A review of published evidence on the impact of specialist dyslexia teaching.* London: The Dyslexia-SpLD Trust.

Singleton, C. H. (2012). Visual stress and its relationship to dyslexia. In J. Stein & Z. Kapoula (Eds.), *Visual aspects of dyslexia* (pp. 91–110). Oxford: Oxford University Press.

Siok, W. T., Perfetti, C. A., Jin, Z., & Tan, L. H. (2004). Biological abnormality of impaired reading is constrained by culture. *Nature, 431*, 71–76.

Skiba, T., Landi, N., Wagner, R., & Grigorenko, E. L. (2011). In search of the perfect phenotype: An analysis of linkage and association studies of reading and reading-related processes. *Behavior Genetics, 41*, 6–30.

Skottun, B. C. (2000). The magnocellular deficit theory of dyslexia: The evidence from contrast sensitivity. *Vision Research, 40*, 111–127.

Skottun, B. C. (2011). On the use of visual motion perception to assess magnocellular integrity. *Journal of Integrative Neuroscience, 10*(1), 15–32.

Skottun, B. C., & Skoyles, J. (2006b). Is coherent motion an appropriate test for magnocelular sensitivity? *Brain and Cognition, 61*, 172–180.

Skottun, B. C., & Skoyles, J. (2011). Dyslexia, magnocellular integrity and rapidly presented stimuli. Nature Procedings. Retrieved June 10, 2012 from http://dx.doi.org/10.1038/npre.2011.6050.1

Skottun, B. C., & Skoyles, J. R. (2006a). Attention, reading and dyslexia. *Clinical & Experimental Optometry, 89*, 241–245.

Skottun, B. C., & Skoyles, J. R. (2008). Dyslexia and rapid visual processing: A commentary. *Journal of Clinical and Experimental Neuropsychology, 30*, 666–673.

Skottun, B. C., & Skoyles, J. R. (2010a). L- and M-cone ratios and magnocellular sensitivity in reading. *International Journal of Neuroscience, 120*, 241–244.

Skottun, B. C., & Skoyles, J. R. (2010b). Temporal order judgment in dyslexia – Task difficulty or temporal processing deficiency? *Neuropsychologia, 48*, 2226–2229.

Skoyles, J. R., & Skottun, B. C. (2004). On the prevalence of magnocellular deficits in the visual system of non-dyslexic individuals. *Brain and Language, 88*, 79–82.

Slavin, R. E., Lake, C., Chambers, B., Cheung, A., & Davis, S. (2009). Effective reading programs for the elementary grades: A best-evidence synthesis. *Review of Educational Research, 79*, 1391–1466.

Slavin, R. E., Lake, C., Davis, S., & Madden, N. A. (2011). Effective programs for struggling readers: A best-evidence synthesis. *Educational Research Review, 6*, 1–26.

Smith, F. (1971). *Understanding reading: A psycholinguistic analysis of reading and learning to read.* New York: Holt, Rinehart & Winston.

Smith, S. D. (2007). Genes, language development, and language disorders. *Mental Retardation and Developmental Disabilities, 13*, 95–105.

Smith, S. D., Gilger, J. W., & Pennington, B. F. (2001). Dyslexia and other specific learning disorders. In D. L. Rimoin, J. M. Conner, & R. E. Pyeritz (Eds.), *Emery and Rimoin's principles and practice of medical genetics* (pp. 2827–2865). New York: Churchill Livingstone.

Smith, S. D., Kimberling, W. J., Pennington, B. F., & Lubs, H. A. (1983). Specific reading disability: Identification of an inherited form through linkage analyses. *Science, 219*, 1345–1347.

Smith-Spark, J. H., & Fisk, J. E. (2007). Working memory functioning in developmental dyslexia. *Memory, 15*(1), 34–56.

Smith-Spark, J. H., Fisk, J. E., Fawcett, A. J., & Nicolson, R. I. (2003). Central executive impairments in adult dyslexics: Evidence from visuospatial working memory performance. *European Journal of Cognitive Psychology, 15*, 567–587.

Snow, C. E., Burns, M. S., & Griffin, P. (1998). *Preventing reading difficulties in young children.* Washington, DC: National Academy Press.

Snow, C. E., & Juel, C. (2005). Teaching children to read: What do we know about how to do it? In M. J. Snowling & C. Hulme (Eds.), *The science of reading: A handbook* (pp. 501–520). Oxford: Blackwell.

Snowling, M. J. (2000). *Dyslexia.* Oxford: Blackwell.

Snowling, M. J. (2008). Specific disorders and broader phenotypes: The case of dyslexia. *Quarterly Journal of Experimental Psychology, 61*, 142–156.

Snowling, M. J. (2010). *Dyslexia.* In C. L. Cooper, J. Field, U. Goswami, R. Jenkins, & B. J. Sahakian (Eds.), *Mental capital and mental wellbeing* (pp. 775–783). Oxford: Blackwell.

Snowling, M. J. (2011). Beyond phonological deficits: Sources of individual differences in reading disability. In S. A. Brady, D. Braze, & C. A. Fowler (Eds.), *Explaining individual differences in reading: Theory and evidence* (pp. 121–136). New York: Psychology Press.

Snowling, M. J. (2013). Early identification and interventions for dyslexia: A contemporary view. *Journal of Research in Special Educational Needs, 13*(1), 7–14.

Snowling, M. J., Duff, F., Petrou, A., Schiffeldrin, J., & Bailey, A. M. (2011). Identification of children at risk of dyslexia: The validity of teacher judgements using 'Phonic Phases'. *Journal of Research in Reading, 34*, 157–170.

Snowling, M. J., & Hulme, C. (1994). The development of phonological skills in children. *Philosophical Transactions of the Royal Society B, 346*, 21–26.

Snowling, M. J., & Hulme, C. (2003). A critique of claims from Reynolds, Nicolson & Hambly (2003) that DDAT is an effective treatment for reading problems: "Lies, damned lies and (inappropriate) statistics." *Dyslexia, 9*, 1–7.

Snowling, M. J., & Hulme, C. (2011). Evidence-based interventions for reading and language difficulties: Creating a virtuous circle. *British Journal of Educational Psychology, 81*, 1–23.

Snowling, M. J., & Hulme, C. (2012). Annual research review: The nature and classification of reading disorders – commentary on proposals for DSM-5. *Journal of Child Psychology and Psychiatry, 53*, 593–607.

Soler, J. (2009). The historical construction of dyslexia: Implications for higher education. In J. Soler, F. Fletcher-Campbell, & G. Reid (Eds.), *Understanding difficulties in literacy development: Issues and concepts* (pp. 39–50). London: Sage.

Soler, J. (2010). Dyslexia lessons: The politics of dyslexia and reading problems. In K. Hall, U. Goswami, C. Harrison, S. Ellis, & J. Soler (Eds.), *Interdisciplinary perspectives on learning to read* (pp. 179–192). London: Routledge.

Song, M., & Miskel, C. (2002). *Interest groups in national reading policy: Perceived influence and beliefs on teaching reading.* Ann Arbor: University of Michigan, Center for the Improvement of Early Reading Achievement.

Song, R., Zhang, J., Wang, B., Zhang, H., & Wu, H. (2013). A near-infrared brain function study of Chinese dyslexic children. *Neurocase: The Neural Basis of Cognition, 19*(4), 382–389.

Soroli, E., Szenkovits, G., & Ramus, F. (2010). Exploring dyslexics' phonological deficit III: Foreign speech perception and production. *Dyslexia, 16*, 318–340.

Spear-Swerling, L. (2004). A road map for understanding reading disability and other reading problems: Origins, intervention and prevention. In R. Ruddell & N. Unrau (Eds.), *Theoretical models and processes of reading* (Vol. 5). Newark, DE: International Reading Association.

Spear-Swerling, L. (2011). Patterns of reading disabilities across development. In R. Allington & A. McGill-Franzen (Eds.), *Handbook of research on reading disabilities* (pp. 149–161). New York: Routledge.

Spear-Swerling, L., & Sternberg, R. J. (1994). The road not taken: An integrative theoretical model of reading disability. *Journal of Learning Disabilities, 27*, 91–103.

Speece, D. L. (2005). Hitting the moving target known as reading development: Some thoughts on screening children for secondary interventions. *Journal of Learning Disabilities, 38*, 487–493.

Speece, D. L., Ritchey, K. D., Silverman, R., Schatsneider, C., Walker, C. Y., & Andrusik, K. N. (2010). Identifying children in middle childhood who are at risk for reading problems. *School Psychology Review, 39*, 258–276.

Speece, D. L., & Shekitka, L. (2002). How should reading disabilities be operationalized? A survey of experts. *Learning Disabilities Research & Practice, 17*, 118–123.

Spencer, S., & Manis, F. (2010). The effects of a fluency intervention program on fluency and comprehension outcomes of middle-school students with severe reading deficits. *Learning Disabilities Research & Practice, 25*, 76–86.

Spinelli, D., De Luca, M., Judica, A., & Zoccolotti, P. (2002). Crowding effects on word identification in developmental dyslexia. *Cortex, 38*, 179–200.

Spironelli, C., & Angrilli, A. (2006). Language lateralization in phonological, semantic and orthographic tasks: A slow evoked potential study. *Behavioural Brain Research, 175*, 296–304.

Spironelli, C., Angrilli, A., & Pertile, M. (2008). Language plasticity in aphasics after recovery: Evidence from slow evoked potentials. *Neuroimage, 40*, 912–922.

Spironelli, C., Penolazzi, B., & Angrilli, A. (2008). Dysfunctional hemispheric asymmetry of theta and beta EEG activity during linguistic tasks in developmental dyslexia. *Biological Psychology, 77*, 123–131.

Spironelli, C., Penolazzi, B., Vio, C., & Angrilli, A. (2010). Cortical reorganization in dyslexic children after phonological training: Evidence from early evoked potentials. *Brain, 133*, 3385–3395.

Stackhouse, J., & Wells, B. (1997). *Children's speech and literacy difficulties: A psycholinguistic framework*. London: Whurr.

Stahl, S. A., & Miller, P. D. (1989). Whole language and language experience approaches for beginning reading: A quantitative research synthesis. *Review of Educational Research, 59*, 87–116.

Stainthorp, R., Stuart, M., Powell, D., Quinlan, P., & Garwood, H. (2010). Visual processing deficits in children with slow RAN performance. *Scientific Studies of Reading, 14*, 266–292.

Stankiewicz, P., & Lupski, J. R. (2010). Structural variation in the human genome and its role in disease. *Annual Review of Medicine, 61*, 437–455.

Stanovich, K. E. (1980). Toward an interactive-compensatory model of individual differences in the development of reading fluency. *Reading Research Quarterly, 16*, 32–71.

Stanovich, K. E. (1986). Matthew effects in reading: Some consequences of individual differences in the acquisition of literacy. *Reading Research Quarterly, 21*, 360–407.

Stanovich, K. E. (1988). Explaining the differences between the dyslexic and the garden-variety poor reader: The phonological-core variable-difference model. *Journal of Learning Disabilities, 21*, 590–604.

Stanovich, K. E. (1992). Response to Christensen. *Reading Research Quarterly, 27*, 279–280.

Stanovich, K. E. (1994). Annotation: Does dyslexia exist? *Journal of Child Psychology and Psychiatry, 35*, 579–595.

Stanovich, K. E. (1996). Toward a more inclusive definition of dyslexia. *Dyslexia, 2*, 154–166.

Stanovich, K. E. (1998). Twenty-five years of research on the reading process: The grand synthesis and what it means for our field. In T. Shanahan & F. Rodriguez-Brown (Eds.), *Forty-seventh yearbook of the National Reading Conference* (pp. 44–58). Chicago: National Reading Conference.

Stanovich, K. E. (2000). *Progress in understanding reading: Scientific foundations and new frontiers*. New York: Guilford Press.

Stanovich, K. E. (2005). The future of a mistake: Will discrepancy measurement continue to make the learning disabilities field a pseudoscience? *Learning Disability Quarterly*, *28*, 103–106.

Stanovich, K. E., & Siegel, L. S. (1994). Phenotypic performance profile of children with reading disabilities: A regression-based test of the phonological-core variable-difference model. *Journal of Educational Psychology*, *86*, 24–53.

Stanovich, K. E., & Stanovich, P. J. (1997). Further thoughts on aptitude/achievement discrepancy. *Educational Psychology in Practice*, *13*, 3–8.

Stein, J. (2008). The neurobiological basis of dyslexia. In H. Reid, A. Fawcett, F. Manis, & L. Siegel (Eds.), *The Sage handbook of dyslexia* (pp. 53–76). London: Sage.

Stein, J. (2012a). The magnocellular theory of dyslexia. In A. A. Benasich & R. H. Fitch (Eds.), *Developmental dyslexia: Early precursors, neurobehavioral markers, and biological substrates* (pp. 32–45). Baltimore, MD: Paul H. Brookes Publishing.

Stein, J. (2012b). Visual contributions to reading difficulties: The magnocellular theory. In J. Stein & Z. Kapoula (Eds.), *Visual aspects of dyslexia* (pp. 171–197). Oxford: Oxford University Press.

Stein, J., & Kapoula, Z. (Eds.). (2012). *Visual aspects of dyslexia*. Oxford: Oxford University Press.

Stein, J., & Talcott, J. B. (1999). Impaired neuronal timing in developmental dyslexia – The magnocellular hypothesis. *Dyslexia*, *5*, 59–77.

Stein, J., Talcott, J. B., & Walsh, V. (2000). Controversy about the visual magnocellular deficit in developmental dyslexics. *Trends in Cognitive Science*, *4*, 209–211.

Stein, J., & Walsh, V. (1997). To see but not to read: The magnocellular theory of dyslexia. *Trends in Neuroscience*, *20*, 147–152.

Steinberg, E., & Andrist, C. G. (2012). Dyslexia comes to Congress: A call to action. Retrieved April 17, 2012 from http://www.interdys.org/DyslexiaComesToCongress.htm?utm_source=April+2012+eXaminer&utm_campaign=April+eXaminer&utm_medium=email.

Steinbrink, C., Vogt, K., Kastrup, A., Muller, H. P., Juengling, F. D., Kassubek, J., et al. (2008). The contribution of white and gray matter differences to developmental dyslexia: Insights from DTI and VBM at 3.0 T. *Neuropsychologia*, *46*, 3170–3178.

Stenneken, P., Egetemeir, J., Schulte-Körne, G., Müller, H. J., Schneider, W. X., & Finke, K. (2011). Slow perceptual processing at the core of developmental dyslexia: A parameter-based assessment of visual attention. *Neuropsychologia*, *49*, 3454–3465.

Stephenson, J. (2009). A case study of unfounded concepts underpinning controversial practices: Lost in "Space Dyslexia". *International Journal of Disability, Development and Education*, *56*, 37–47.

Stephenson, S. (1904). Congenital word blindness. *Lancet*, *2*, 827–828.

Stephenson, S. (1907). Six cases of congenital word-blindness affecting three generations of one family. *Ophthalmoscope*, *5*, 482–484.

Sternberg, R. J., & Grigorenko, E. L. (1999a). Myths in psychology and education regarding the gene-environment debate. *Teachers College Record*, *100*, 536–553.

Sternberg, R. J., & Grigorenko, E. L. (1999b). *Our labeled children. (What every parent and teacher needs to know about learning disabilities)*. Reading, MA: Perseus Publishing Group.

Sternberg, R. J., & Grigorenko, E. L. (2002a). Difference scores in the identification of children with learning disabilities: It's time to use a different method. *Journal of School Psychology, 40*, 65–83.

Sternberg, R. J., & Grigorenko, E. L. (2002b). *Dynamic testing.* New York: Cambridge University Press.

Stevens, C., Harn, B., Chard, D., Currin, J., Parisi, D., & Neville, H. (2013). Examining the role of attention and instruction in at-risk kindergarteners: Electrophysiological measures of selective auditory attention before and after an early literacy intervention. *Journal of Learning Disabilities, 46*(1), 73–86.

Stevenson, J. (2011). Commentary: A contribution to evidence-informed education policy – reflections on Strong, Torgerson, Torgerson, and Hulme. *Journal of Child Psychology and Psychiatry, 52*, 236–237.

Stoodley, C. J., Fawcett, A. J., Nicolson, R. I., & Stein, J. F. (2006). Balancing and pointing tasks in dyslexic and control adults. *Dyslexia, 12*, 276–288.

Stoodley, C. J., & Stein, J. F. (2011). The cerebellum and dyslexia. *Cortex, 47*, 101–116.

Stoodley, C. J., & Stein, J. F. (2013). Cerebellar function in developmental dyslexia. *Cerebellum, 12*(2), 267–276.

Strauss, A. A., & Lehtinen, L. E. (1947). *Psychopathology and education of the brain-injured child.* New York: Grune & Stratton.

Strong, G. K., Torgerson, C. J., Torgerson, D., & Hulme, C. (2011). A systematic meta-analytic review of evidence for the effectiveness of the "Fast ForWord" language intervention program. *Journal of Child Psychology and Psychiatry, 52*(3), 224–235.

Studdert-Kennedy, M. (2002). Deficits in phoneme awareness do not arise from failures in rapid auditory processing. *Reading and Writing, 15*, 5–14.

Studdert-Kennedy, M., & Mody, M. (1995). Auditory temporal perception deficits in the reading impaired: A critical review of the evidence. *Psychonomic Bulletin and Review, 2*, 508–514.

Stuebing, K. K., Barth, A. E., Molfese, P. J., Weiss, B., & Fletcher, J. M. (2009). IQ is not strongly related to response to reading instruction: A meta-analytic interpretation. *Exceptional Children, 76*, 31–51.

Stuebing, K. K., Fletcher, J. M., Branum-Martin, L., & Francis, D. J. (2012). Evaluation of the technical adequacy of three methods for identifying specific learning disabilities based on cognitive discrepancies. *School Psychology Review, 41*, 3–22.

Stuebing, K. K., Fletcher, J. M., & Hughes, L. C. (2012). Meta-analysis and inadequate responders to intervention: A response. *Journal of Learning Disabilities, 45*(6), 565–569.

Stuebing, K. K., Fletcher, J. M., LeDoux, J. M., Lyon, R. G., Shaywitz, S. E., & Shaywitz, B. A. (2002). Validity of IQ-discrepancy classifications of reading disabilities: A meta-analysis. *American Educational Research Journal, 39*, 469–518.

Sumner, C. R., Gathercole, S., Greenbaum, M., Rubin, R., Williams, D., Hollandbeck, M., et al. (2009). Atomoxetine for the treatment of attention-deficit/hyperactivity disorder (ADHD) in children with ADHD and dyslexia. *Child and Adolescent Psychiatry and Mental Health, 3*, 40.

Sunseth, K., & Bowers, P. G. (2002). Rapid naming and phonemic awareness: Contributions to reading, spelling, and orthographic knowledge. *Scientific Studies of Reading, 6*, 401–429.

Surányi, Z., Csépe, V., Richardson, U., Thomson, J. M., Honbolygó, F., & Goswami, U. (2009). Sensitivity to rhythmic parameters in dyslexic children: A comparison of Hungarian and English. *Reading and Writing, 22*, 41–56.

Swanson, H. L. (1978). Memory development in learning disabled children: Evidence from nonverbal tasks. *Journal of Psychology: Interdisciplinary and Applied, 100*, 9–12.

Swanson, H. L. (1999). Reading research for students with LD: A meta-analysis of intervention outcomes. *Journal of Learning Disabilities, 32*, 504–532.

Swanson, H. L. (2003). Age-related differences in learning disabled and skilled readers' working memory. *Journal of Experimental Child Psychology, 85*, 1–31.

Swanson, H. L. (2006). Working memory and reading disabilities: Both phonological and executive processing deficits are important. In T. P. Alloway & S. E. Gathercole (Eds.), *Working memory and neurodevelopmental disorders* (pp. 59–88). New York: Psychology Press.

Swanson, H. L. (2012). Meta-analysis and inadequate responders to intervention: A reply. *Journal of Learning Disabilities, 45*(6), 570–575.

Swanson, H. L. (2013). Meta-analysis of research on children with learning disabilities. In H. L. Swanson, K. R. Harris, & S. Graham (Eds.), *Handbook of learning disabilities* (pp. 627–642). New York: Guilford Press.

Swanson, H. L., Ashbaker, M. H., & Lee, C. (1996). Learning disable readers' working memory as a function of processing demands. *Journal of Experimental Child Psychology, 61*, 242–275.

Swanson, H. L., Hoskyn, M., & Lee, C. (1999). *Interventions for students with learning disabilities: A meta-analysis of treatment outcomes.* New York: Guilford.

Swanson, H. L., Howard, C. B., & Sáez, L. (2006). Do different components of working memory underlie different subgroups of reading disabilities? *Journal of Learning Disabilities, 39*, 252–269.

Swanson, H. L., & Howell, M. (2001). Working memory, short-term memory, and speech rate as predictors of children's reading performance at different ages. *Journal of Educational Psychology, 93*, 720–734.

Swanson, H. L., & Hsieh, C.-J. (2009). Reading disabilities in adults: A selective meta-analysis of the literature. *Review of Educational Research, 79*, 1362–1390.

Swanson, H. L., & O'Connor, R. (2009). The role of working memory and fluency practice on the reading comprehension of students who are dysfluent readers. *Journal of Learning Disabilities, 42*, 548–575.

Swanson, H. L., Trainin, G., Necoechea, D. M., & Hammill, D. D. (2003). Rapid naming, phonological awareness, and reading: A meta-analysis of the correlation evidence. *Review of Educational Research, 73*, 407–440.

Swanson, H. L., & Zheng, X. (2013). Memory difficulties in children and adults with learning disabilities. In H. L. Swanson, K. R. Harris, & S. Graham (Eds.), *Handbook of learning disabilities* (pp. 214–238). New York: Guilford Press.

Swanson, H. L., Zheng, X., & Jerman, O. (2009). Working memory, short-term memory, and reading disabilities: A selective meta-analysis of the literature. *Journal of Learning Disabilities, 42*, 260–287.

Szenkovits, G., & Ramus, F. (2005). Exploring dyslexics' phonological deficit I: Lexical vs. sub-lexical and input vs. output processes. *Dyslexia, 11*, 253–268.

Szwed, M., Ventura, P., Querido, L., Cohen, L., & Dehaene, S. (2012). Reading acquisition enhances an early visual process of contour integration. *Developmental Science, 15*, 139–149.

Taipale, M., Kaminen, N., Nopola-Hemmi, J., Haltia, T., Myllyluoma, B., Lyytinen, H., et al. (2003). A candidate gene for developmental dyslexia encodes a nuclear tetratricopeptide repeat domain protein dynamically regulated in brain. *Proceedings of the National Academy of Sciences of the United States of America, 100*, 11553–11558.

Talcott. J. B., Hansen, P. C., Willis-Owen, C., McKinnell, I. W., Richardson, A. J., & Stein, J. F. (1998). Visual magnocellular impairment in adult developmental dyslexics. *Neuro-ophthalmology, 20*, 187–201.

Talcott, J. B., Witton, C., Hebb, G. S., Stoodley, C. J., Westwood, E. A., France, S. J., et al. (2002). On the relationship between dynamic visual and auditory processing and literacy skills; results from a large primary-school study. *Dyslexia, 8*, 204–225.

Talcott, J. B., Witton, C., McLean, M. F., Hansen, P. C., Rees, A., Green, G. G. R., et al. (1999). Can sensitivity to auditory frequency modulation predict children's phonological and reading skills? *NeuroReport, 10*, 2045–2050.

Tallal, P. (1980). Auditory temporal perception, phonics, and reading disabilities in children. *Brain and Language, 9*, 182–198.

Tallal, P., & Gaab, N. (2006). Dynamic auditory processing, musical experience and language development. *Trends in Neurosciences, 29*, 382–390.

Tallal, P., Miller, S. L., Bedi, G., Byma, G., Wang, X., Nagarajan, S. S., et al. (1996). Language comprehension in language-learning impaired children improved with acoustically modified speech. *Science, 271*, 81–84.

Tan, L. H., Spinks, J. A., Eden, G., Perfetti, C. A., & Siok, W. T. (2005). Reading depends on writing, in Chinese. *Proceedings of the National Academy of Sciences, 102*, 8781–8785.

Tanaka, H., Black, J. M., Hulme, C., Stanley, L. M., Kesler, S. R., Whitfield-Gabrieli, S., et al. (2011). The brain basis of the phonological deficit in dyslexia is independent of IQ. *Psychological Science, 22*, 1442–1451.

Tannock, R. (2013). Rethinking ADHD and LD in *DSM-5*: Proposed changes in diagnostic criteria. *Journal of Learning Disabilities, 46*(1), 5–25.

Tansey, M. (1991). Wechsler (WISC-R) changes following treatment of learning disabilities via EEG biofeedback training in a private practice setting. *Australian Journal of Psychology, 34*, 147–153.

Taylor, E. (2011). Commentary: Reading and attention problems – how are they connected? Reflections on reading McGrath et al. (2011). *Journal of Child Psychology and Psychiatry, 52*, 558–559.

Taylor, E., & Rutter, M. (2008). Classification. In M. Rutter, D. Bishop, D. Pine, S. Scott, J. Stevenson, E. Taylor & E. Thapar (Eds.), *Rutter's child and adolescent psychiatry* (5th ed., pp. 18–31). Oxford: Wiley-Blackwell.

Taylor, J., Roehrig, A. D., Soden Hensler, B., Connor, C. M., & Schatschneider, C. (2010). Teacher quality moderates the genetic effects on early reading. *Science, 328*, 512–514.

Temple, E. (2002). Brain mechanisms in normal and dyslexic readers. *Current Opinion in Neurobiology, 12*, 178–183.

Temple, E., Deutsch, G. K., Poldrack, R. A., Miller, S. L., Tallal, P., Merzenich, M. M., et al. (2003). Neural deficits in children with dyslexia ameliorated by behavioral remediation: evidence from functional MRI. *Proceedings of the National Academy of Sciences of the United States of America, 100*, 2860–2865.

Temple, E., Poldrack, R. A., Salidis, J., Deutsch, G. K., Tallal, P., Merzenich, M. M., et al. (2001). Disrupted neural responses to phonological and orthographic processing in dyslexic children: An fMRI study. *Neuroreport, 12*, 299–307.

Thomas, C. J. (1905). Congenital "word-blindness" and its treatment. *Ophthalmoscope, 3*, 380–385.

Thompson, T. M., Sharfi, D., Lee, M., Yrigollen, C. M., Naumova, O. Yu., & Grigorenko, E. L. (2013). Comparison of whole-genome DNA methylation patterns in whole blood, saliva, and lymphoblastoid cell lines. *Behavior Genetics, 43*, 168–176.

Thomson, J. M., Leong, V., & Goswami, U. (2013). Auditory processing interventions and developmental dyslexia: A comparison of phonemic and rhythmic approaches. *Reading and Writing, 26*(2), 139–161.

Thomson, M. (1990). *Developmental dyslexia*. London: Whurr.

Thomson, M. (2002). Dyslexia and diagnosis. *The Psychologist, 15*, 151.

Thomson, M. (2003). Monitoring dyslexics' intelligence and attainments: A follow-up study. *Dyslexia, 9*, 3–17.

Thomson, M. (2009). *The psychology of dyslexia: A handbook for teachers* (2nd ed.). Oxford: Wiley-Blackwell.

Thornton, K. E., & Carmody, D. P. (2005). Electroencephalogram biofeedback for reading disability and traumatic brain injury. *Child and Adolescent Psychiatric Clinics of North America, 14*, 137–162.

Tønnessen, F. E. (1995). On defining 'dyslexia'. *Scandinavian Journal of Educational Research, 39*, 139–156.

Tønnessen, F. E. (1997). How can we best define 'dyslexia'? *Dyslexia, 3*, 78–92.

Torgerson, C. J., Brooks, G., & Hall, G. (2006). *A systematic review of the research literature on the use of systematic phonics in the teaching of reading and spelling*. London: Department for Education and Skills.

Torgesen, J. K. (2000). Individual differences in response to early interventions in reading: The lingering problem of treatment resisters. *Learning Disabilities Research and Practice, 15*, 55–64.

Torgesen, J. K. (2002). The prevention of reading difficulties. *Journal of School Psychology, 40*, 7–26.

Torgesen, J. K. (2004). Lessons learned from research on interventions for students who have difficulty learning to read. In P. McCardle & V. Chhabra (Eds.), *The voice of evidence in reading research* (pp. 355–382). Baltimore, MD: Brookes.

Torgesen, J. K. (2005). Recent discoveries on remedial interventions for children with dyslexia. In M. J. Snowling & C. Hulme (Eds.), *The science of reading: A handbook* (pp. 521–537). Oxford: Blackwell.

Torgesen, J. K. (2007). Using an RTI model to guide early reading instruction: Effects on identification rates for students with learning disabilities. Retrieved February 26, 2012 from http://www.fcrr.org/TechnicalReports/Response_to_intervention_Florida .pdf.

Torgesen, J. K., Alexander, A. W., Wagner, R. K., Rashotte, C. A., Voeller, K. K., & Conway, T. (2001). Intensive remedial instruction for children with severe reading disabilities: Immediate and long-term outcomes from two instructional approaches. *Journal of Learning Disabilities, 34*, 33–58.

Torgesen, J. K., Foorman, B. R., & Wagner, R. K. (n.d.). Dyslexia: A Brief for Educators, Parents, and Legislators in Florida – FCRR Technical Report #8. Florida Center for Reading Research. Retrieved August 9, 2012 from http://www.fcrr.org/TechnicalReports/Dyslexia_Technical_Assistance_Paper-Final.pdf.

Torgesen, J. K., Rashotte, C. A., & Alexander, A. W. (2001). Principles of fluency instruction in reading: Relationships with established empirical outcomes. In M. Wolf (Ed.), *Dyslexia, fluency, and the brain* (pp. 333–355). Parkton, MD: York.

Torgesen, J. K., Wagner, R.K., Rashotte, C.A., Herron, J., & Lindamood, P. (2010). Computer-assisted instruction to prevent early reading difficulties in students at risk for dyslexia: Outcomes from two instructional approaches. *Annals of Dyslexia, 60*(1), 40–56.

Torgesen, J. K., Wagner, R. K., Rashotte, C. A., Rose, E., Lindamood, P., Conway, T., et al. (1999). Preventing reading failure in young children with phonological processing disabilities: Group and individual responses to instruction. *Journal of Educational Psychology, 91*, 579–593.

Torppa, M., Lyytinen, P., Erskine, J., Eklund, K., & Lyytinen, H. (2010). Language development, literacy skills, and predictive connections to reading in Finnish children with and without familial risk for dyslexia. *Journal of Learning Disabilities, 43*, 308–321.

Torppa, M., Parrila, R., Niemi, P., Lerkkanen, M.-K., Poikkeus, A.-M., & Nurmi, J.-E. (2013). The double deficit hypothesis in the transparent Finnish orthography: a longitudinal study from kindergarten to Grade 2. *Reading and Writing, 26*, 1353–1380.

Townend, J. (2000). Phonological awareness and other foundational skills of literacy. In J. Townend & M. Turner (Eds.), *Dyslexia in practice: A guide for teachers* (pp. 1–29). London: Kluwer.

Tran, L., Sanchez, T., Arellano, B., & Swanson, H. L. (2011). A meta-analysis of the RTI literature for children at risk of reading disabilities. *Journal of Learning Disabilities, 44*(3), 283–295.

Tree, J. J., & Kay, J. (2006). Phonological dyslexia and phonological impairment: An exception to the rule? *Neuropsychologia, 44*, 2861–2873.

Tressoldi, P. E., Lonciari, I., & Vio, C. (2000). Treatment of specific developmental reading disorders, derived from single- and dual-route models. *Journal of Learning Disabilities, 33*, 278–285.

Troia, G. A., & Whitney, S. D. (2003). A close look at the efficacy of Fast ForWord Language for children with academic weaknesses. *Contemporary Educational Psychology, 28*, 465–494.

Tunmer, W. (2011). Foreword. In S. A. Brady, D. Braze, & C. A. Fowler (Eds.), *Explaining individual differences in reading: Theory and evidence* (pp. ix–xiii). New York: Psychology Press.

Tunmer, W. E. (2008). Recent developments in reading intervention research: Introduction to the special issue. *Reading and Writing: An Interdisciplinary Journal, 21*, 299–316.

Tunmer, W. E., & Chapman, J. W. (2003). The reading recovery approach to preventive early intervention. As good as it gets? *Reading Psychology, 24*, 337–360.

Tunmer, W. E., & Greaney, K. (2010). Defining dyslexia. *Journal of Learning Disabilities, 43*, 229–243.

Tunmer, W. E., & Nicholson, T. (2011). The development and teaching of word recognition skill. In M. L. Kamil, P. D. Pearson, E. B. Moje, & P. Afflerbach (Eds.), *Handbook of reading research* (Vol. 4, pp. 405–431). London: Routledge.

Tunmer, W. E., & Prochnow, J. E. (2009). Cultural relativism and literacy education: Explicit teaching based on specific learning needs is not deficit theory. In R. Openshaw & E. Rata (Eds.), *Thinking inside the square: Political and cultural conformity in New Zealand* (pp. 154–190). Auckland: Pearson Education.

Turkeltaub, P. E., Eden, G. F., Jones, K. M., & Zeffiro, T. A. (2002). Meta-analysis of the functional neuroanatomy of single-word reading: method and validation. *Neuroimage, 16*, 765–780.

Turner, D. A. (2012). Education and neuroscience. *Contemporary Social Science, 7*(2), 167–179.

U.S. Department of Education (2004). *Individuals with Disabilities Education Improvement Act of 2004 (IDEA)*, Pub. L. No. 108–446, 118 Stat. 2647.

Vadasy, P. F., & Sanders, E. A. (2010). Efficacy of supplemental phonics-based instruction for low-skilled kindergarteners in the context of language minority status and classroom phonics instruction. *Journal of Educational Psychology, 102*, 786–803.

Vadasy, P. F., Sanders, E. A., & Abbott, R. D. (2008). Effects of supplemental early reading intervention at 2-year follow-up: Reading skill growth patterns and predictors. *Scientific Studies of Reading, 12*, 51–89.

Vaessen, A., & Blomert, L. (2010). Long-term cognitive dynamics of fluent reading development. *Journal of Experimental Child Psychology, 105*, 213–231.

Vaessen, A., Gerretsen, P., & Blomert, L. (2009). Naming problems do not reflect a second independent core deficit in dyslexia: Double deficits explored. *Journal of Experimental Child Psychology, 103*, 202–221.

Valdois, S., Bidet-Ildei, C., Lassus-Sangosse, D., Reilhac, C., N'guyen-Morel, M., Guinet, E., et al. (2011). A visual processing but no phonological disorder in a child with mixed dyslexia. *Cortex, 47*, 1197–1218.

Valdois, S., Lassus-Sangosse, D., & Lobier, M. (2012a). The visual nature of the visual attention span disorder in developmental dyslexia. In J. Stein & Z. Kapoula (Eds.), *Visual aspects of dyslexia* (pp. 111–121). Oxford: Oxford University Press.

Valdois, S., Lassus-Sangosse, D., & Lobier, M. (2012b). Impaired letter-string processing in developmental dyslexia: What visual-to-phonology code mapping disorder? *Dyslexia, 18*, 77–93.

Valencia, S. W. (2011). Reader profiles and reading disabilities. In R. Allington & A. McGill-Franzen (Eds.), *Handbook of research on reading disabilities* (pp. 25–35). New York: Routledge.

van Atteveldt, N., Formisano, E., Goebel, R., & Blomert, L. (2004). Integration of letters and speech sounds in the human brain. *Neuron, 43*, 271 282.

van Bergen, E., de Jong, P. F., Maassen, B., Krikhaar, E., Plakas, A., & van der Leij, A. (2012). Child and parental literacy levels within families with a history of dyslexia. *Journal of Child Psychology and Psychiatry, 53*, 28–36.

van Bergen, E., de Jong, P. F., Plakas, A., Maassen, B., & van der Leij, A. (in press). IQ of four-year-olds who go on to develop dyslexia. *Journal of Learning Disabilities*,

van der Leij, A. (2013). Dyslexia and early intervention: What did we learn from the Dutch Programme? *Dyslexia, 19*, 241–255.

van der Leij, A., van Bergen, E., van Zuijen, T., de Jong, P., Maurits, N., & Maassen, B. (2013). Precursors of developmental dyslexia: An overview of the Longitudinal Dutch Dyslexia Programme Study. *Dyslexia, 19*, 191–213.

van der Sluis, S., Verhage, M., Posthuma, D., & Dolan, C. V. (2010). Phenotypic complexity, measurement bias, and poor phenotypic resolution contribute to the missing heritability problem in genetic association studies. *PLoS ONE, 5*(11), e13929. doi:10.1371/journal.pone.0013929.

Van Ingelghem, M. C. A., van Wieringen, A. W. J., Vandenbussche, E., Onghena, P., & Ghesquiere, P. (2001). Psychophysical evidence for a general temporal processing deficit in children with dyslexia. *Neuroreport, 12*, 3603–3607.

VanDerHeyden, A. M. (2011). Technical adequacy of response to intervention decisions. *Exceptional Children, 77*(3), 335–350.

Vandermosten, M., Boets, B., Luts, H., Poelmans, H., Golestani, N., Wouters, J., et al. (2010). Adults with dyslexia are impaired in categorizing speech and nonspeech sounds on the basis of temporal cues. *Proceedings of the National Academy of Sciences, 107*, 10389–10394.

Vandermosten, M., Boets, B., Wouters, J., & Ghesquière, P. (2012). A qualitative and quantitative review of diffusion tensor imaging studies in reading and dyslexia. *Neuroscience & Biobehavioral Reviews, 36*, 1532–1552.

van Zuijen, T., Plakas, A., Maassen, B., Maurits, N. M., & van der Leij, A. (2013). Infant ERPs separate children at risk of dyslexia who become good readers from those who become poor readers. *Developmental Science, 16*(4), 554–563.

Vargo, F. E., Grossner, G. S., & Spafford, C. S. (1995). Digit span and other WISC-R scores in the diagnosis of dyslexic children. *Perceptual and Motor Skills, 80*, 1219–1229.

Vaughn, S., Cirino, P. T., Wanzek, J., Wexler, J., Francis, D. J., Fletcher, J. M., et al. (2010). Response to intervention for middle school students with reading difficulties: Effects of a primary and secondary intervention. *School Psychology Review, 39*, 3–21.

Vaughn, S., Denton, C. A., & Fletcher, J. M. (2010). Why intensive interventions are necessary for students with severe reading difficulties. *Psychology in the Schools, 47*, 432–444.

Vaughn, S., & Fletcher, J. M. (2010). Thoughts on rethinking response to intervention with secondary students. *School Psychology Review, 39*, 296–299.

Vaughn, S., & Fletcher, J. M. (2012). Response to intervention with secondary school students with reading difficulties. *Journal of Learning Disabilities, 45*, 244–256.

Vaughn, S., Fletcher, J. M., Francis, D. J., Denton, C. A., Wanzek, J., Wexler, J., et al. (2008). Response to intervention with older students with reading difficulties. *Learning and Individual Differences, 18*, 338–345.

Vaughn, S., & Linan-Thompson, S. (2003). What is special about special education for students with learning disabilities? *Journal of Special Education, 37*, 140–147.

Vaughn, S., & Roberts, G. (2007). Secondary interventions in reading: Providing additional instruction for students at risk. *Teaching Exceptional Children, 39*, 40–46.

Vaughn, S., Wanzek, J., Murray, C. S., Scammacca, N., Linan-Thompson, S., & Woodruff, A. L. (2009). Response to early reading intervention: Examining higher and lower responders. *Exceptional Children, 75*, 165–183.

Vaughn, S., Wanzek, J., Wexler, J., Barth, A., Cirino, P. T., Fletcher, J., et al. (2010). The relative effects of group size on reading progress of older students with reading difficulties. *Reading and Writing, 23*, 931–956.

Vaughn, S., Wexler, J., Leroux, A, Roberts, G., Denton, C., Barth, A., & Fletcher, J. (2012). Effects of intensive reading intervention for eighth-grade students with persistently inadequate response to intervention. *Journal of Learning Disabilities, 45*(6), 515–525.

Vaughn, S., Wexler, J., Roberts, G., Barth, A., Cirino, P. T., Romain, M. A., et al. (2011). Effects of individualized and standardized interventions on middle school students with reading disabilities. *Exceptional Children, 77*, 391–407.

Vellutino, F. R. (1979). *Dyslexia: Theory and research*. Cambridge, MA: MIT Press.

Vellutino, F. R. (1987). Dyslexia. *Scientific American, 256*, 34–41.

Vellutino, F. R., & Fletcher, J. M. (2007). Developmental dyslexia. In M. J. Snowling & C. Hulme (Eds.), *The science of reading: A handbook* (pp. 362–378). Malden, MA: Blackwell.

Vellutino, F. R., Fletcher, J. M., Snowling, M. J., & Scanlon, D. M. (2004). Specific reading disability (dyslexia): What have we learned in the past four decades? *Journal of Child Psychology & Psychiatry, 45*, 2–40.

Vellutino, F. R., Scanlon, D. M., & Jaccard, J. (2003). Toward distinguishing between cognitive and experiential deficits as primary sources of difficulty in learning to read: A two year follow-up of difficult to remediate, readily remediated poor readers. In B. R. Foorman (Ed.), *Preventing and remediating reading difficulties: Bringing science to scale* (pp. 73–120). Baltimore, MD: York Press.

Vellutino, F. R., Scanlon, D. M., & Lyon, G. R. (2000). Differentiating between difficult-to-remediate and readily remediated poor readers: More evidence against the IQ-achievement discrepancy definition for reading disability. *Journal of Learning Disabilities, 33*, 223–238.

Vellutino, F. R., Scanlon, D. M., Sipay, E. R., Small, S. G., Pratt, A., Chen, R., et al. (1996). Cognitive profiles of difficult-to-remediate and readily remediated poor readers: Early intervention as a vehicle for distinguishing between cognitive and experiential deficits as basic causes of specific reading disability. *Journal of Educational Psychology, 88*, 601–638.

Vellutino, F. R., Scanlon, D. M., Small, S., & Fanuele, D. P. (2006). Response to intervention as a vehicle for distinguishing between children with and without reading disabilities: Evidence for the role of kindergarten and first grade interventions. *Journal of Learning Disabilities, 39*, 157–169.

Vellutino, F. R., Scanlon, D. M., & Spearing, D. (1995). Semantic and phonological coding in poor and normal readers. *Journal of Experimental Child Psychology, 59*, 76–123.

Vellutino, F. R., Scanlon, D. M., & Tanzman, M. S. (1998). The case for early intervention in diagnosing specific reading disability. *Journal of School Psychology, 36*, 367–397.

Vellutino, F. R., Scanlon, D. M., Zhang, H., & Schatschneider, C. (2008). Using response to kindergarten and first grade intervention to identify children at-risk for long-term reading difficulties. *Reading and Writing, 21*, 437–480.

Vidyasagar, T. R. (1999). A neuronal model of attentional spotlight: Parietal guiding the temporal. *Brain Research Reviews, 30*, 66–76.

Vidyasagar, T. R. (2012). Aetiology of dyslexia: A visual perspective on a phonological marker. In J. Stein & Z. Kapoula (Eds.), *Visual aspects of dyslexia* (pp. 151–170). Oxford: Oxford University Press.

Vidyasagar, T. R., & Pammer, K. (2010a). Dyslexia: A deficit in visuo-spatial attention, not in phonological processing. *Trends in Cognitive Science, 14*, 57–63.

Vidyasagar, T. R., & Pammer, K. (2010b). Letter-order encoding is both bottom-up and top-down: Response to Whitney. *Trends in Cognitive Science, 14*, 238–239.

Vigneau, M., Beaucousin, V., Herve, P. Y., Duffau, H., Crivello, F., Houde, O., et al. (2006). Meta-analyzing left hemisphere language areas: Phonology, semantics, and sentence processing. *Neuroimage, 30*, 1414–1432.

Viholainen, H., Ahonen, T., Cantell, M., Lyytinen, P., & Lyytinen, H. (2002). Development of early motor skills and language in children at risk for familial dyslexia. *Developmental Medicine & Child Neurology, 44*, 761–769.

Vinckenbosch, E., Robichon, F., & Eliez, S. (2005). Gray matter alteration in dyslexia: converging evidence from volumetric and voxel-by-voxel MRI analyses. *Neuropsychologia, 43*, 324–331.

Vineis, P., & Pearce, N. (2010). Missing heritability in genome-wide association study research. *Nature Reviews Genetics, 11*, 589.

von Bastian, C. C., & Oberaver, K. (in press). Effects and mechanisms of working memory training: A review. *Psychological Research*.

von Plessen, K., Lundervold, A., Duta, N., Heiervang, E., Klauschen, F., Smievoll, A., et al. (2002). Less developed corpus callosum in dyslexic subjects – a structural MRI study. *Neuropsychologia, 40*, 1035–1044.

Vourkas, M., Micheloyannis, S., Simos, P. G., Rezaie, R., Fletcher, J. M., Cirino, P. T., et al. (2011). Dynamic task-specific brain network connectivity in children with severe reading difficulties. *Neuroscience Letters, 488*, 123–128.

Vukovic, R. K., Lesaux, N. K., & Siegel, L. S. (2010). The mathematics skills of children with reading difficulties. *Learning and Individual Differences, 20*, 639–643.

Vukovic, R. K., & Siegel, L. S. (2006). The double-deficit hypothesis: A comprehensive analysis of the evidence. *Journal of Learning Disabilities, 39*, 25–47.

Vukovic, R. K., Wilson, A. M., & Nash, K. K. (2004). Naming speed deficits in adults with reading disabilities: A test of the double-deficit hypothesis. *Journal of Learning Disabilities, 37*, 440–450.

Wadlington, E. M., Elliot, C., & Kirylo, J. (2008). The dyslexia simulation: Impact and implications. *Literacy Research and Instruction, 47*, 264–272.

Wadlington, E. M., & Wadlington, P. L. (2005). What educators really believe about dyslexia. *Reading Improvement, 42*, 16–33.

Wadsworth, S. J., Olson, R. K., & DeFries, J. C. (2010). Differential genetic etiology of reading difficulties as a function of IQ: An update. *Behavior Genetics, 40*, 751–758.

Wagner, R. K. (2008). Rediscovering dyslexia: New approaches for identification and classification. In G. Reid, A. Fawcett, F. Manis, & L. Siegel (Eds.), *The Sage handbook of dyslexia* (pp. 174–191). London: Sage.

Wagner, R. K., Brown Waesche, J. B., Schatschneider, C., Maner, J. K., & Ahmed, Y. (2011). Using response to intervention for identification and classification. In P. McCardle, J. Lee, B. Miller, & O. Tzeng (Eds.), *Dyslexia across languages: Orthography and the brain-gene-behavior link* (pp. 202–213). Baltimore: Brookes Publishing.

Wagner, R. K., & Muse, A. (2006). Short-term memory deficits in developmental dyslexia. In T. P. Alloway & S. E. Gathercole (Eds.), *Working memory and neurodevelopmental disorders*. New York: Psychology Press.

Wagner, R. K., & Torgesen, J. K. (1987). The nature of phonological processing and its causal role in the acquisition of reading skills. *Psychological Bulletin, 101*, 192–212.

Wagner, R. K., Torgesen, J. K., & Rashotte, C. A. (1999). *Comprehensive Test of Phonological Processing*. Austin, TX: Pro-Ed.

Wagner, R. K., Torgesen, J. K., Rashotte, C. A., Hecht, S. A., Barker, T. A., Burgess, S. R., et al. (1997). Changing relations between phonological processing abilities and word-level reading as children develop from beginning to skilled readers: A five-year longitudinal study. *Developmental Psychology*, *33*, 468–479.

Walker, J. E. (2010). Recent advances in quantitative EEG as an aid to diagnosis and as a guide to neurofeedback training for cortical hypofunctions, hyperfunctions, disconnections, and hyperconnections: Improving efficacy in complicated neurological and psychological disorders. Applied psychophysiological selective review with implications for neurofeedback remediation and results of treatment in twelve consecutive patients. *Journal of Neurotherapy*, *10*, 45–55.

Walker, J. E., & Norman, C. A. (2006). The neurophysiology of dyslexia: A selective review with implications for neurofeedback remediation and results of treatment in twelve consecutive patients. *Journal of Neurotherapy: Investigations in Neuromodulation Neurofeedback and Applied Neuroscience*, *10*, 45–55.

Walker, K., Hall, S., Klein, R. G., & Phillips, D. (2006). Development of perceptual correlates of reading performance. *Brain Research*, *1124*(1), 126–141.

Wallace, M. T. (2009). Dyslexia: Bridging the gap between hearing and reading. *Current Biology*, *19*, R260–R262.

Wang, J. J., Bi, H. Y., Gao, L. Q., & Wydell, T. N. (2010). The visual magnocellular pathway in Chinese-speaking children with developmental dyslexia. *Neuropsychologia*, *48*, 3627–3633.

Wang, S., & Gathercole, S. E. (2013). Working memory deficits in children with reading difficulties: Memory span and dual task coordination. *Journal of Experimental Child Psychology*, *115*(1), 188–197.

Wanzek, J., & Roberts, G. (2012). Reading interventions with varying instructional emphases for fourth graders with reading difficulties. *Learning Disability Quarterly*, *35*(2), 90–101.

Wanzek, J., & Vaughn, S. (2007). Research-based implications from extensive early reading interventions. *School Psychology Review*, *36*, 541–561.

Wanzek, J., & Vaughn, S. (2008). Response to varying amounts of time in reading intervention for students demonstrating insufficient response to intervention. *Journal of Learning Disabilities*, *41*, 126–142.

Wanzek, J., Vaughn, S., Roberts, G., & Fletcher, J. M. (2011). Efficacy of a reading intervention for middle school students with learning disabilities. *Exceptional Children*, *78*, 73–87.

Wanzek, J., Vaughn, S., Scammacca, N. K., Metz, K., Murray, C. S., Roberts, G., & Danielson, L. (2013). Extensive reading interventions for students with reading difficulties after grade 3. *Review of Educational Research*, *83*(2), 163–195.

Wanzek, J., Wexler, J., Vaughn, S., & Ciullo, S. (2010). Reading interventions for struggling readers in the upper elementary grades: A synthesis of 20 years of research. *Reading and Writing*, *23*, 889–912.

Ward, S. B., Ward, T. J., Hatt, C. V., Young, D. L., & Molner, N. R. (1995). The incidence and utility of the ACID, ACIDS and SCAD profiles in a referred population. *Psychology in the Schools*, *32*, 267–276.

Warnke, A., Schulte-Körne, G., & Ise, E. (2012). Developmental dyslexia. In M. E. Garralda & J. Raynaud (Eds.), *Brain, mind, and developmental psychopathology in childhood* (pp. 173–198). Lanham, MD: Jason Aronson Publishing.

Washburn, E. K., Joshi, R. M., & Cantrell, E. B. (2011). Are preservice teachers prepared to teach struggling readers? *Annals of Dyslexia*, *61*, 21–43.

Watkins, E. (1922). *How to teach silent reading to beginners*. Philadelphia and London: Lippincott.

Watkins, M. W., Kush, J. C., & Glutting, J. J. (1997). Discriminant and predictive validity of the WISC-III ACID profile among children with learning disabilities. *Psychology in the Schools*, *34*, 309–319.

Watson, C., & Willows, D. M. (1995). Information-processing patterns in specific reading disability. *Journal of Learning Disabilities*, *28*, 216–231.

Westendorp, M., Hartman, E., Houwen, S., Smith, J., & Visscher, C. (2011). The relationship between gross motor skills and academic achievement in children with learning disabilities. *Research in Developmental Disabilities*, *32*, 2773–2779.

Wexler, J., Vaughn, S., Edmonds, M., & Reutebuch, C. L. (2008). A synthesis of fluency interventions for secondary struggling readers. *Reading and Writing*, *21*, 317–347.

Wexler, J., Vaughn, S., Roberts, G., & Denton, C. A. (2010). The efficacy of repeated reading and wide reading practice for high school students with severe reading disabilities. *Learning Disabilities Research & Practice*, *25*, 2–10.

What Works Clearinghouse (2007). Fast ForWord. Retrieved February 7, 2012 from http://ies.ed.gov/ncee/wwc/interventionreport.aspx?sid=172.

White, S., Milne, E., Rosen, S., Hansen, P., Swettenham, J., Frith, U., et al. (2006). The role of sensorimotor impairments in dyslexia: A multiple case study of dyslexic children. *Developmental Science*, *9*, 237–269.

Whitney, C. (2010). Serial letter encoding is bottom-up, not top-down: Comment on Vidyasagar and Pammer. *Trends in Cognitive Sciences*, *14*, 237–238.

Wilkins, A., Garside, S., & Enfield, M. L. (1993). *Basic facts about dyslexia: What everyone ought to know*. Baltimore, MD: The Orton Dyslexia Society.

Wilkins, A. J. (1995). *Visual stress*. Oxford: Oxford University Press.

Wilkins, A. J. (2003). *Reading through colour*. London: Wiley.

Wilkins, A. J. (2012). Origins of visual stress. In J. Stein & Z. Kapoula (Eds.), *Visual aspects of dyslexia* (pp. 63–77). Oxford: Oxford University Press.

Willburger, E., & Landerl, K. (2010). Anchoring the deficit of the anchor deficit: Dyslexia or attention? *Dyslexia*, *16*, 175–182.

Willcutt, E. G., Betjemann, R. S., McGrath, L. M., Chhabildas, N. A., Olson, R. K., DeFries, J. C., et al. (2010). Etiology and neuropsychology of comorbidity between RD and ADHD: The case for multiple-deficit models. *Cortex*, *46*, 1345–1361.

Willcutt, E. G., & Pennington, B. F. (2000). Comorbidity of reading disability and attention-deficit/hyperactivity disorder: Differences by gender and subtype. *Journal of Learning Disabilities*, *33*, 179–191.

Willcutt, E. G., Pennington, B. F., Olson, R. K., & DeFries, J. C. (2007). Understanding comorbidity: A twin study of reading disability and attention-deficit/hyperactivity disorder. *American Journal of Medical Genetics Part B: Neuropsychiatric Genetics*, *144B*, 709–714.

Willcutt, E. G., Petrill, S. A., Wu, S., Boada, R., DeFries, J. C., Olson, R. K., & Pennington, B. F. (2013). Comorbidity between reading disability and math disability: Concurrent psychopathology, functional impairment, and neuropsychological functioning. *Journal of Learning Disabilities*, *46*(6), 500–516.

Willcutt, E. G., Sonuga-Barke, E. J. S., Nigg, J. T., & Sergeant, J. A. (2008). Recent developments in neuropsychological models of childhood disorders. *Advances in Biological Psychiatry*, *24*, 195–226.

Wimmer, H., & Mayringer, H. (2001). Is the reading-rate problem of German dyslexic children caused by slow visual processes? In M. Wolf (Ed.), *Dyslexia, fluency, and the brain* (pp. 93–102). Timonium, MD: York.

Wimmer, H., Mayringer, H., & Landerl, K. (2000). The double-deficit hypothesis and difficulties in learning to read a regular orthography. *Journal of Educational Psychology, 92,* 668–680.

Wimmer, H., Schurz, M., Sturm, D., Richlan, F., Klackl, J., Kronbichler, M., et al. (2010). A dual-route perspective on poor reading in a regular orthography: An fMRI study. *Cortex, 46,* 1284–1298.

Wise, B. W., Ring, J., & Olson, R. K. (1999). Training phonological awareness with and without explicit attention to articulation. *Journal of Experimental Child Psychology, 72,* 271–304.

Wolf, M. (2007). *Proust and the squid: The story and science of the reading brain.* New York: HarperCollins.

Wolf, M., & Bowers, P. G. (1999). The double-deficit hypothesis for the developmental dyslexia. *Journal of Educational Psychology, 91,* 415–438.

Wolf, M., Bowers, P. G., & Biddle, K. (2000). Naming-speed processes, timing, and reading: A conceptual review. *Journal of Learning Disabilities, 33,* 387–407.

Wolf, M., Gottwald, S., Galante, W., Norton, E., & Miller, L. (2009). How the origins of the reading brain instruct our knowledge of reading intervention. In K. Pugh & P. McCardle (Eds.), *How children learn to read: Current issues and new directions in the integration of cognition, neurobiology and genetics of reading and dyslexia research and practice* (pp. 289–299). New York: Psychology Press.

Wolf, M., & Katzir-Cohen, T. (2001). Reading fluency and its intervention. *Scientific Studies of Reading, 5,* 211–238.

Wolf, M., Miller, L., & Donnelly, K. (2000). Retrieval, Automaticity, Vocabulary Elaboration, Orthography (RAVE-O): A comprehensive, fluency-based reading intervention program. *Journal of Learning Disabilities, 33,* 375–386.

Wolf, M., O'Brien, B., Adams, K. D., Joffe, T., Jeffrey, J., Lovett, M., et al. (2003). Working for time: Reflections on naming speed, reading fluency, and intervention. In I. B. R. Foorman (Ed.), *Preventing and remediating reading difficulties* (pp. 355–380). Baltimore, MD: York Press.

Wolf, M., O'Rourke, A. G., Gidney, C., Lovett, M., Cirino, P., & Morris, R. (2002). The second deficit: An investigation of the independence of phonological and naming-speed deficits in developmental dyslexia. *Reading & Writing, 15,* 43–72.

Wolff, P. H., & Melngailis, I. (1994). Family patterns of developmental dyslexia. *American Journal of Medical Genetics (Neuropsychiatric Genetics), 54,* 122–131.

Wolff, P. H., Melngailis, I., Obregon, M., & Bedrosian, M. (1995). Family patterns of developmental dyslexia, part II: Behavioral phenotypes. *American Journal of Medical Genetics, 60,* 494–505.

Wood, C. (2006). Metrical stress sensitivity in young children and its relationship to phonological awareness and reading. *Journal of Research in Reading, 29,* 270–287.

Woodcock, R. W. (1987). *Woodcock Reading Mastery Tests-Revised.* Circle Pines, MN: American Guidance Service.

World Federation of Neurology. (1968). *Report of research group on dyslexia and world illiteracy.* Dallas, TX: World Federation of Neurology.

Wright, C. M., & Conlon, E. G. (2009). Auditory and visual processing in children with dyslexia. *Developmental Neuropsychology, 34,* 330–355.

Wright, C. M., Conlon, E. G., & Dyck, M. (2012). Visual search deficits are independent of magnocellular deficits in dyslexia. *Annals of Dyslexia, 62,* 53–69.

Yeatman, J. D., Ben-Shachar, M., Bammer, R., & Feldman, H. M. (2009). Using diffusion tensor imaging and fiber tracking to characterize diffuse perinatal white matter injury: A case report. *Journal of Child Neurology, 24,* 795–800.

Yeatman, J. D., Dougherty, R. F., Ben-Shachar, M., & Wandell, B. A. (2012). Development of white matter and reading skills. *Proceedings of the National Academy of Sciences of the United States of America, 109*(44), E3045–E3053.

Yule, W. (1976). Dyslexia. *Psychological Medicine, 6,* 165–167.

Zane, T. (2005). Fads in special education: An overview. In J. W. Jacobson, R. M. Foxx, & J. A. Mulick (Eds.), *Controversial therapies for developmental disabilities: Fad, fashion and science in professional practice* (pp. 175–191). Mahwah, NJ: Lawrence Erlbaum.

Zappulla, D. C., & Cech, T. R. (2006). RNA as a flexible scaffold for proteins: Yeast telomerase and beyond. *Cold Spring Harbor Symposia on Quantitative Biology, 71,* 217–224.

Zeri, F., De Luca, M., Spinelli, D., & Zoccolotti, P. (2011). Ocular dominance stability and reading skill: A controversial relationship. *Optometry & Vision Science, 88*(11), 1353–1362.

Zhang, J., & McBride-Chang, C. (2010). Auditory sensitivity, speech perception, and reading development and Impairment. *Educational Psychology Review, 22,* 323–338.

Ziegler, J. C. (2008). Better to lose the anchor than the whole ship. *Trends in Cognitive Sciences, 12,* 244–245.

Ziegler, J. C., Bertrand, D., Tóth, D., Csépe, V., Reis, A., Faísca, L., et al. (2010). Orthographic depth and its impact on universal predictors of reading. *Psychological Science, 21,* 551–559.

Ziegler, J. C., Pech-Georgel, C., Dufau, S., & Grainger, J. (2010). Rapid processing of letters, digits and symbols: What purely visual-attentional deficit in developmental dyslexia? *Developmental Science, 13,* F8–F14.

Zirkel, P. A. (2013). The trend in SLD enrollments and the role of RTI. *Journal of Learning Disabilities, 46*(5), 473–479.

Zoccolotti, P., De Luca, M., Di Filippo, G., Judica, A., & Martelli, M. (2009). Reading development in an orthographically regular language: Effects of length, frequency, lexicality and global processing ability. *Reading and Writing, 22,* 1053–1079.

Zoccolotti, P., & Friedmann, N. (2010). From dyslexia to dyslexias, from dysgraphia to dysgraphias, from a cause to causes: A look at current research on developmental dyslexia and dysgraphia. *Cortex, 46,* 1211–1215.

Zorzi, M., Barbiero, C., Facoetti, A., Lonciari, I., Carrozzi, M., et al. (2012). Extra-large letter spacing improves reading in dyslexia. *Proceedings of the National Academy of Sciences, 109,* 11455–11459.

Zumeta, R. O., Compton, D. L., & Fuchs, L. S. (2012). Using word identification fluency to monitor first-grade reading development. *Exceptional Children, 78,* 201–220.

Index

abnormal crowding hypothesis, visual deficits and, 78

academic achievement
intervention strategies based on, 142
IQ levels and, 19
risk identification for reading disability and, 135
working memory intervention and, 62–63

academic skills
dyslexia diagnosis and, 21
working memory intervention and, 62–63

ACID profile (arithmetic, coding, information, and digit span subtests), 20–21

Adi, Y., 155–156

advocacy groups, definitions of dyslexia and, 6–7

age-based dynamics
dyslexia and, 6–7
genetics of dyslexia and, 111, 119–121
genetics of reading disability and, 111, 115
interventions in reading disability and, 137–138
rapid automatized naming and, 50
resistance to intervention and, 139–149
in risk identification for reading disability, 131–132

Ahissar, M., 12–13, 64–65, 78–79, 83–85

Albion, E., 155–156

allophonic perception, reading disability and, 67–68

Al Otaiba, S., 131–132, 135

alphabetic principle, risk identification for reading disability, 133–134

alphanumeric systems, rapid automatized naming and, 50–51

alternative interventions for dyslexia, 152–160

American Academy of Ophthalmology, 155–156

American Academy of Pediatric Ophthalmology and Strabismus, 155–156

American Academy of Pediatrics, 155–156
on visual stress, 73–74

American Association of Certified Orthoptists, 155–156

American Psychiatric Association (APA), dyslexia classification and, 8

American Psychological Association, resistance to reform in, 23

analytical validity, genetics of dyslexia and, 111, 115, 119–121

anchoring deficit hypothesis, dyslexia and, 78–79

Andrist, C. G., 177

Anglocentric focus in dyslexia research, 7

angular gyrus
dyslexia linked to, 2–3
reading-brain model research and, 91–93

assessment of dyslexia
overview of, 123–165
specialist skills for, 149–151

assistive listening devices
auditory processing training and, 68
reading disability remediation, 151–152

asymmetric tonic neck reflex, dyslexia linked to, 152–155

"attentional blink" phenomenon, 74–81

attentional factors
in dyslexia, 86–87
in reading disability, 74–81

attention-deficit hyperactivity disorder (ADHD)
auditory processing and, 66
dyslexia and, 12–13
reading disability and, 160–164

auditory cortex ectopias
functional magnetic resonance imaging studies, 99–101
reading-brain model research and, 91–93
voxel-based morphometry of, 95–96

auditory interventions, for dyslexia management, 157–158

auditory processing
causal relationships in, 66–67
current research issues in, 81